Pulmonary Pathology

Editor

KIRK D. JONES

SURGICAL PATHOLOGY CLINICS

www.surgpath.theclinics.com

Consulting Editor
JASON L. HORNICK

March 2020 • Volume 13 • Number 1

ELSEVIER

1600 John F. Kennedy Boulevard • Suite 1800 • Philadelphia, Pennsylvania, 19103-2899

http://www.theclinics.com

SURGICAL PATHOLOGY CLINICS Volume 13, Number 1
March 2020 ISSN 1875-9181, ISBN-13: 978-0-323-71138-8

Editor: Katerina Heidhausen
Developmental Editor: Donald Mumford

Surgical Pathology Clinics (ISSN 1875-9181) is published quarterly by Elsevier Inc., 360 Park Avenue South, New York, NY 10010. Months of issue are March, June, September, and December. Business and Editorial Office: Elsevier Inc., 1600 John F. Kennedy Blvd., Ste. 1800, Philadelphia, PA 19103-2899. Accounting and Circulation Offices: Elsevier Inc., 3251 Riverport Lane, Maryland Heights, MO 63043. Periodicals postage paid at New York, NY and at additional mailing offices. Subscription prices are $219.00 per year (US individuals), $294.00 per year (US institutions), $100.00 per year (US students/residents), $272.00 per year (Canadian individuals), $335.00 per year (Canadian Institutions), $263.00 per year (foreign individuals), $335.00 per year (foreign institutions), and $120.00 per year (international students/residents), $100.00 per year (Canadian students/residents). Foreign air speed delivery is included in all *Clinics'* subscription prices. All prices are subject to change without notice. **POSTMASTER:** Send address changes to *Surgical Pathology Clinics*, Elsevier, 3251 Riverport Lane, Maryland Heights, MO 63043. **Customer Service: 1-800-654-2452 (US). From outside the United States, call 1-314-447-8871. Fax: 1-314-447-8029. E-mail: JournalsCustomerServiceusa@elsevier.com (for print support)** and **JournalsOnlineSupport-usa@elsevier.com (for online support).**

Reprints. For copies of 100 or more, of articles in this publication, please contact the Commercial Reprints Department, Elsevier Inc., 360 Park Avenue South, New York, NY 10010-1710. Tel. 212-633-3874; Fax: 212-633-3820; E-mail: reprints@elsevier.com.

Surgical Pathology Clinics of North America is covered in *MEDLINE/PubMed (Index Medicus)*.

Contributors

CONSULTING EDITOR

JASON L. HORNICK, MD, PhD
Director of Surgical Pathology and
Immunohistochemistry, Brigham and Women's
Hospital, Professor of Pathology, Harvard
Medical School, Boston, Massachusetts, USA

EDITOR

KIRK D. JONES, MD
Clinical Professor, Department of Pathology,
University of California, San Francisco, San
Francisco, California, USA

AUTHORS

ALAIN C. BORCZUK, MD
Professor, Department of Pathology, Weill
Cornell Medicine, New York, New York, USA

ALBERTO CAVAZZA, MD
Pathology Unit, Azienda USL/IRCCS di Reggio
Emilia, Reggio Emilia, Italy

THOMAS V. COLBY, MD
Department of Pathology and Laboratory
Medicine (Emeritus), Mayo Clinic, Scottsdale,
Arizona, USA

WALTER PATRICK DEVINE, MD, PhD
Assistant Clinical Professor, Department of
Pathology, University of California, San
Francisco, San Francisco, California, USA

ALESSANDRA DUBINI, MD
Pathology Unit, Azienda USL Romagna, GB
Morgagni Hospital, Forlì, Italy

**DAFFOLYN RACHAEL FELS ELLIOTT, MD,
PhD**
Department of Pathology, University of
California, San Francisco, San Francisco,
California, USA

JUNYA FUKUOKA, MD, PhD
Chair, Department of Pathology, Nagasaki
University Hospital, Professor and Chair,
Department of Pathology, Nagasaki University
Graduate School of Biomedical Sciences,
Nagasaki, Japan; Chair, Department of
Pathology, Kameda Medical Center,
Kamogawa, Japan

JENS GOTTLIEB, MD
Member of the German Center for Lung
Research (DZL), Biomedical Research in
Endstage and Obstructive Lung Disease
Hannover (BREATH); Department of
Pneumology, Hannover Medical School,
Hannover, Germany

ALIYA N. HUSAIN, MD
Professor, Department of Pathology, University
of Chicago, Chicago, Illinois, USA

JIAN JING, MD, PhD
Assistant Professor, Department of Pathology,
University of Colorado Anschutz Medical
Center, Aurora, Colorado, USA

KIRK D. JONES, MD
Clinical Professor, Department of Pathology, University of California, San Francisco, San Francisco, California, USA

DANNY JONIGK, FRCPath
Member of the German Center for Lung Research (DZL), Biomedical Research in Endstage and Obstructive Lung Disease Hannover (BREATH); Institute for Pathology, Hannover Medical School, Hannover, Germany

KRISTINE E. KONOPKA, MD
Assistant Professor, Department of Pathology, University of Michigan, Ann Arbor, Michigan, USA

LEILA KUTOB, MD
Department of Pathology and Laboratory Medicine, Emory University School of Medicine, Emory University Hospital, Atlanta, Georgia, USA

FLORIAN LAENGER, MD
Member of the German Center for Lung Research (DZL), Biomedical Research in Endstage and Obstructive Lung Disease Hannover (BREATH); Institute for Pathology, Hannover Medical School, Hannover, Germany

MARIA CECILIA MENGOLI, MD
Pathology Unit, Azienda USL/IRCCS di Reggio Emilia, Reggio Emilia, Italy

VENERINO POLETTI, MD
Department of Diseases of the Thorax, Azienda USL Romagna, GB Morgagni Hospital, Forlì, Italy

CLAUDIA RAVAGLIA, MD
Department of Diseases of the Thorax, Azienda USL Romagna, GB Morgagni Hospital, Forlì, Italy

GIULIO ROSSI, MD
Pathology Unit, Azienda USL Romagna, St. Maria delle Croci Hospital, Ravenna, Italy

ROBERTO RUIZ-CORDERO, MD
Assistant Clinical Professor, Department of Pathology, University of California, San Francisco, San Francisco, California, USA

FRANK SCHNEIDER, MD
Department of Pathology and Laboratory Medicine, Emory University School of Medicine, Emory University Hospital, Atlanta, Georgia, USA

JEFREE J. SCHULTE, MD
Fellow, Department of Pathology, University of Chicago, Chicago, Illinois, USA

ALLISON SEIDEL
Member of the German Center for Lung Research (DZL), Biomedical Research in Endstage and Obstructive Lung Disease Hannover (BREATH); Institute for Pathology, Hannover Medical School, Hannover, Germany

ELENA TAGLIAVINI, MD
Pathology Unit, Azienda USL/IRCCS di Reggio Emilia, Reggio Emilia, Italy

SARA TOMASSETTI, MD
Department of Diseases of the Thorax, Azienda USL Romagna, GB Morgagni Hospital, Forlì, Italy

ANATOLY URISMAN, MD, PhD
Department of Pathology, University of California, San Francisco, San Francisco, California, USA

GREGOR WARNECKE, MD
Member of the German Center for Lung Research (DZL), Biomedical Research in Endstage and Obstructive Lung Disease Hannover (BREATH); Department of Cardiac, Thoracic, Transplantation and Vascular Surgery, Hannover Medical School, Hannover, Germany

CHRISTOPHER WERLEIN
Physician, Institute for Pathology, Hannover Medical School, Hannover, Germany

YOSHIAKI ZAIZEN, MD
Fellow, Department of Pathology, Nagasaki University Hospital, Nagasaki, Japan; Assistant Professor, Division of Respirology, Neurology and Rheumotology, Department of Medicine, Kurume University School of Medicine, Kurume, Japan

Contents

Given the growing desire in clinical practice to detect lung carcinoma early, small biopsies are becoming more common and vital to the diagnostic process. Accurately diagnosing lung carcinoma on small biopsies is challenging but can significantly affect patient management. The challenge is due in part to the overlapping features between benign, reactive, and malignant processes and the lack of discriminating biomarkers. Specimen preservation for ancillary tests is also increasingly important to provide targeted precision medicine. We focuses on the morphologic features and diagnostic pitfalls of the most common lung carcinoma seen in small biopsies and the appropriate specimen handling practice.

Lung cancer is the leading cause of cancer mortality. It is classified into different histologic subtypes, including adenocarcinoma, squamous carcinoma, and large cell carcinoma (commonly referred as non–small cell lung cancer) and small cell lung cancer. Comprehensive molecular characterization of lung cancer has expanded our understanding of the cellular origins and molecular pathways affected in each of these subtypes. Many of these genetic alterations represent potential therapeutic targets for which drugs are constantly under development. This article discusses the molecular characteristics of the main lung cancer subtypes and discusses the current guidelines and novel targeted therapies, including checkpoint immunotherapy.

Pulmonary neuroendocrine tumors represent a morphologic spectrum of tumors from the well-differentiated typical carcinoid tumor, to the intermediate-grade atypical carcinoid tumor, to the high-grade neuroendocrine carcinomas composed of small-cell carcinoma and large-cell neuroendocrine carcinoma. The addition of immunohistochemistry in diagnostics is helpful and often essential, especially in the classification of large-cell neuroendocrine carcinoma. The importance of the intermediate-grade atypical carcinoid group is underscored by the impact of this diagnosis on therapy. The distinction of pulmonary small-cell carcinoma from large-cell neuroendocrine carcinoma, despite both being in the high-grade group, is of relevance to the therapeutic approach to these tumor types.

Lung cancer staging is a foundation of patient care, informing management decisions and prognosis. This comprehensive overview of the current 8th edition

American Joint Committee on Cancer Cancer Staging Manual addresses common difficulties in staging, such as measuring the invasive component of adenocarcinomas and staging multiple lung nodules.

Mesothelioma is a rare neoplasm that arises from mesothelial cells lining body cavities including the pleura, pericardium, peritoneum, and tunica vaginalis. Most malignant mesotheliomas occur in the chest and are frequently associated with a history of asbestos exposure. The diagnosis of malignant mesothelioma is challenging and fraught with pitfalls, particularly in small biopsies. This article highlights what the pathologist needs to know regarding the clinical and radiographic presentation of mesothelioma, histologic features including subtypes and variants, and recent advances in immunohistochemical markers and molecular testing.

This review discusses diagnostic pathology in idiopathic interstitial pneumonias (IIPs). Accurate understanding of basic structure of lung lobules is critical because the location of abnormalities inside the lobule is an important effector of pathology diagnosis. Depending on the method of obtaining tissue, recognition of the location may be difficult or impossible. Cryobiopsy is a new technology and its coverage of lung lobules is limited. This article discusses fundamental anatomy and approach to interstitial pneumonia. In addition, most histologic types of IIPs are covered, but the focus is on diagnosis of usual interstitial pneumonia because of its clinical importance.

Alloimmune reactions are, besides various infections, the major cause for impaired lung allograft function following transplant. Acute cellular rejection is not only a major trigger of acute allograft failure but also contributes to development of chronic lung allograft dysfunction. Analogous to other solid organ transplants, acute antibody-mediated rejection has become a recognized entity in lung transplant pathology. Adequate sensitivity and specificity in the diagnosis of alloimmune reactions in the lung can only be achieved by synoptic analysis of histopathologic, clinical, and radiological findings together with serologic and microbiologic findings.

Cystic diseases of the lung encompass a fairly broad variety of different diseases with causes including genetic abnormalities, smoking-related problems, developmental disorders, malignant neoplasms, and inflammatory processes. In addition, there are several diagnoses that closely resemble cystic lung disease, including cavitary diseases, cystic bronchiectasis, emphysema, and cystic changes in fibrosing interstitial lung disease. This article provides a review of cystic lung disease and its gross and histologic mimics.

> Patients with connective tissue diseases may have pulmonary involvement, including interstitial lung disease. Various patterns of interstitial lung disease have been classically described in certain connective tissue diseases. It is now recognized that there is significant overlap between patterns of interstitial lung disease observed in the various connective tissue diseases. Differentiating idiopathic from connective tissue disease-related interstitial lung disease is challenging but of clinical importance. New concepts in the diagnosis of connective tissue disease related interstitial lung disease may prove useful in making the diagnosis.

> Three major histologic patterns of bronchiolitis: obliterative bronchiolitis, follicular bronchiolitis, and diffuse panbronchiolitis, are reviewed in detail. These distinct patterns of primary bronchiolar injury provide a useful starting point for formulating a differential diagnosis and considering possible causes. In support of the aim toward a cause-based classification system of small airway disease, a simple diagnostic algorithm is provided for further subclassification of the above 3 bronchiolitis patterns according to the major associated etiologic subgroups.

> Transbronchial cryobiopsy, a new diagnostic procedure in patients with diffuse lung disease, provides larger and better-preserved lung specimens compared to forceps biopsy. The diagnostic yield of cryobiopsy is much better than that of forceps biopsy and slightly lower than that of surgical lung biopsy, but with a lower complication rate compared to the latter. Literature suggests that, in the multidisciplinary approach to patients with diffuse lung disease cryobiopsy provides diagnostic and prognostic information similar to surgical lung biopsy. Cryobiopsy can also be performed in some patients unsuitable for surgical biopsy, yet in whom histologic input is needed.

SURGICAL PATHOLOGY CLINICS

SERIES OF RELATED INTEREST

Clinics in Laboratory Medicine

THE CLINICS ARE AVAILABLE ONLINE!
Access your subscription at:
www.theclinics.com

Preface
Pulmonary Pathology: Providing Practical Answers for Busy Pathologists

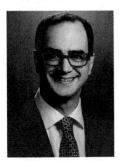

Kirk D. Jones, MD
Editor

There have been several developments in the decade since the last pulmonary-centered issue of *Surgical Pathology Clinics:* new molecular testing methods, a new cancer staging system, new diagnostic entities, and new diagnostic modalities. Many pathologists find the lung interesting, but often lack the volume of cases to feel comfortable when confronted with pulmonary pathology. In assembling this issue of *Surgical Pathology Clinics*, I have tried to consider which questions I have been asked in my daily consultation practice. My hope is that the issue will provide practical answers for the working pathologist.

Drs Konopka and Jing provide an introduction to the articles on neoplastic disease with an approach to small biopsies. As personalized medicine continues to develop and expand, understanding how to provide adequate information on limited tissue has become a salient issue. In a similar vein, many diagnostic pathologists find the molecular testing nomenclature and reasoning to be mysterious. Drs Ruiz-Cordero and Devine pull back the curtain to reveal the simplified underpinnings of these tests. As different organ systems have moved to more standardized neuroendocrine tumor grading schema, understanding the pulmonary system has become more necessary. Dr Borczuk provides a practical approach to these neoplasms, elaborating on pertinent clinical

issues. Drs Schneider and Kotub break down the recently introduced TNM staging system, focusing on several issues that are often encountered in general practice. The final article in the neoplastic section is provided to assist in diagnosis of mesothelioma. Dr Fels-Elliott and I communicate several of the developments that have arisen since the last pulmonary issue of *Surgical Pathology Clinics* in 2010.

Drs Fukuoka and Zaizen start the nonneoplastic articles, with a detailed overview on diagnosis and classification of the idiopathic interstitial pneumonias. Recognition of these patterns provides the basis of nonneoplastic lung disease. The number of lung transplant cases has increased nearly every year for the past decade, and Dr Jonigk and colleagues have produced a state-of-the-art review of lung transplant pathology that covers the histologic and molecular findings observed in these patients. Drs Husain and Schulte elucidate the variegated findings observed in autoimmune connective tissue disease, a group of diseases in which the vigilant pathologist often makes the initial diagnosis. In a tip of the hat to my colleagues in radiology, I have provided an article on interpretation of cystic lung disease. Dr Urisman and I venture into the diagnosis of small airway disease and discuss the importance of multidisciplinary discussion in accurate recognition and classification of

Surgical Pathology 13 (2020) ix–x
https://doi.org/10.1016/j.path.2019.12.001
1875-9181/20/© 2019 Published by Elsevier Inc.

surgpath.theclinics.com

these cases. Finally, the issue concludes with a discussion of cryobiopsy. Dr Cavazza and colleagues represent one of the most experienced groups working with this technique, and they share their expertise in the diagnosis of diffuse lung diseases.

It is my hope that pathologists in general practice will find this issue of *Surgical Pathology Clinics* to be a useful aid when lung biopsies pass across their microscope stages. I am extremely thankful for the work that my colleagues across the globe have done in putting their knowledge down on these pages.

Kirk D. Jones, MD
Department of Pathology
University of California San Francisco
505 Parnassus Avenue, Room M545
San Francisco, CA 94143, USA

E-mail address:
kirk.jones@ucsf.edu

Diagnosis of Lung Carcinoma on Small Biopsy

Jian Jing, MD, PhD[a], Kristine E. Konopka, MD[b],*

KEYWORDS

- Lung nodule • Core needle biopsy • Fine needle aspiration • Small biopsies
- Specimen management

Key points

- Early detection of lung cancer significantly reduces mortality, and small biopsies play a key part in allowing for early medical and/or surgical intervention.
- Pathologists are encouraged to build awareness for appropriate tissue triage of small biopsies to preserve material for possible ancillary molecular testing.
- Differentiating benign from malignant epithelial changes on small biopsies may require correlation with the clinical and radiographic context to avoid an erroneous overcall of malignancy.

ABSTRACT

Given the growing desire in clinical practice to detect lung carcinoma early, small biopsies are becoming more common and vital to the diagnostic process. Accurately diagnosing lung carcinoma on small biopsies is challenging but can significantly affect patient management. The challenge is due in part to the overlapping features between benign, reactive, and malignant processes and the lack of discriminating biomarkers. Specimen preservation for ancillary tests is also increasingly important to provide targeted precision medicine. We focuses on the morphologic features and diagnostic pitfalls of the most common lung carcinoma seen in small biopsies and the appropriate specimen handling practice.

OVERVIEW

In the past decade, there has been significant progress in early diagnosis and treatment of lung cancer. Nonetheless, lung and bronchial cancers remain one of the leading causes of cancer-related death, with up to 25% mortality and 5-year relative survival rate ranked the second worst after pancreatic cancer.[1] According to the most recent edition of the Cancer Staging Manual (American Joint Committee on Cancer 8th edition), the 5-year overall survival rate is 92% for clinical-stage IA, but decreases to 53% for stage IIB, indicating that early-stage lesions can be successfully treated.[2] Improved outcomes have been accomplished in part through the National Lung Screening Trial (NLST), which has shown a reduction in mortality through the use of low-dose screening computed tomography (CT).[3] Despite that, the implementation of high-quality screening guidelines for lung cancer still has major challenges, including insufficient published data to establish reproducible and evidence-based criteria.[4] Another difficulty for early detection and diagnosis is the inherently complex nature of lung cancer with overlapping radiographic and pathologic features in benign and malignant processes. Accurate diagnosis of early-stage lung cancer on small biopsies can benefit patients by reducing unnecessary procedures and facilitating appropriate early interventions. Although NLST has well-established imaging protocols and target populations, there are still no well-defined pathologic criteria for lung carcinoma in small biopsies, leading to imprecise diagnoses and suboptimal treatment. Therefore, there is an urgent need for better diagnostic precision on small biopsies obtained from tissue or cytology sampling.

[a] Department of Pathology, University of Colorado Anschutz Medical Center, Aurora, CO, USA; [b] Department of Pathology and Clinical Laboratories, Michigan Medicine, University of Michigan, 2800 Plymouth Road, Building 35, Ann Arbor, MI 48109, USA
* Corresponding author.
E-mail address: krkonopk@med.umich.edu

Surgical Pathology 13 (2020) 1–15
https://doi.org/10.1016/j.path.2019.11.001

In this review, we discuss the role of pathology in diagnosis, and the further clinical applications of small biopsies based on current guidelines for incidental pulmonary nodules detected on CT imaging.[5] We will review currently accepted terminology and diagnostic criteria for the most common malignant epithelial entities encountered on small biopsies, and discuss in detail the morphologic features of lung carcinoma and its histologic mimickers in samples obtained through imaging-guided methods, including core needle biopsy (CNB) and fine needle aspiration (FNA).

SMALL BIOPSIES IN LUNG CANCER DIAGNOSIS AND STAGING

As our understanding of the molecular mechanisms of lung cancer and the application of targeted therapy continues to expand, high-quality biopsy methods are becoming increasingly important. Early diagnosis of lung cancer is mostly the result of lung cancer screening programs for patients with a smoking history or incidental discoveries on chest CT scans performed for other reasons. The decision to sample and send nodules for pathologic evaluation is complex and based in part on radiographic findings, such as lesion size, shape, and density.[6–8]

As an organ protected by the chest wall and surrounded by complex anatomic structures, biopsies of lung tissue or mediastinal lymph nodes are most effectively performed through minimally invasive, low-risk, and low-cost procedures.[9] According to updated National Comprehensive Cancer Network guidelines version 4.2019, the tumor size feasible for biopsy is at least 6 mm for subsolid nodules and 8 mm for solid nodules. For central lesions, ultrasound-guided transbronchial biopsy is commonly applied for both diagnosis and staging. CT-guided transthoracic biopsy is more commonly reserved for peripheral lesions.

Based on the bore diameter of the needle, specimens are examined by either a surgical pathologist or cytopathologist. At present, there is no sufficient evidence to favor CNB or FNA based on the overall diagnostic rate for malignancies or the rate of complications (eg, pneumothorax or hemoptysis).[10,11] Therefore, the method selected largely depends on anatomic location, local practice, resources, and expertise (procedure and pathology interpretation). Smaller-bore needles tend to be more flexible and can reach more lesions, whereas larger-bore needles are better suited for peripheral lesions and can obtain larger tissue samples. FNA provides tissue for evaluation by cytomorphology, whereas CNB evaluates both cytomorphology and histologic structures. Generally, the cell morphology is better preserved in FNA specimens, which are appropriate for "cellular lesions" with less fibrosis, and which are often seen as subsolid lesions on CT. A complicated malignant lesion affiliated with inflammation and fibrosis is better evaluated by CNB, which offers architectural information. Although the 2 biopsy modalities are considered complementary,[12] in practice it is not uncommon to see diagnostic material in only 1 modality (ie, FNA or CNB) when both are used concurrently.

Besides the benefit of offering immediate, actionable preliminary diagnoses, the tissue obtained through small biopsies can be used for tumor classification and molecular testing. For advanced-stage lung cancers, the tissue provided in these samples may be the only available tissue for ancillary testing and should, therefore, be used prudently. For this reason, numerous techniques have been suggested to maximize tissue preservation for later examination. One study from the University of Colorado summarizes techniques and strategies to implement at the time of biopsy procurement and processing.[13] These techniques include improving interdepartmental communication before biopsy, splitting samples into multiple blocks and avoiding decalcification during processing, and superficial facing of blocks. Methods for tissue preservation include trimming the cell block of small biopsies without skipping levels. In addition, a better understanding of the purpose of immunohistochemistry (IHC) should be advocated because of the many unfortunate circumstances in which the diagnostic tissue is exhausted by unnecessary stains.

Rapid on site evaluation (ROSE) is a method used to ensure adequate tissue harvest. It is the process of examining the cytomorphology of an FNA biopsy or touch preparations of a CNB at the time of the procedure. This process can guide the operator to efficiently collect tissue and apply proper specimen triage.[14] One of the standard sampling preparations of ROSE is the creation of high-quality mono-layer smears. Although ROSE is helpful in ensuring adequate tumor sampling, it is not without drawbacks. It has been noted that vigorous touch preparation can lead to depletion of CNB cellularity and DNA content.[15] In our consultation practice, it is not uncommon to see the diagnostic material completely transferred from the core biopsy to cytology slides during the process of making touch preparations, resulting in suboptimal smears with poor visible quality, and paucicellular core biopsy samples, both of which hinder interpretation and the ability to perform ancillary studies. When used appropriately, ROSE has been shown to have significant advantages of cost-effectiveness and reduced morbidity due to fewer overall needle passes.[16] Ultimately, the decision to implement ROSE should be based on the individual circumstances of the institution.

TERMINOLOGIES FOR LUNG CANCER DIAGNOSIS IN SMALL BIOPSIES

Guidelines for respiratory cytology reporting terminology have been suggested by the Papanicolaou Society of Cytopathology (PSC). These include nondiagnostic, negative for malignancy, atypical, neoplastic, suspicious, and malignant.[17] The nondiagnostic category is particularly important in providing important feedback that the sample tissue is not representative of the radiographic abnormality and repeat biopsies may be indicated if clinically warranted and feasible. Although the terminology is widely accepted and applied, the interobserver agreement for the assessment of respiratory cytology using the PSC categorization has been shown to be fair at best.[18] This has led some to call for changes to the classification system that include more stringent diagnostic criteria and updates to better reflect estimates of risk of malignancy.

A major update in the 2015 World Health Organization classification of lung tumors was the standardization of terminologies and diagnostic criteria for small biopsies in the context of radiological imaging.[19] This change was driven partly by the advances in therapeutic options. Besides the driver mutation-based targeted therapy for lung adenocarcinoma, the chemotherapeutic strategy differs based on tumor classification and the incorrect therapy can result in catastrophic harm.[20] With smaller tissue samples, the classification of carcinoma should be rendered under light microscopy with support from IHC stains. **Table 1** shows the recommended terminologies and classifications for small biopsies. Because of the heterogeneity in lung carcinoma, we focus on the most common tumors that represent over 99% of those seen on small biopsies.

SMALL CELL LUNG CARCINOMA

The diagnosis of small cell lung carcinoma (SCLC) is based on the combination of cellular morphology and IHC. These lesions are commonly centrally located and at the time of discovery have often metastasized to regional lymph nodes. Small biopsies present extra challenges by frequently presenting anemic diagnostic material with crush artifact. IHC is often necessary to differentiate SCLC from other entities with mimicking

Table 1
Terminology and interpretation in small biopsies

Small Biopsies Terminology	Morphology/Stains
Small cell carcinoma	Morphologic small cell carcinoma pattern with positive cytokeratin markers
Adenocarcinoma of the lung origin/ adenocarcinoma	Morphologic adenocarcinoma patterns clearly present with/without TTF-1/napsin A-positive stain
NSCC, favor adenocarcinoma of the lung origin	Morphologic adenocarcinoma patterns not present but supported by TTF-1/napsin A-positive stain
Squamous cell carcinoma	Morphologic squamous cell patterns clearly present
NSCC, favor SqCC	Morphologic squamous cell patterns not present but supported by p63/p40-positive stains
NSCC NOS	No clear adenocarcinoma, squamous or neuroendocrine morphology or staining pattern

Abbreviations: NOS, not otherwise specified; NSCC, non-small cell carcinoma; SqCC, squamous cell carcinoma.

morphologies, such as lymphoma and low-grade neuroendocrine tumor. Commonly used markers to support a diagnosis of SCLC include TTF-1 and neuroendocrine markers (CD56, chromogranin, synaptophysin), and a Ki-67 can be helpful in excluding a low-grade neuroendocrine tumor.

ADENOCARCINOMA

The diagnosis of adenocarcinoma on small biopsies can be made morphologically with definite gland formation or intracytoplasmic mucin vacuole. For the purpose of tissue preservation, minimal IHC stains should be used to confirm lung origin or to support the diagnosis of poorly differentiated adenocarcinoma. TTF-1 or napsin A expression in neoplastic cells in conjuncture with a history of solitary lung mass is sufficient to label the lesion as a lung primary. Subclassification of adenocarcinoma by the predominant pattern is not required in small biopsies due to intratumoral heterogeneity.

SQUAMOUS CELL CARCINOMA

The diagnosis of keratinizing squamous cell carcinoma (SqCC) can be made by morphology alone through the identification of keratin pearls or intercellular bridges. For nonkeratinizing SqCC, diffuse positivity for p63 or p40 is supportive for the diagnosis in small biopsies. Differentiating primary pulmonary from metastatic SqCC cannot be determined by histology alone and should be correlated with clinical history and imaging.

NON-SMALL CELL LUNG CARCINOMA

The diagnosis of non-small cell lung carcinoma (NSCLC) on small biopsies is reserved for cases whereby there is (1) an absence of differentiating morphologic features of small cell carcinoma, adenocarcinoma, or SqCC, and (2) ambiguous or negative IHC staining pattern.

DIAGNOSIS AND CLASSIFICATION WITH SMALL BIOPSIES

Malignant histologic features can be best described as "clonal cells with malignant nuclear features." It is more challenging to identify malignant cells in small biopsies in the presence of obscuring artifacts or an inflammatory background. In this section, we use the rule of "clonal cells with malignant nuclear features" and discuss morphologic features to differentiate benign versus malignant, classify the lesion, and distinguish mimickers (Table 2).

BENIGN VERSUS MALIGNANT

There is no single golden criterion that can distinguish between benign and malignant epithelial lesions; a constellation of features must be used to judge a mass lesion to be benign or malignant. For CNB, both architecture and cytology are evaluated. At low magnification, the growth pattern of a malignant tumor is likely to show a complex architectural arrangement. On closer inspection, clonal cells commonly have the following characteristics: high nucleus to cytoplasm (N/C) ratio, nuclear hyperchromasia, coarse chromatin, irregular nuclear contours, and prominent nucleoli (Fig. 1A, B). The cytologic features can overlap between reactive cells and well-differentiated tumor cells. This difficult scenario is commonly seen in reactive pneumocytes and bronchial cells in the setting of acute lung injury. In FNA preparations, only cytology may be evaluated. Similar to the features described in CNB, neoplastic cells are seen on FNA as clusters of epithelial cells with high N/C ratio, hyperchromatic nuclei, prominent nucleoli, and irregular nuclear membranes. In the proper clinical context, these features are considered highly suspicious for malignancy even in specimens with low cellularity (Fig. 1C–E).

By morphology, reactive pneumocytes are usually arranged as a single cell layer with homogenous space between the cells appearing as "shoulders." Unfortunately, similar features can be seen in well-differentiated adenocarcinoma. A diagnosis of malignancy is favored, however, when there is no other reactive cause and a clear abrupt transition from benign cells to malignant cells on histology (Fig. 1F-1, G). One should be cautious for rare atypical cells or atypical cells mixed with inflammatory cells, because this feature can be frequently seen in acute lung injury (Fig. 1H, I). Recognizing clonal cells with a complex growth pattern in a background of inflammation is particularly valuable even if the tumor cells are partially obscured by inflammatory cells (Fig. 1J).

Reactive bronchial cells can commonly cause confusion with malignant cells on cytologic specimens. The presence of cilia can be particularly helpful in supporting a benign process. Ciliated cells can be present at the periphery of a cluster or buried in the middle. Frustratingly, cilia may be lost in some reactive pathologic conditions or during the collection process. A close comparison of the nuclear features is the key to distinguish between benign versus malignant cells.

Although the cytomorphology is better presented in cytology specimens, the limited architectural information is one of the reasons why cytopathologists tend to use less-specific diagnostic terminologies (eg, atypical/suspicious categories), depending on the quality and the quantity of tumor cells. The clinical history and imaging studies can be helpful and should be correlated in these uncertain situations. The clinical findings that would favor malignancy are solitary nodule or mass with lymphadenopathy or subsolid lesion with increasing size or density changes. Caution should be applied to avoid overinterpretation of a reactive process as malignant when there is a history of acute lung injury, chemoradiotherapy, or ambiguous mass lesion.

The use of IHC stains to separate benign from malignant processes has limited value since there are no specific "benign or malignant" markers. Reactive benign cells are often embedded in the collapsed lung parenchyma or fibrotic tissue, leading to misinterpretation with positive TTF-1/napsin A staining.

Table 2
Diagnostic features and pitfalls of common lung carcinomas in small biopsies

	Major Criterion	Minor Criterion	Pitfalls	Comments
SCLC	Fine chromatin (salt and pepper), high N/C ratio, high Ki-67 index (>60%), sign of increased cell proliferation (necrosis, apoptosis, or mitosis)	Crush artifacts, areas of necrosis, cellular molding	Focal conspicuous nucleoli or moderate cytoplasm do not exclude SCLC, differentials to consider due to sampling error and crushing artifacts include lymphoma, low-grade neuroendocrine tumor, basaloid SqCC, metastatic melanoma, metastatic small round blue cell tumor, Merkel cell carcinoma	Use IHC stains to support and rule out mimickers Correlate clinically
Adeno	Glandular formation, cytoplasmic mucin vacuole, mucin pool, "honeycomb"-like cytomorphology	3D cellular clusters, overlapping, eccentric nuclei, fine cytoplasm, pleomorphic nuclei, prominent nucleoli	Reactive pneumocytes with similar morphology Differentials include poorly differentiated adeno and SqCC Aggregations of macrophages and clusters of mesothelial cells	Correlate for possible reactive condition; IHC support; TTF-1/napsin A stain is required for poorly diff. carcinoma
SqCC	Keratin pearls, intercellular bridges, orangeophilic cytoplasm in Pap smear	2D sheets of cells with some scattered in the background, dense cytoplasm, blue waxy in Diff-Quik smear	Overlapping morphology between squamous metaplasia and SqCC due to sampling error; differentials include poorly differentiated adeno Primary vs metastatic SqCC	Correlate clinically

Abbreviations: IHC, immunohistochemistry; SqCC, squamous cell carcinoma.

SMALL CELL LUNG CARCINOMA

The classic histologic features of SCLC are a hyperchromatic population of tumor cells, arranged in sheets or a nested growth pattern, commonly accompanied by crush artifact and coagulative tumor necrosis. The tumor cells are small to intermediate size with hyperchromatic nuclei, finely dispersed chromatin, inconspicuous nucleoli, scant cytoplasm, nuclear molding, and easily identified mitoses and apoptotic bodies (**Fig. 2**A). Occasionally, conspicuous nucleoli and a moderate amount of cytoplasm may appear in focal areas, which should not exclude the diagnosis of SCLC when other classic features are present and IHC stains are supportive (see **Fig. 2**A). In cytologic smear preparations, SCLC is usually present as hyperchromatic crowded clusters or single cells with mechanical distortion or smear crushing artifact. The "salt and pepper" nuclear features are prominent in Pap smears with para-nuclear blue bodies in a background of necrotic debris. The main differential diagnostic considerations for SCLC in small biopsies include lymphoma, the basaloid variant of SqCC, metastatic melanoma, metastatic small round blue cell tumor, and low-grade neuroendocrine tumor (**Fig. 2**B–F). The cytokeratin markers often show a perinuclear dot staining pattern, which helps to exclude nonepithelial-derived tumors. The absence of diffuse staining

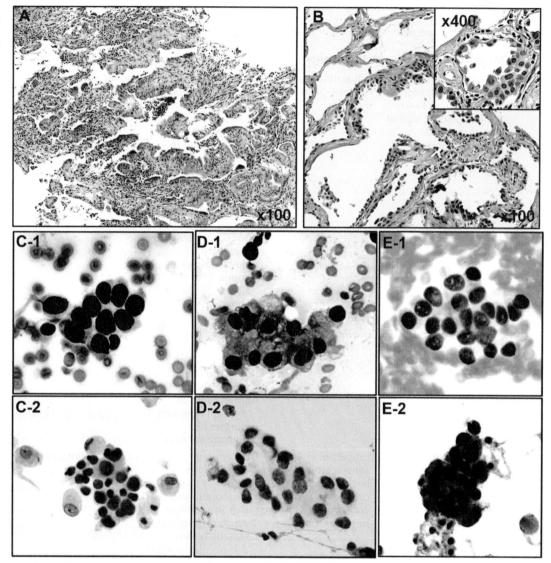

Fig. 1. (*A, B*) Adenocarcinoma. Complex structure with bland cytology in (*A*) OR marked atypical cells with less complex structure and abrupt transition from benign cells to malignant cells in (*B*) is sufficient to make malignancy diagnosis in small biopsies. (*C–E*) Adenocarcinoma, 3 cases with one Diff-Quik (DQ, 1) and Pap smear (2) in each case. Cytomorphology range from cuboidal (*C*) to columnar (*D*) cells with prominent nucleoli (*E-2*). A cluster of enlarged overlapping epithelial cells with pleomorphism, irregular nuclear membrane, hyperchromia (*C-1–E-1, C-2–E-2*), conspicuous to prominent nucleoli (*E-2*) (DQ and Pap ×400). (*F, G*) Contrast between benign tissue and adenocarcinoma. The benign tissue has bland cytology with even intracellular space ("shoulder" appearance) and areas of complex structure. (*F-2*) Area of higher magnification of (*F-1*). (*H, I*) Reactive pneumocytes. Rare marked atypical cells present in organizing pneumonia (*H*) and acute lung injury (*I*) with fibroblast foci and fibrinous secretion in air space. (*H-2*) Area of higher magnification of (*H-1*). (*J*) Adenocarcinoma. Clonal dysplastic epithelial cells with mild to moderate cellular atypia and focal complex structure in a background of inflammatory cells and fibrosis. (*J-2*) Area of higher magnification of (*J-1*).

for p63/p40 by immunohistochemistry is most helpful in excluding the possibility of basaloid SqCC. The Ki-67 index can be used to differentiate low-grade neuroendocrine tumors from small cell carcinoma by lower expression level (<20%).[15] Another minor feature of low-grade neuroendocrine tumors is the strong chromogranin stain, whereas it is usually focal and weak in SCLC (see **Fig. 2**B). Finally, expression of neuroendocrine markers are supportive, but not required for the diagnosis because approximately 10% of SCLC have negative neuroendocrine IHC stains.[15]

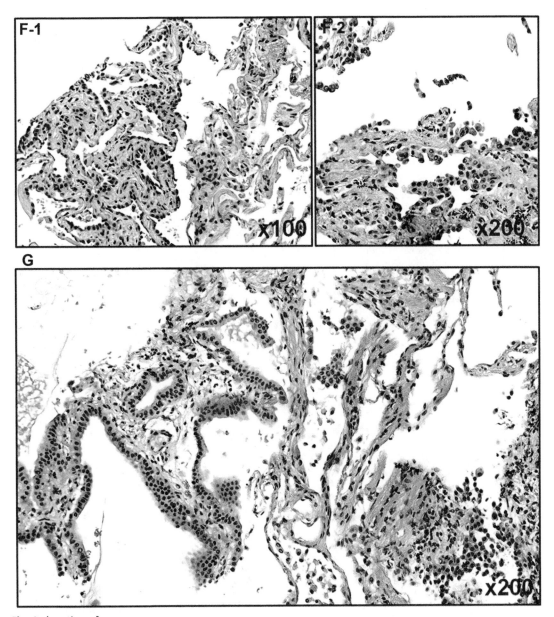

Fig. 1. (*continued*)

ADENOCARCINOMA

The most specific features for diagnosis of adenocarcinoma using routine light microscopy are glandular differentiation and cytoplasmic mucin. A classic morphology for gland formation is a lumen surrounded by cuboidal or columnar epithelial cells with an apically accentuated border. The lining cells in adenocarcinoma are at least focally crowded, overlapped, or sloughed off into the lumen, forming the growth patterns, such as lepidic, acinar, papillary, and micropapillary (**Fig. 3A–D**). The solid growth pattern often requires IHC stains to differentiate from SqCC, which can be seen in up to 30% to 40% of NSCLC in small biopsies.[21] Intracytoplasmic mucin can be subtle and easy to miss in small biopsies, particularly in cases with small amounts of tissue, and in cases of invasive mucinous adenocarcinoma, which typically shows bland cytology (**Fig. 3E**). In cytology specimens, the cytoplasmic mucin is light pale, and one may see specific "drunken honeycomb"-like cell clusters with clear intercellular borders, which are a nearly diagnostic feature of mucinous adenocarcinoma (**Fig. 3F**).[22] Sometimes, a cytoplasmic vacuole with a well-defined border and a dense dot in the center (targetoid appearance) can present in both histology and

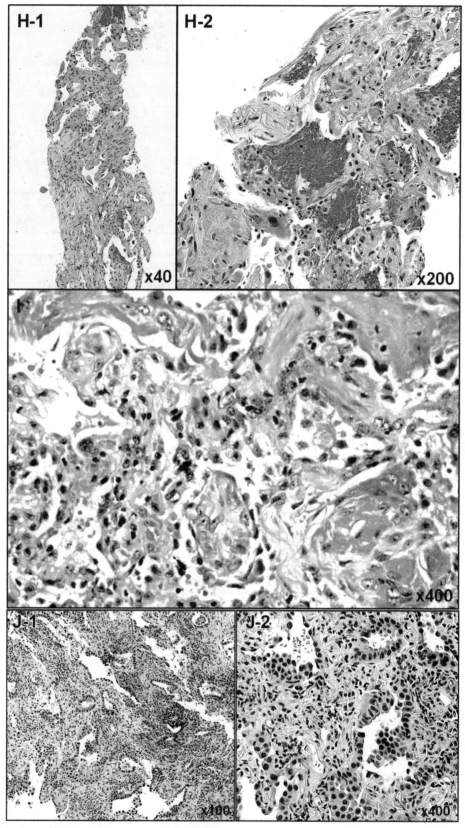

Fig. 1. (*continued*)

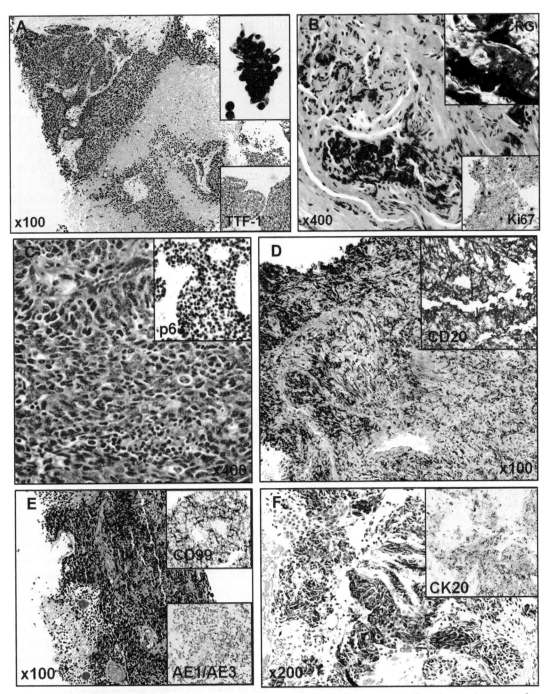

Fig. 2. (*A*) Small cell carcinoma. Sheets of hyperchromatic cells with high N/C ratio, fine chromatin, areas of necrosis, and apoptotic bodies. Conspicuous nucleoli can occasionally present in SCLC (*arrows* in Pap smear). (*B*) Carcinoid tumor. Crushing artifacts in biopsy with strong chromogranin (CRG) stain and low Ki-67 index. (*C–F*) Mimickers of SCLC in biopsies. (*C*) Basaloid SqCC. (*D*) Large B cell lymphoma with strong and diffuse CD20 staining. (*E*) Metastatic Ewing sarcoma. Sheets of hyperchromatic cells with high N/C ratio, and extensive necrosis; they are negative for pancytokeratin and positive for CD99 (membrane). The fluorescence in situ hybridization test was positive for the EWSR1 translocation. (*F*) Metastatic Merkel cell carcinoma. Sheets of cells with high N/C ratio, crush artifact, and positive stain for CD20 (perinuclear dot staining pattern).

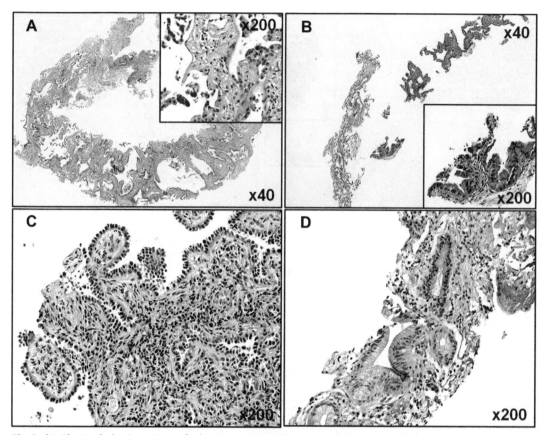

Fig. 3. (*A–D*) Morphologic variants of adenocarcinoma. (*A*) Cuboidal cells in a lepidic growth pattern. (*B*) Nonmucinous columnar cells in lepidic growth pattern. (*C*) Cuboidal to columnar cells with papillary and acinar growth pattern. (*D*) Mucinous adenocarcinoma in lepidic and acinar growth pattern. (*E–H*) Mucinous adenocarcinoma. (*E*) Small fragments of bland epithelial cells with intra- and extra-mucinous materials. (*F* and *H*) Specific "drunken honeycomb"-like cell clusters and well-defined intercellular boarder in Pap smears. (*G* and *H*) A targetoid lesion (indicated by the *red arrow*) in mucinous adenocarcinoma. (*I–M*) Mimickers and pitfalls in small biopsy. (*I*) Nonmucinous columnar adenocarcinoma cells with apical cytoplasmic snout (*red arrow*). (*J*) Peribronchial metaplasia (PBM) with hyperchromatic columnar cells and areas of dedicated cilia (*black arrow*). (*K*) Clusters of sloughed bland malignant cells in the air space, confirmed by epithelial marker AE1/AE3. (*L*) Mild atypical aggregated macrophages confirmed by CD68 staining. (*M*) Benign mesothelial cells. Specimens from CT-guided transthoracic FNA. A cluster of uniform cells with the streaming pattern.

cytology specimens, and is a marker for adenocarcinoma (red arrow in **Fig. 3**G, H). The minor cytologic features of adenocarcinoma include 3-dimensional overlapping cellular clusters, eccentric nuclei with prominent nucleoli, and delicate cytoplasm. The minimum IHC stain panel for adenocarcinoma of lung origin are TTF-1 (nuclear) or napsin A (granular cytoplasmic). In poorly differentiated NSCLC, focal and weak TTF-1 reactivity is sufficient to support the diagnosis of adenocarcinoma.[23,24] Application of IHC stains should be based on morphology since there are no IHC markers to differentiate benign from malignant processes. To better preserve limited tissue, clinical information should be used when there is a question of primary versus metastatic process,

rather than a predetermined application of immunostains. For example, neither cytokeratin 7 nor 20 is specific for adenocarcinoma of lung origin. For mucinous adenocarcinoma, there are no IHC markers to differentiate primary lung adenocarcinoma from metastatic adenocarcinoma, which is common but usually limited to the upper gastrointestinal system, including the pancreas.[24]

Besides previously discussed reactive pneumocytes, other mimickers of malignancy are peribronchiolar metaplasia (PBM), macrophages, and mesothelial cells.[25] PBM is commonly seen in diffuse lung diseases. However, it can occasionally be seen in a nodule or mass lesion. The cells of PBM are often columnar shaped with a hyperchromatic nucleus and delicate cilia. Although

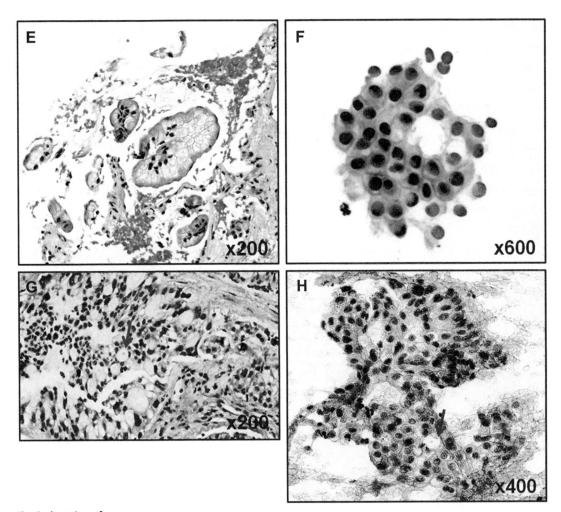

Fig. 3. (continued)

the cilia can be reassuring, they may be lost in PBM or be confused with fuzzy apical cytoplasmic snouts in malignant cells (**Fig. 3I, J**). Macrophages and mesothelial cells can have variable morphologies and be easily misinterpreted as malignant cells and vice versa. These difficult scenarios are commonly seen as aggregates of intraluminal macrophages in core or resection biopsies and clusters of mesothelial cells in CT-guided FNA specimens where they represent a contaminant from the needle passing through the parietal and visceral pleurae. Morphologically, the clusters are composed of uniform oval to spindle cells with regular intracellular spaces (**Fig. 3M**). IHC stains are often helpful in resolving this problem and identify cell lineage (**Fig. 3K, L**).

SQUAMOUS CELL CARCINOMA

For keratinizing SqCC, the presence of keratin pearls or intercellular bridges defines the

squamous origin, and are best appreciated in histology specimens including cell blocks. The major evidence for squamous differentiation in cytology specimens is orangeophilic cytoplasm in Pap smears (**Fig. 4A-1, B-1**). Minor cytomorphology features are dense cytoplasm or pale-blue waxy appearance in Diff-Quik smears (**Fig. 4B-2**). For poorly differentiated SqCC, IHC stain (p63 or p40) is recommended. The supportive staining pattern is diffuse (>50%) and strong nuclear immunoreactivity.[24] Cytokeratin 5/6 is another sensitive marker for SqCC with diffuse and strong cytoplasmic staining and high negative predictive value. Occasionally, TTF-1, p63, and p40 are coexpressed in the same population of malignant cells. In this scenario, a diagnosis of "NSCLC favor adenocarcinoma" is recommended due to low frequency of TTF-1 positivity in SqCC and relative higher frequency of p63/p40 positive adenocarcinoma.[21] If TTF-1 and p63/p40 are positive in a different population of malignant cells, the

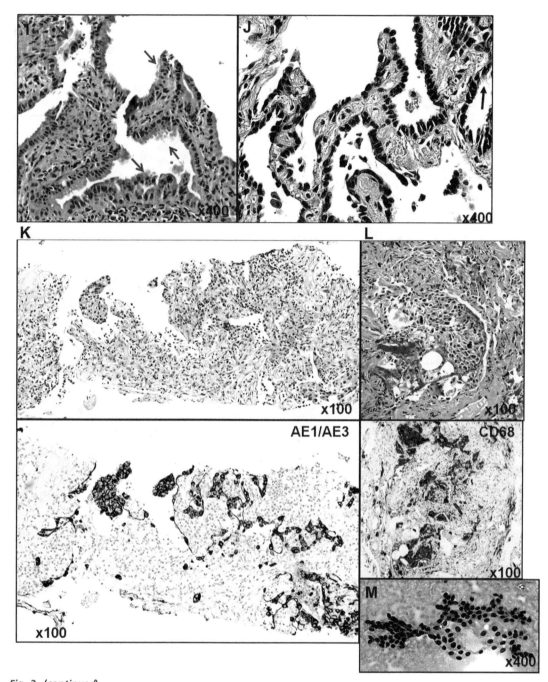

Fig. 3. (continued)

diagnosis of adenosquamous carcinoma is possible, but should be reserved for large resection specimen as the final definite diagnosis.[23]

Squamous metaplasia in small biopsies can have the same morphology as SqCC, and may show squamous cells with mild atypia, orangeophilic cytoplasm with mild dysplastic nuclei in Pap-stained samples, and a necrotic background (**Fig. 4**A, B). Both SqCC and squamous metaplasia can present as cavitary lesions on imaging, and it is not uncommon that only the keratin debris or necrotic materials are biopsied due to sampling issues. Because of this limitation, additional work up should be suggested when only keratin debris is observed.

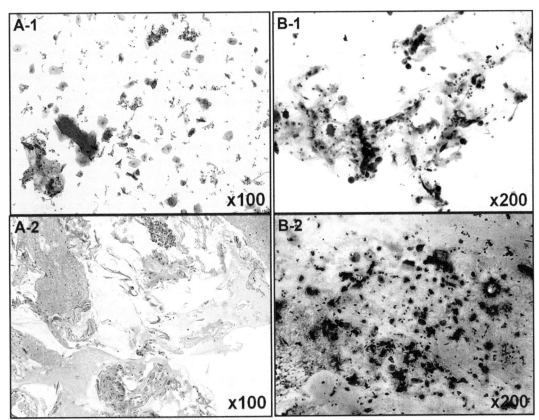

Fig. 4. (*A, B*) SqCC versus squamous metaplasia. (*A-1*) In a Pap smear, orangeophilic, keratinized, and isolated squamous cells in a background of necrosis; (*A-2*) in the cell block, a small cluster of malignant epithelial cells in a background of keratin debris. (*B*) Squamous metaplasia in a background of necrosis; (*B-1*) (Pap), (*B-2*) (DQ), squamous cells with blue waxy dense cytoplasm.

THE ROLE OF SMALL BIOPSIES IN CLINIC

Outside of diagnosis and classification, small biopsies also play an important role in staging and ancillary test management. Endobronchial ultrasound-guided transbronchial needle aspiration is used in staging and is commonly applied to paratracheal (station 2, 4), subcarinal (station 7), hilar (station 10), and lobar (station 11, 12) lymph nodes. ROSE (see above) is performed as an efficient form of biopsy. Malignant cells, lymphocyte density, or microscopic anthracotic pigment are suggested as the adequacy criteria for ROSE.[26] Presence of metastatic lung carcinoma in mediastinal or contralateral lymph nodes indicates at least N2 disease or pathology stage III or worse,[2,27] which will require ancillary tests for more therapy options, including targeted tyrosine kinase inhibitors and PD-L1 immunotherapy.

The updated molecular testing guidelines for the selection of patients with lung cancer for treatment with targeted tyrosine kinase inhibitors recommends that advanced-stage lung cancer with an adenocarcinoma component should be tested. Pathologists may use either cell blocks or other cytologic preparations as suitable specimens for lung cancer biomarker molecular testing.[28] Besides the epidermal growth factor receptor mutation tested by Next Generation Sequencing, other required molecular tests in the current guidelines, such as 2 driver gene translocations (ALK and ROS1) and PD-L1, can also be tested in cytologic specimens.[29] A recent study with a large number of specimens has shown PD-L1 IHC testing in cytology cell blocks to be effective with no significant difference from other modalities.[30] Any cytology sample with adequate cellularity and preservation could be made available for molecular testing, but appropriate validation is required.

The management of a lung nodule or mass can be best achieved by a multidisciplinary team that includes pulmonologist, thoracic radiologist, thoracic surgeon, and pathologist. We have observed that false-positive and -negative cases involving small biopsies are often those with a discrepancy between radiology and pathology. Many cases are the result of lack of communication and consensus. In summary, the pathologist's role in lung cancer is not only as diagnostician and tumor classifier, but also as consultant for specimen management, especially for small biopsies.

ACKNOWLEDGMENTS

Thanks to Keluo Yao for proofreading the article.

DISCLOSURE

The authors have no relevant commercial or financial conflicts of interest in the products or companies described in this article.

REFERENCES

1. Siegel RL, Miller KD, Jemal A. Cancer statistics, 2019. CA Cancer J Clin 2019;69(1):7–34.
2. Goldstraw P, Chansky K, Crowley J, et al. The IASLC lung cancer staging project: proposals for revision of the TNM stage groupings in the forthcoming (eighth) edition of the TNM classification for lung cancer. J Thorac Oncol 2016;11(1):39–51.
3. National Lung Screening Trial Research Team, Aberle DR, Adams AM, et al. Reduced lung-cancer mortality with low-dose computed tomographic screening. N Engl J Med 2011;365(5):395–409.
4. Chin J, Syrek Jensen T, Ashby L, et al. Screening for lung cancer with low-dose CT—translating science into Medicare coverage policy. N Engl J Med 2015;372(22):2083–5.
5. MacMahon H, Naidich DP, Goo JM, et al. Guidelines for management of incidental pulmonary nodules detected on CT images: from the Fleischner Society 2017. Radiology 2017;284(1):228–43.
6. Kim H, Park CM, Koh JM, et al. Pulmonary subsolid nodules: what radiologists need to know about the imaging features and management strategy. Diagn Interv Radiol 2014;20(1):47.
7. Gould MK, Donington J, Lynch WR, et al. Evaluation of individuals with pulmonary nodules: when is it lung cancer? Diagnosis and management of lung cancer: American College of Chest Physicians evidence-based clinical practice guidelines. Chest 2013;143(5):e93S–120.
8. Ettinger DS, Wood DE, Aisner DL, et al. Non–small cell lung cancer, version 5.2017, NCCN clinical practice guidelines in oncology. J Natl Compr Canc Netw 2017;15(4):504–35.
9. Stamatis G. Staging of lung cancer: the role of noninvasive, minimally invasive and invasive techniques. Eur Respir J 2015;46(2):521–31.
10. Yao X, Gomes MM, Tsao MS, et al. Fine-needle aspiration biopsy versus core-needle biopsy in diagnosing lung cancer: a systematic review. Curr Oncol 2012;19(1):e16.
11. Coley SM, Crapanzano JP, Saqi A. FNA, core biopsy, or both for the diagnosis of lung carcinoma: obtaining sufficient tissue for a specific diagnosis and molecular testing. Cancer Cytopathol 2015;123(5):318–26.
12. Lee Y, Park C-K, Oh Y-H. Diagnostic performance of core needle biopsy and fine needle aspiration separately or together in the diagnosis of intrathoracic lesions under C-arm guidance. J Belg Soc Radiol 2018;102(1):78.
13. Aisner DL, Rumery MD, Merrick DT, et al. Do more with less: tips and techniques for maximizing small biopsy and cytology specimens for molecular and ancillary testing: the University of Colorado experience. Arch Pathol Lab Med 2016;140(11):1206–20.
14. Jain D, Allen TC, Aisner DL, et al. Rapid on-site evaluation of endobronchial ultrasound-guided transbronchial needle aspirations for the diagnosis of lung cancer: a perspective from members of the pulmonary pathology society. Arch Pathol Lab Med 2017;142(2):253–62.
15. Rekhtman N. Neuroendocrine tumors of the lung: an update. Arch Pathol Lab Med 2010;134(11):1628–38.
16. Schmidt RL, Walker BS, Cohen MB. When is rapid on-site evaluation cost-effective for fine-needle aspiration biopsy? PLoS One 2015;10(8):e0135466.
17. Layfield LJ, Baloch Z, Elsheikh T, et al. Standardized terminology and nomenclature for respiratory cytology: the Papanicolaou Society of Cytopathology guidelines. Diagn Cytopathol 2016;44(5):399–409.
18. Layfield LJ, Esebua M, Dodd L, et al. The Papanicolaou Society of Cytopathology guidelines for respiratory cytology: reproducibility of categories among observers. Cytojournal 2018;15:22.
19. Travis WD, Brambilla E, Nicholson AG, et al. The 2015 World Health Organization classification of lung tumors: impact of genetic, clinical and radiologic advances since the 2004 classification. J Thorac Oncol 2015;10(9):1243–60.
20. Hellmann MD, Chaft JE, Rusch V, et al. Risk of hemoptysis in patients with resected squamous cell and other high-risk lung cancers treated with adjuvant bevacizumab. Cancer Chemother Pharmacol 2013;72(2):453–61.
21. Thunnissen E, Boers E, Heideman DAM, et al. Correlation of immunohistochemical staining p63 and TTF-1 with EGFR and K-ras mutational spectrum and diagnostic reproducibility in non small cell lung carcinoma. Virchows Arch 2012;461(6):629–38.
22. Morency E, Rodriguez Urrego PA, Szporn AH, et al. The "drunken honeycomb" feature of pulmonary mucinous adenocarcinoma: a diagnostic pitfall of bronchial brushing cytology. Diagn Cytopathol 2013;41(1):63–6.
23. Travis WD, Brambilla E, Noguchi M, et al. Diagnosis of lung cancer in small biopsies and cytology:

implications of the 2011 International Association for the Study of Lung Cancer/American Thoracic Society/European Respiratory Society classification. Arch Pathol Lab Med 2012;137(5):668–84.

24. Yatabe Y, Dacic S, Borczuk AC, et al. Best practices recommendations for diagnostic immunohistochemistry in lung cancer. J Thorac Oncol 2019;14(3):377–407.

25. Idowu MO, Powers CN. Lung cancer cytology: potential pitfalls and mimics—a review. Int J Clin Exp Pathol 2010;3(4):367.

26. Choi SM, Lee A-R, Choe J-Y, et al. Adequacy criteria of rapid on-site evaluation for endobronchial ultrasound-guided transbronchial needle aspiration: a simple algorithm to assess the adequacy of ROSE. Ann Thorac Surg 2016;101(2):444–50.

27. Kassis ES, Vaporciyan AA. Defining N2 disease in non–small cell lung cancer. Thorac Surg Clin 2008; 18(4):333–7.

28. Lindeman NI, Cagle PT, Aisner DL, et al. Updated molecular testing guideline for the selection of lung cancer patients for treatment with targeted tyrosine kinase inhibitors: guideline from the College of American Pathologists, the International Association for the Study of Lung Cancer, and the Association for Molecular Pathology. J Thorac Oncol 2018; 13(3):323–58.

29. Bubendorf L, Lantuejoul S, de Langen AJ, et al. Non-small cell lung carcinoma: diagnostic difficulties in small biopsies and cytological specimens: number 2 in the series "Pathology for the clinician" Edited by Peter Dorfmüller and Alberto Cavazza. Eur Respir Rev 2017;26(144):170007.

30. Wang H, Agulnik J, Kasymjanova G, et al. Cytology cell blocks are suitable for immunohistochemical testing for PD-L1 in lung cancer. Ann Oncol 2018; 29(6):1417–22.

Targeted Therapy and Checkpoint Immunotherapy in Lung Cancer

Roberto Ruiz-Cordero, MD[a],*, Walter Patrick Devine, MD, PhD[b]

KEYWORDS

- Lung cancer • Non–small cell lung cancer • Molecular landscape • Targeted therapy
- Immunotherapy • Checkpoint inhibitors • Resistance mechanisms

Key points

- Lung cancer transitioned from a rare disease into the main cause of cancer-related death in humans over the past 100 years.

- Increasing understanding of the molecular underpinnings driving lung carcinogenesis have allowed therapies to be developed that target specific genomic alterations.

- Multigene panel testing decreases cost and can have a faster turnaround time than single-gene testing.

- Immunotherapy, mainly through the use of checkpoint inhibitors, has shown promising results in lung cancer treatment.

- Despite tremendous efforts and progress against lung cancer, the overall survival remains dismal and the mortalities high.

ABSTRACT

Lung cancer is the leading cause of cancer mortality. It is classified into different histologic subtypes, including adenocarcinoma, squamous carcinoma, and large cell carcinoma (commonly referred as non–small cell lung cancer) and small cell lung cancer. Comprehensive molecular characterization of lung cancer has expanded our understanding of the cellular origins and molecular pathways affected in each of these subtypes. Many of these genetic alterations represent potential therapeutic targets for which drugs are constantly under development. This article discusses the molecular characteristics of the main lung cancer subtypes and discusses the current guidelines and novel targeted therapies, including checkpoint immunotherapy.

OVERVIEW

The first text book on malignant lung tumors was published in 1912 by Dr. I. Adler.[1] At the time, he questioned the utility of writing a monograph on an entity that was among the rarest forms of cancer, with only 374 verifiable cases published in the literature worldwide.[1,2] Since then, lung cancer has transitioned from an exceedingly rare disease into the main cause of cancer-related mortality in both men and women, accounting for approximately 142,670 deaths in the United States in 2019.[3] Similarly, lung cancer therapy has undergone dramatic changes, initially starting with only supportive care in the first half of the twentieth century, followed by the empiric use of cytotoxic therapy. Single-agent chemotherapy in the 1970s was rapidly replaced by platinum-based

[a] Department of Pathology, University of California San Francisco, 1825 4th Street Room L2181A, San Francisco, CA 94158, USA; [b] Department of Pathology, University of California San Francisco, 1600 Divisadero Street Room B-620, San Francisco, CA 94115, USA

* Corresponding author.

E-mail address: Roberto.Ruiz-Cordero@ucsf.edu

Twitter: @drruizcor (R.R.-C.)

Surgical Pathology 13 (2020) 17–33

https://doi.org/10.1016/j.path.2019.11.002

combination therapy (eg, cisplatin plus another cytotoxic therapy) in the 1980s as standard therapy for patients with advanced disease[4] (**Fig. 1**). In more recent years, the identification of subgroups of tumors harboring distinct genetic alterations has transformed the landscape of lung cancer therapy and propelled thoracic oncology to the forefront of personalized oncology. Lung cancer encompasses several subgroups with distinct morphologic features, mutation and transcriptomic profiles, therapeutic indications, and prognoses (**Figs. 2** and **3**). Although the overall survival still remains dismal for most patients with lung cancer, particularly those with advanced stages (5-year survival ranging from 5% to 17.7%),[5,6] several key discoveries have defined some of the basic mechanisms driving oncogenesis. These discoveries have been translated into targeted therapies that have now become standard of care in the clinical management of patients with lung cancer. Along with these advances, survival for a subset of patients with lung cancer has modestly but steadily increased[7] (see **Fig. 1**).

CONTENT

Although the broad histologic classification of lung cancer into small cell lung cancer (SCLC) and non–

small cell lung cancer (NSCLC) is still widely used, molecular classification of lung cancer suggests that there are vastly different diseases that can no longer be broadly grouped and should be recognized as distinct entities[8] (see **Fig. 3**). In this era of targetable molecular therapies, NSCLC and SCLC are no longer valid diagnostic choices to adequately guide therapy.[8,9] To this end, pathologists now need to not only differentiate among cell types but to perform a complex set of tests with smaller samples in a timely manner while fostering communication with clinical colleagues so that patients fully benefit from molecularly selected therapies. Current molecular testing guidelines follow the standards recommended by the National Comprehensive Cancer Network[10] in order for oncologists to commence therapy (**Table 1**). Given that the size of the tissue samples continues to decrease with more and more minimally invasive procedures but the number of potential molecular targets in lung cancer continues to increase, prioritization of the limited tissue becomes key. This article discusses the major molecular subtypes of lung cancer as they relate to the classic histotypes, the molecular targets for which therapies have been and are under development, the most common mechanisms of resistance to these therapies, the current

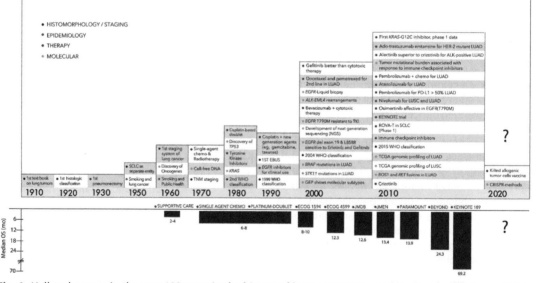

Fig. 1. Hallmark events in the past 100 years in the history of lung cancer grouped by decade. The legend highlights 4 categories: purple indicates histomorphology/staging events, orange shows epidemiologic events, red highlights therapeutic advances, and many key molecular discoveries are shown in blue. The bottom portion indicates the increase in overall survival shown in months. ALK, anaplastic lymphoma kinase; ECOG, Eastern Cooperative Oncology Group; EGFR, epidermal growth factor receptor; LUAD, lung adenocarcinoma; LUSC, lung squamous carcinoma; OS, overall survival; SCLC, small cell lung cancer; TCGA, The Cancer Genome Atlas; TKI, tyrosine kinase inhibitor; TNM, tumor, node, metastasis; WHO, World Health Organization. (*Data from* Refs.[2,4,12,98,99]; and *Courtesy of* Marisa Ruiz.)

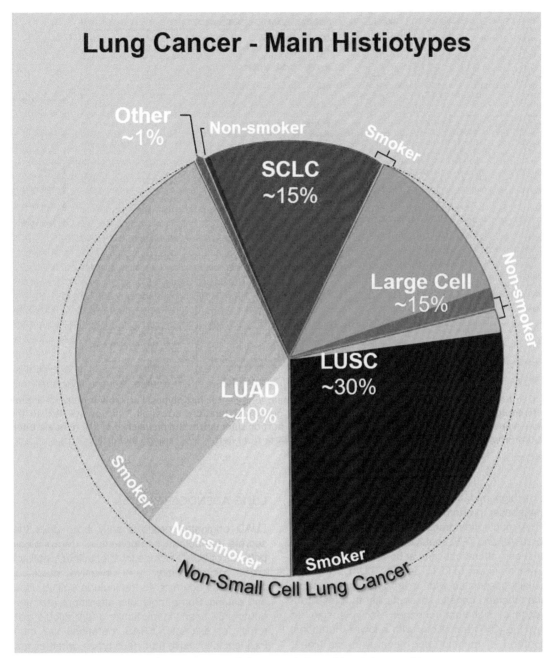

Fig. 2. The main histiotypes of lung cancer and their association with tobacco smoking.

guidelines and recommendations for molecular testing, the challenges and opportunities in the field, and future directions.

NON–SMALL CELL LUNG CANCER

NSCLC encompasses the following histotypes (see **Fig. 2**):

- Lung adenocarcinoma (LUAD): accounts for 40% of all lung cancers.

- Lung squamous carcinoma (LUSC): accounts for 25% to 30% of all lung cancers.
- Large cell carcinoma: accounts for 15% of all lung cancers.
- Mixed histotypes: rare.[11]

Tobacco smoking accounts for more than 80% of lung cancer cases and is associated with all major histotypes, predominantly LUSC and SCLC but also LUAD[12] (see **Fig. 2**). The mutational signature caused by tobacco carcinogens is characterized

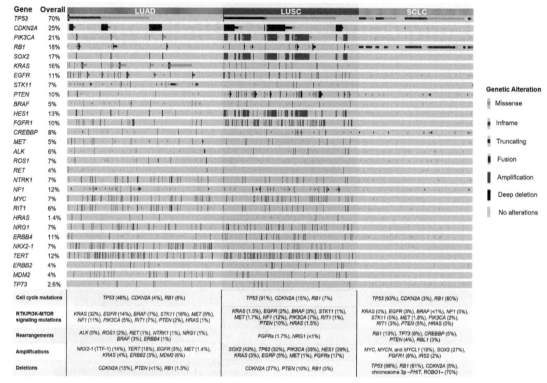

Fig. 3. Key molecular alterations occurring in the 3 main lung cancer histiotypes. Each row represents a gene referenced to the left with the overall frequency of genomic alterations across all 3 histiotypes next to the gene name. Each column indicates a case. The bottom portion summarizes the prevalence of key genomic alterations grouped by type of alteration and histiotype. (*Data from* Refs.[7,13,76,84] using cBioPortal.[100,101])

by a high mutation burden (~10 mutations per megabase), predominance of cytosine to adenine (C>A) nucleotide transversions, and enrichment for *KRAS* and *TP53* mutations.[5,12] To date, neither of these alterations are actionable. In contrast, never smokers tend to develop LUADs that are usually associated with environmental exposures and inherited genetic susceptibility that lead to a genomic signature enriched for cytosine to thymine (C>T) transitions with a lower mutational burden (~1 mutation per megabase) and higher prevalence of actionable alterations, including epidermal growth factor receptor (*EGFR*) mutations and anaplastic lymphoma kinase (*ALK*) and *ROS1* fusions (discussed later) as well as *PIK3CA* and *RB1* mutations.[5,12,13]

In contrast with SCLCs, a subset of patients with NSCLCs are more frequently diagnosed at a localized stage when tumors can undergo surgery or radiotherapy with curative intent.[8] For patients with advanced disease and unresectable tumors for whom surgery is not an option, pharmacologic therapy becomes the mainstay of treatment.

LUNG ADENOCARCINOMA

LUAD originates predominantly from cells that secrete surfactant components.[14] Morphologic patterns of LUAD include lepidic, acinar, papillary, solid, micropapillary, and invasive mucinous types. Less common forms include colloid, fetal, and enteric. Some molecular alterations are more commonly seen, in particular morphologic patterns; for example, *KRAS* mutations are more frequent in invasive mucinous types, whereas mutations in *TP53* are associated with solid growth.[13,15] Although LUAD occurs in smokers, it is the most common type of lung cancer seen in nonsmokers. It is more common in women, particularly of Asian descent, than in men and is more likely to occur in younger individuals than other types of lung cancer.[5,12,13,16] In the past 20 to 30 years, LUAD has replaced LUSC as the most frequent histotype. This epidemiologic shift is thought to be a reflection of smoking behavior trends and cigarette manufacturing, whereby wide adoption of filter and light cigarettes has led to deeper smoke aspirations that help carcinogens

Table 1 Recommended molecular markers based on tiers			
Tier 1 Must Test	**Tier 2 Should Test**	**Tier 3 May Test/ Emerging**	**Extra Genes**
EGFR	ERBB2	MEK1	TP53
ALK	MET	MAP2K1	STK11
ROS1	RET	FGFR1	PRKACA
BRAF	KRAS	FGFR2	PRKCA
		FGFR3	PRKCB
		FGFR4	
		NTRK1	
		NTRK2	
		NTRK3	
		RIT1	
		NF1	
		PIK3CA	
		AKT1	
		NRAS	
		MTOR	
		TSC1	
		TSC2	
		KIT	
		PDGFRA	
		DDR2	
		NRG1	

reach the more distal parts of the bronchial tree, including the alveoli where many LUADs arise.[5]

Genomic alterations, including gene amplification, mutations, or translocations, can cause aberrant activation of signaling pathways involved in cellular growth and differentiation, ultimately leading to uncontrolled cell proliferation, resistance to apoptotic signals, tumor formation, and eventually metastasis (**Fig. 4**). Comprehensive molecular profiling of LUAD identified *TP53*, *KRAS*, *KEAP1*, *STK11*, *EGFR*, *NF1*, *BRAF*, *SETD2*, *RMB10*, and *MGA* as the 10 most commonly mutated genes.[7,13] Significant copy number alterations (CNAs) include amplifications in *NKX2-1*, the gene encoding thyroid transcription factor 1 (TTF-1), *TERT*, *MDM2*, *KRAS*, *EGFR*, *MET*, *CCNE1*, and *CCND1*, and deletion of *CDKN2A* in a subset of patients[7,13] (see **Fig. 3**). Transcriptional analysis identified 3 main subgroups of LUAD: (1) a subgroup that presents more commonly in women who never smoked. These tumors are characterized by acinar, papillary, or lepidic histomorphology and harbor mutations or CNAs in *EGFR* and kinase fusions. (2) A second subgroup of tumors with variable histology characterized by mutations and CNAs in *KRAS* and *STK11*. (3) A third subgroup of tumors showing primarily solid architecture with enrichment for *TP53* and *NF1* mutations in addition to p16 methylation.[13] These findings confirm the presence of the 3 molecular subtypes (ie, terminal respiratory unit, proximal proliferative, and proximal inflammatory, respectively) previously identified by gene expression profiling.[13,17–20] Although only 2 of the top 10 genes (ie, *EGFR* and *BRAF*) can be pharmacologically targeted at present in LUAD, other actionable mutations that drive oncogenesis and can be specifically targeted are observed in a minority

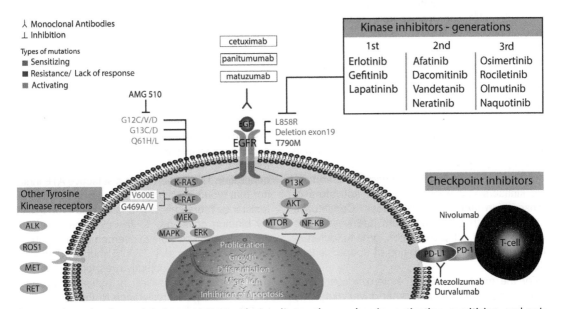

Fig. 4. Main molecules and their association with signaling pathways showing activating, sensitizing, and resistance mutations as well as available targeted therapies for key molecular targets. (*Courtesy of* Marisa Ruiz.)

of patients. Nevertheless, the unprecedented benefits observed in this small subset of patients have led to a large increase in drug development and approvals presaging the era of personalized medicine.

MOLECULAR ALTERATIONS WITH APPROVED TARGETED THERAPIES AND MECHANISMS OF RESISTANCE

Epidermal Growth Factor Receptor

The epidermal growth factor (EGF) receptor gene maps to the short arm of chromosome 7q22, spans 110 kb of DNA, and is divided into 28 exons.[21] It encodes a receptor tyrosine kinase also known as ErbB1/HER1 and is the prototype of the ErbB family of tyrosine kinase receptors comprising ErbB2/HER2/Neu, ErbB3/HER3, and ErbB4/HER4. After cleavage at the N-terminal domain, the final transmembrane EGFR consists of 1186 amino acid residues encompassing 3 domains, including the N-terminal domain with an extracellular ligand binding and dimerization arm (exons 1–16), a hydrophobic transmembrane domain (exon 17), and the intracellular tyrosine kinase and C-terminal domains (exons 18–28).[21,22] EGFR mutations can occur across all domains, although mutations in the transmembrane region are uncommon. Most mutations occur at specific mutational hotspots that seem to be cancer dependent. For example, EGFR mutations in LUAD occur in ~14% of patients and cluster almost exclusively to the ATP-binding pocket of the tyrosine kinase domain, whereas most glioblastomas harbor mutations in the ectodomain and colorectal cancers contain mainly EGFR gene amplification.[23–27]

Under regular circumstances, normal cells, including pulmonary epithelial cells, can express around 40,000 to 100,000 EGF receptors per cell and up to 10,000,000 receptors per cancer cell,[28] each promoting the constitutive and ligand-independent activation of EGFR-associated pathways, including the extracellular signal–regulated kinase (ERK), mitogen-activated protein kinase (MAPK), phosphatidylinositol 3-kinase (PI3K)-AKT, SRC, c-Jun N-terminal kinase (JNK), and Janus kinase/signal transducers and activators of transcription (JAK-STAT) pathways. Constitutive activation of these downstream pathways leads to uncontrolled cell proliferation, growth, differentiation, migration, and inhibition of apoptosis (see Fig. 4).

For the most part, EGFR heterozygous mutations do not co-occur with other driver mutations such as KRAS or ALK rearrangements. They occur early in the pathogenesis of LUAD and more than 80% involve in-frame deletions in exon 19 (E746-A750) (Fig. 5A), a point mutation change of leucine for asparagine in codon 858 (L858R) within exon 21 (Fig. 5B), or substitutions in exon 18 (G719C/S/A).[16,21,23,25,26,29–32] The impact of these mutations occurring in the tyrosine kinase domain is reflected in the 50-fold increase in kinase activity compared with wild-type EGFR caused by a stabilized active conformation.[26]

The connection between the development of tyrosine kinase inhibitors (TKIs) in the 1980s and the discovery of specific genomic alterations in NSCLC allowed the implementation of molecularly targeted therapies in the late 1990s (see Fig. 1). First-generation EGFR TKIs, including erlotinib and gefitinib, were designed to reversibly bind to the ATP-binding site in EGFR exclusively, whereas afatinib and dacomitinib, second-generation TKIs, are irreversible inhibitors that also target HER2 and HER4[12,32] (see Fig. 4). First-generation and second-generation TKIs showed increased frequency of responses and improved survival, with both afatinib and dacomitinib showing improved progression-free survival compared with gefitinib in patients with NSCLC, mainly LUAD. Afatinib was shown to provide significant overall survival improvement in patients with exon 19 deletion but not in patients with the L858R mutation.[5,12,32] It has been shown that each of these common sensitizing EGFR mutations confers different conformational changes to the mutated ATP-binding pocket protein that lead to variability in autophosphorylation and could explain the difference in patient outcomes.[25]

Additional EGFR mutations such as the exon 20 insertion is not inhibited by TKIs. Furthermore, the substitution of threonine to methionine on codon 790 (T790M), also in exon 20, is the most common cause of acquired resistance to first-generation TKI therapy. This mutation is thought to increase the affinity of the tyrosine kinase domain for ATP.[5,12,21,33] Genetic mechanisms of acquired resistance have been shown to arise in a subclonal fashion by conferring resistance to a subclone that expands gradually under the selective pressure of the first-generation EGFR TKI.[5,33] The third-generation TKI osimertinib is a selective ATP inhibitor that works on both the sensitizing and T790M resistance mutations, and spares wild-type EGFR. By binding covalently to the cysteine on codon 797, osimertinib is able to overcome the enhanced ATP affinity from the T790M mutation, thereby showing increased objective response rates and progression-free survival in patients harboring T790M.[33] Acquired resistance to third-generation EGFR TKIs has been reported to occur secondary to the C797S mutation.[32,34] Patients with a

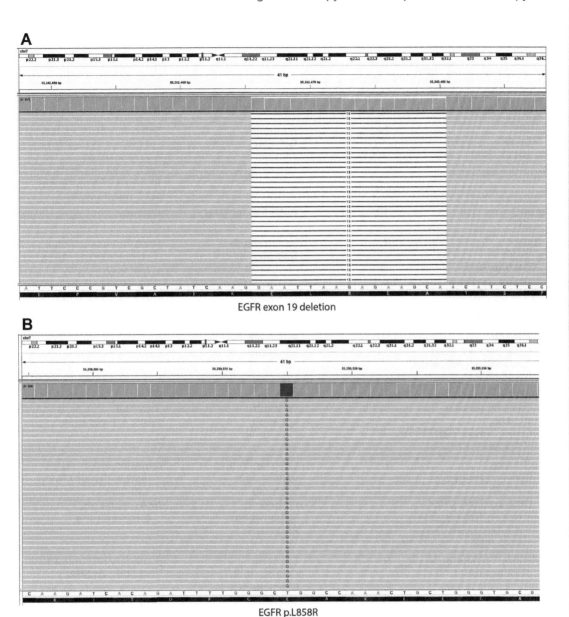

Fig. 5. Most common activating *EGFR* mutations showing (*A*) the exon 19 deletion and (*B*) the L858R missense mutation, which are sensitive to tyrosine kinase inhibitors.

sensitizing mutation and C797S but without T790M show resistance to osimertinib but not to gefitinib or afatinib. However, patients with triple-mutant tumors (sensitizing mutation, T790M, and C797S) are resistant to all 3 generations of EGFR TKIs.[12,35] Additional mechanisms of resistance include *HER2* amplification; mutations in *MET*, *BRAF*, *PIK3CA*; and SCLC transformation[5,12,32,33] (**Table 2**). Because cases with C797S are rare and the mutation is poorly studied and not currently treatable, routine molecular testing for C797S is not recommended for management at this time.[36,37]

Anaplastic Lymphoma Kinase

The *ALK* gene encodes a transmembrane tyrosine kinase receptor whose function in humans remains poorly understood. *ALK* is rearranged in approximately 5% of patients with LUAD with multiple possible partners.[32,38–40] The most common alteration occurs as a result of a small inversion in chromosome 2p that leads to the fusion of the N-terminal end of the echinoderm microtubule-associated protein–like 4 (*EML4*) gene with the C-terminal kinase domain of *ALK* (**Fig. 6**). ALK is not normally transcribed

Table 2
Summary of oncogenic drivers, frequency, targeted therapies and most common resistance mechanism in lung adenocarcinoma

Genomic Alteration	Frequency (%)	Approved or Emerging Targeted Therapies	Main Mechanisms of Resistance
EGRF • L858R • Del exon 19	14	Erlotinib Gefitinib Afatinib Osimertinib	Secondary *EGFR* mutations: T790M, C797S, D761Y, L747S, T854A *MET, HER2* amplification BRAF, PIK3CA mutations SCLC transformation
KRAS • G12	30	AMG 510 for G12C	Unknown
BRAF • V600E • G469A/V/R • G466V	7	Vemurafenib Dabrafenib	Mutation-independent reactivation of MAPK pathway
ALK rearrangements Common partners: • *EML4* • *KIF5B* Other partners: *ASXL2, ATP6V1B1, PRKAR1A, SPDYA*	5	Crizotinib Alectinib Ceritinib Brigatinib Lorlatinib	Secondary *ALK* mutations: G1202R, I1171T
ROS1 fusion Common partner: • *CD74* Other partners: *EZR, SLC34A2, SDC4*	2	Crizotinib Ceritinib Lorlatinib Entrectinib	Secondary *ROS1* mutations: G2032R *KRAS, KIT* mutations
RET fusion Common partner: • *KIF5B* Other partners: *CCDC6, NCOA, TRIM33, CUX1, KIAA1217, FRMD4A, KIAA1468*	2	Cabozantinib Vandetanib Sunitinib Pralsetinib Selpercatinib RXDX-105	Mutation-independent reactivation of MAPK pathway *NRAS* mutation, overexpression
MET exon 14 alteration or amplification	5	Crizotinib Cabozantinib Capmatinib Tepotinib Savolitinib	Secondary *MET* mutations: Y1248H, D1246N
ERBB2/HER2 mutations	3	Trastuzumab deruxtecan Poziotinib Pyrotinib	Secondary *ERBB2* mutations: G776YVMAins *PIK3CA* mutations
NTRK1/2/3 fusion	<1	Larotrectinib Entrectinib	Secondary *NTRK1* mutations: G595R IGF1R bypass pathway–mediated resistance

in the adult human lung; however, EML4 is expressed at high levels and the translocation event results in the overexpression of the chimeric protein that includes the C-terminal kinase domain of *ALK*.[40] The resulting chimeric EML4-ALK fusion protein has increased tyrosine kinase activity but is highly responsive to TKIs.

Patients with *ALK* rearrangement are often of younger age and nonsmokers or light smokers.[39] Crizotinib was designed as an ATP-competitive kinase inhibitor to specifically target human ALK, MET, and ROS1 tyrosine kinase receptors (see **Fig. 4**); it has shown tumor response rates of 60% in ALK-positive tumors.[38–40] Similar to EGFR TKIs,

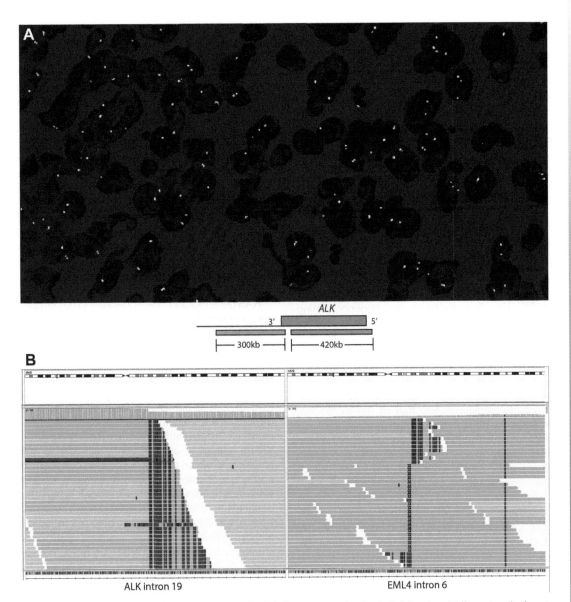

Fig. 6. *ALK*-rearranged case of LUAD as shown by (*A*) fluorescence in situ hybridization. Yellow signals denote intact ALK gene locus, whereas separate green signals occur as a result of an inversion event on chromosome 2p between *ALK* and *EML4*. (*B*) Next-generation sequencing confirms the inversion and shows breakpoints in intron 19 of *ALK* and intron 6 of *EML4*.

resistance to ALK inhibitors is commonly acquired mainly caused by mutations in *ALK*, including L1152R, C1156Y, I1171T, L1196M G1202R, S1206Y, and G1269A. These mutations lead to non-canonical activation of EGFR, KRAS, and KIT pathways[5,38–40] (see **Table 2**). Second-generation ALK inhibitors, ceritinib, alectinib, and brigatinib, have shown promising results in patients with acquired resistance to ALK inhibitors. The third-generation ALK inhibitor lorlatinib has shown activity against most ALK resistance mutations, including the common G1202R mutation.[12]

There is currently insufficient evidence to support a recommendation for or against routine testing for *ALK* mutational status for patients with LUAD with sensitizing *ALK* mutations who have progressed after treatment with an ALK-targeted TKI.[37]

ROS Proto-Oncogene 1 (ROS1)

ROS proto-oncogene 1 (*ROS1*) is a member of the insulin receptor family that also encodes a receptor tyrosine kinase. Gene rearrangements with different partners such as *CD74* lead to constitutive activation.[41] *ROS1* fusions are rare, seen in approximately 1% of patients with LUAD, and they are also associated with younger age and never smokers.[32,39] ROS1-positive tumors respond well to the ALK inhibitors crizotinib, ceritinib, and lorlatinib because of the high homology between *ROS1* and *ALK* kinase domains.[32,42] Similarly, mechanisms of acquired resistance include secondary *ROS1* mutations, most commonly G2032R, mutations in *KRAS* and *KIT*, and wild-type EGFR signaling activation (see **Table 2**).

B-Raf Proto-oncogene, Serine/Threonine Kinase

B-Raf proto-oncogene, serine/threonine kinase (*BRAF*) encodes a protein that belongs to a family of serine-threonine kinases that mediate the MAPK signaling pathway by phosphorylating different proteins involved in the activation of MEK.[43] Although rare, *BRAF* mutations develop in 3% of patients with LUAD, commonly associated with tobacco exposure.[5,12,32,44,45] The hotspot transversion at exon 15 in which valine is replaced by glutamate at residue 600 (V600E) accounts for approximately half of the mutations, whereas the other mutations occur at different positions also within the kinase domain. *BRAF* mutations usually do not co-occur with other oncogenic alterations such as *EGFR* or *ALK* rearrangements.[43,45]

Vemurafenib, a BRAF inhibitor, has been shown to provide clinical efficacy in selected cases. Anecdotal cases of LUAD harboring *BRAF* V600E mutation have developed resistance to vemurafenib mainly via mutation-independent reactivation of the MAPK pathway.[46] More recently dabrafenib, another BRAF inhibitor, in combination with the MEK inhibitor trametinib, has yielded promising results and the combination has been approved by the US Food and Drug Administration (FDA) and European Medicines Agency for LUAD with *BRAF* V600E mutations.[47]

MOLECULAR ALTERATIONS WITH POTENTIAL TARGETED THERAPIES

Kirsten Rat Sarcoma Viral Oncogene Homolog

The *RAS* oncogenes include 2 rat sarcoma (RAS)–inducing viruses named after their respective discoverers, Harvey RAS (*H-RAS*) and Kirsten RAS (*K-RAS*), in the 1960s, with the human homolog genes isolated in the early 1980s, and the neuroblastoma RAS (*N-RAS*) that was subsequently identified.[48] These genes encode the 21-kDa RAS family proteins, which share high sequence homology and are key signaling molecules that regulate cell growth, survival, and differentiation. The different isoforms have discrepant sequences in the carboxy-terminal region, also known as the hypervariable domain, which is essential for the localization of RAS to the plasma membrane.[48] Despite their similarities and interaction with common molecules, RAS isoforms generate different biological effects. Nevertheless, RAS activates the MAPK cascade, PI3K, and Ral factors through the Raf kinases effector proteins (see **Fig. 4**). All 3 RAS isoforms can activate the 3 Raf serine/threonine kinases, A-RAF, B-RAF, and RAF1, which phosphorylate the serine/threonine kinases Mek1 and Mek2, which in turn activate ERK kinases. Through a series of steps, ERK then leads to the expression of proteins that control cell-cycle progression, such as cyclin D.[48–51]

RAS gene mutations are prevalent in human cancers, occurring in approximately 30% of all cancers and 32% of LUAD (see **Fig. 3**). The most frequent somatic missense mutations introduce amino acid substitutions at codons 12 (>80% of the time), 13, and 61 and can be observed in all *RAS* genes. Substitution of glutamine 61 with any amino acid except glutamic acid as well as replacing glycine 12 with any other amino acid except proline leads to a constitutively active RAS protein.[48,49] *KRAS* mutations are frequently associated with smoking, in which they occur early in oncogenesis and show characteristic substitutions of a purine with a pyrimidine (G-T transversion); when they occur in nonsmokers they usually show G-A transitions.[51] Notably, the frequency of *KRAS* mutations among current or former smokers and never smokers can be as high as 26% versus 6%, respectively (hazard ratio, 4.36; $P<.01$).[52] Furthermore, the frequency of *KRAS* mutations varies among different ethnic groups, with lower frequency in east Asians and higher frequency in black people compared with white people. *KRAS* mutations are mutually exclusive with *EGFR* mutations and confer resistance to EGFR TKIs.[50,52,53] Recent reports have shown that the co-occurrence of *KRAS* mutations with *TP53* mutations is associated with a worse prognosis; however, increased response to immunotherapy has also been reported in these co-mutated tumors.[15,54]

Although *KRAS* remains a frustrating oncogenic driver to pharmacologically attack, a novel small molecule inhibitor of the *KRAS* G12C mutation has shown partial response in half of the patients with NSCLC studied in a phase I trial.[55] Additional targeted therapies for *KRAS* mutations are in development and could potentially usher in a new era of therapy for patients with lung cancer.

MET Proto-oncogene, Receptor Tyrosine Kinase

MET encodes a tyrosine kinase known as the hepatocyte growth factor receptor. MET is amplified in different tumors and in 2% to 4% of NSCLCs. In addition, 3% of LUADs harbor splice site mutations around exon 14 that lead to deletion of exon 14, a process also known as exon skipping.[56] Exon skipping leads to enhanced ligand-mediated proliferation of cancer cells. Patients whose tumors show high-level amplification of MET benefit from crizotinib, and those with MET exon 14 skipping mutations also respond to capmatinib and cabozantinib in addition to crizotinib.[56–58] Potential resistance mechanisms include a secondary MET mutation.[59,60]

RET Proto-oncogene, Receptor Tyrosine Kinase

RET encodes a receptor tyrosine kinase focused on cell growth and differentiation.[61,62] The most common alteration includes an inversion on chromosome 10, inv(10) (p11q11), that results in a fusion between RET and KIF5B genes.[63,64] However, other fusion partners include CCDC6, ELE1, KIAA1217, NCOA4, and TRIM33. RET fusions occur in 1% to 2% of LUAD, are associated with never smokers, but do not occur in conjunction with EGFR, KRAS, BRAF, and ERBB2 mutations.[39] Recent preliminary data on newer selective RET inhibitors, including pralsetinib and selpercatinib, showed greater activity and more favorable safety profiles compared with previous multikinase agents.[65,66] Both of these new drugs have received FDA breakthrough therapy designation for patients with RET fusion–positive NSCLC. Resistance mechanisms include mutation-independent reactivation of MAPK pathway, NRAS mutation, or overexpression.[67]

Erb-B2 Receptor Tyrosine Kinase 2 (ERBB2/HER-2/Neu)

HER-2/Neu is amplified in 2% and mutated in 2% to 4% of NSCLCs. Mutations are exclusively seen in LUAD and cluster in exon 20.[68–70] Mutations and amplifications of ERBB2 portray a distinct subset of LUAD associated with nonsmokers and showing mutual exclusivity with mutations in EGFR and KRAS and ALK rearrangements.[68] Recent data show promising clinical results in patients with NSCLC with oncogenic ERBB2 alterations treated with the ERBB inhibitor neratinib and the anti-HER2 antibody trastuzumab emtansine.[71,72]

Neurotrophic Receptor Tyrosine Kinases 1 to 3

Neurotrophic receptor tyrosine kinases (NTRK) 1, 2, and 3 code for tropomyosin receptor kinase (TRK) A, B, and C, respectively. Rearrangements are exceedingly rare, occurring in 0.1% of patients with NSCLC and in up to 3% in those with no known driver mutation. These patients respond well to selective TRK inhibitors regardless of histology.[42,73]

Fibroblast Growth Factor Receptors 1 to 4

All 4 receptors are tyrosine kinase receptors. FGFR1 is amplified in 20% of LUSC where fusions such as FGFR1-TACC3 or FGFR3-TACC3 are also seen.[32] LUSC with FGFR1 amplification have shown better prognosis independent of treatment; however, clinical trials to confirm the clinical relevance are ongoing.[74]

RECOMMENDATION GUIDELINES

Historically, molecular testing of lung cancer has been performed on formalin-fixed paraffin-embedded tissue from surgical resections. However, validation of current molecular testing assays on cytology samples, including cell block material and alcohol-fixed smears, has recently been accepted in current guidelines as substrates for molecular testing.[37] Molecular testing can also be performed in tumors with histologies other than adenocarcinoma given tumor heterogeneity and potential sampling bias. In addition, across a spectrum of lung carcinomas, light (1–10 packs per year) or absent tobacco exposure should be sufficient to perform testing, particularly in younger patients.[37]

A key new recommendation includes testing for ROS1 mutations for all patients with lung cancer regardless of clinical characteristics. For laboratories performing next-generation sequencing (NGS) panels, the inclusion of additional genes (ERBB2, MET, BRAF, KRAS, and RET) is recommended, given the emerging role for targeted therapies for alterations in these genes as well as potential cost savings.[9,37,44,75] Immunohistochemistry remains an acceptable alternative to fluorescence in situ hybridization for ALK mutation testing.

Recommendations for molecular testing in the setting of relapse or progression following targeted therapy are emerging. For patients who have sensitizing EGFR mutations and have progressed following EGFR-targeted TKI, testing for the EGFR T790M resistance mutation is recommended in order to guide selection for third-generation EGFR-targeted therapy.[37]

LUNG SQUAMOUS CARCINOMA

In contrast with LUAD, LUSC originates from cells that line the inside of the lung airways. LUSC is classified into keratinizing, nonkeratinizing, and basaloid subtypes.[8] LUSCs are linked to a history of smoking and are frequently found in the main bronchi, in central regions of the lungs. No significant differences have been detected across LUSC subtypes for clinicopathologic features, location, pleural involvement, lymphovascular invasion, age, molecular lesions (eg, EGFR), or prognosis.[8,74,76]

The common genomic alterations in LUSC are summarized in **Table 2**.

LARGE CELL LUNG CARCINOMA

Large cell lung carcinoma (LCLC) is a rare subtype with poorly differentiated morphology that lacks cytologic, architectural, and immunohistochemical features of SCLC, LUAD, or LUSC and shows resistance to chemotherapy.[77,78] NGS studies have shown genomic alterations in LCLC reminiscent of LUAD (eg, ATM, BRAF, CDKN2A, EGFR, KRAS, STK11) in most cases and other alterations more in keeping with LUSC (eg, TP53 only or with SOX2, FGFR1, and/or AKT1).[77,78] However, approximately 40% of cases have a genetic profile devoid of recognizable lineage-specific alterations that seem to show high expression of programmed death ligand (PD-L).[77]

SMALL CELL LUNG CARCINOMA

Initially described in 1926 by Barnard,[6,79] SCLC shows neuroendocrine features and is the most aggressive type of lung cancer with a dismal 5-year survival rate of less than 5%.[80] Although the cell of origin has not been formally identified, pulmonary neuroendocrine cells and their neuroendocrine progenitors in the lung are thought to give rise to SCLC and large cell neuroendocrine carcinoma (LCNEC).[81,82] These tumors account for approximately 15% of lung cancers[6,83,84] (see **Fig. 2**). Key molecular findings are shown in **Fig. 3** and include:

- Neuroendocrine features
- Rapid growth
- Strong association with smoking and older age
- Metastatic at presentation; therefore, most SCLC are managed primarily by chemotherapy and radiotherapy
- Association with paraneoplastic syndromes (eg, Eaton-Lambert or inappropriate secretion of antidiuretic hormone)

- Mutations in TP53 and RB1 with loss of CDKN2A in most cases
- PTEN loss and activation of PI3K pathway in a subset of cases
- Extrathoracic metastatic disease is found at autopsy in more than 95% of patients

Based on current testing guidelines, there is no evidence for routine molecular testing in SCLC or LCNEC. However; recent studies using whole-transcriptome data from isolated populations of SCLC and LCNEC tumor cells showed increased deltalike protein 3 (DLL3) gene and protein expression at the tumor cell surface.[85] These findings led to the development of an antibody drug conjugate directed against DLL3 called rovalpituzumab tesirine (Rova-T).[86] Initial results in patients with relapsed or refractory SCLC have shown longer median progression-free survival (4.3 months) and overall survival (5.8 months) compared with the overall population.[86] Also recently, lurbinectedin, a novel drug that blocks transcription and leads to apoptosis by inducing DNA double-strand breaks, showed promising results as second-line therapy for SCLC.[87] However, these therapies have not yet matured into approved treatments.

IMMUNOTHERAPY

It has been well documented that for some tumors, including LUAD, the mutation profile favors the creation of neoantigens that can be recognized by cytotoxic T cells infiltrating the tumor.[88–90] Because the tumor microenvironment is a reflection, to a certain degree, of the mutational burden and profile of some tumors, a portion of LUADs are associated with inflammatory backgrounds rich in activated effector T cells and increased expression of proteins that participate in antigen presentation, T-cell migration, and function as well as overexpression of negative regulators of T-cell cytotoxic activity such as programmed death-1 (PD-1), its ligand (PD-L1) and lymphocyte activation gene-3 (LAG-3).[91]

Immunomodulatory therapies focus on disrupting inhibitory signaling between tumor cells and immune cells (typically T cells), which occurs when tumor cells express proteins that induce immunologic tolerance and prevent the immune system from attacking the tumor. In lung cancer, it involves the interaction between PD-L1 on tumor cells and programmed death receptor-1 (PD-1) on T cells (see **Fig. 4**). This interaction effectively silences the T-cell response to a tumor. By blocking PD-1 with so-called immune checkpoint inhibitors, T cells become enabled to recognize and respond to foreign antigens presented on the cancer cells. Because most lung cancer cells contain many mutations beyond their oncogenic drivers, they typically express many neoantigens, some of which are displayed on the cell surface and recognized as foreign by host immune cells. The higher the mutational burden in a tumor cell, the more neoantigens that can be expressed, and the more likely the immune system is to destroy the cells, provided that the tolerance mechanisms, such as PD-L1/PD-1, are not activated.[88–90]

Immunomodulatory therapies have been approved as second-line agents for patients with advanced lung cancer as well as first-line therapy for patients with high level (>50%) of PD-L1 expression and absence of sensitizing *EGFR* mutations or *ALK* rearrangements. Nivolumab, a monoclonal antibody that blocks PD-1 proteins, was recently approved by the FDA for use in patients with advanced LUSC.[89] Pembrolizumab, an anti–PD-1 antibody, in combination with pemetrexed, and platinum chemotherapy was recently approved as first-line treatment of metastatic LUAD.[88] Atezolizumab in combination with carboplatin/paclitaxel/bevacizumab was recently granted FDA approval in patients with untreated LUAD. The addition of atezolizumab to bevacizumab plus chemotherapy significantly improved progression-free survival and overall survival among patients with metastatic LUAD, regardless of PD-L1 expression and *EGFR* or *ALK* genetic alteration status.[90]

Despite these significant results, unlike the targeted therapies, the number of eligible patients is limited; moreover, the frequency with which patients respond, even in biomarker-selected populations, is closer to 20% to 30% in the second line and 50% in the first line (as opposed to 80% for targeted therapies).[88–90,92]

FUTURE DIRECTIONS

CELL-FREE DNA

Lung cancer cells shed their DNA into the circulation at detectable concentrations.[93] This event enables testing of plasma cell-free DNA (cfDNA) obtained from peripheral blood samples to identify mutations occurring in patients with lung cancer. There is currently insufficient evidence to support the use of circulating plasma cfDNA molecular methods for establishing a primary diagnosis of LUAD.[37] However, in some clinical settings, in which tissue is limited and/or insufficient for molecular testing, physicians may use a cfDNA assay to identify *EGFR* mutations.[37] Current methods for cfDNA have high analytical specificity; however,

because of a lower sensitivity, the absence of a mutation does not exclude its presence in the tumor.[94]

There is an enormous clinical potential for cfDNA in the near future given its ability to be used for the detection of minimal residual disease, treatment monitoring, measurement of tumor mutational load, potential identification of drug targets, and possibly early cancer detection.[95]

CIRCULATING TUMOR CELLS AND EXOSOMES

The direct isolation of circulating tumor cells from the blood as well as exosomes (secreted extracellular vesicles that contain RNA and protein cargo) is more challenging technically than isolation of cfDNA and these have not been sufficiently studied in lung cancer to warrant consideration in this article.

TUMOR MUTATIONAL BURDEN

Varying definitions exist for tumor mutation burden (TMB) making direct comparison among assays challenging. However, as a biomarker, TMB generally serves as a proxy for the presence of neoantigens and has emerged as a complementary marker to PD-L1 expression for predicting response to checkpoint inhibitors.[96,97]

SUMMARY

Lung cancer has evolved from broad histologic subtypes to a complex disease comprising many different molecular subtypes, each with its own prognostic and therapeutic implications. Along with a better understanding of the tumor biology, targeted therapies have emerged that prolong survival in a select group of patients, and testing for these alterations has now become standard of care.

The role of the pathologist has evolved in parallel with the understanding of the disease process. In addition to morphologic classification, pathologists are now responsible for triaging a host of ancillary tests and incorporating these results back into the report in order to guide diagnostic and therapeutic decisions.

Despite major advances in the understanding of the molecular mechanisms driving lung cancer progression, several challenges still remain, including (1) the need to identify unknown driver gene alterations in the population of patients for whom targeted therapies are not currently available, (2) a more detailed understanding of resistance mechanisms and a sensitive and specific way to monitor for resistance, (3) development of additional biomarkers to select those patients that will benefit the most from targeted therapies and immunotherapy, and (4) rational development of new drugs and combinations of therapies that can target multiple molecular pathways that are critical for lung cancer survival and progression.

Pathologists will continue to play a critical role in the management of patients with lung cancer in the future. In the molecular era, pathologists will be responsible for early diagnosis of disease as well as monitoring for tumor response and progression. To this end, pathologists must continue to incorporate new diagnostic tools and do more with less to enable personalized oncology.

DISCLOSURE

The authors have nothing to disclose.

REFERENCES

1. Adler I. Primary malignant growths of the lungs and bronchi; a pathological and clinical study. London: Longmans, Green; 1912.
2. Spiro SG, Silvestri GA. One hundred years of lung cancer. Am J Respir Crit Care Med 2005;172(5):523–9.
3. Siegel RL, Miller KD, Jemal A. Cancer statistics, 2019. CA Cancer J Clin 2019;69(1):7–34.
4. Lee SH. Chemotherapy for lung cancer in the era of personalized medicine. Tuberc Respir Dis (Seoul) 2019;82(3):179–89.
5. Gridelli C, Rossi A, Carbone DP, et al. Non-small-cell lung cancer. Nat Rev Dis Primers 2015;1: 15009.
6. Haddadin S, Perry MC. History of small-cell lung cancer. Clin Lung Cancer 2011;12(2):87–93.
7. Swanton C, Govindan R. Clinical implications of genomic discoveries in lung cancer. N Engl J Med 2016;374(19):1864–73.
8. Relli V, Trerotola M, Guerra E, et al. Abandoning the notion of non-small cell lung cancer. Trends Mol Med 2019;25(7):585–94.
9. Brainard J, Farver C. The diagnosis of non-small cell lung cancer in the molecular era. Mod Pathol 2019;32(Suppl 1):16–26.
10. Network NCC. Clinical practice guidelines in oncology: non-small cell lung cancer. 2019, 2019 Version 7.2019. Available at: http://www.nccn.org/professionals/physician_gls/pdf/nscl.pdf. Accessed October 1, 2019.
11. Borczuk AC. Uncommon types of lung carcinoma with mixed histology: sarcomatoid carcinoma, adenosquamous carcinoma, and mucoepidermoid carcinoma. Arch Pathol Lab Med 2018;142(8):914–21.
12. Herbst RS, Morgensztern D, Boshoff C. The biology and management of non-small cell lung cancer. Nature 2018;553(7689):446–54.
13. Cancer Genome Atlas Research Network. Comprehensive molecular profiling of lung adenocarcinoma. Nature 2014;511(7511):543–50.
14. Kim CF, Jackson EL, Woolfenden AE, et al. Identification of bronchioalveolar stem cells in normal lung and lung cancer. Cell 2005;121(6):823–35.
15. Skoulidis F, Heymach JV. Co-occurring genomic alterations in non-small-cell lung cancer biology and therapy. Nat Rev Cancer 2019;19(9):495–509.
16. Paez JG, Janne PA, Lee JC, et al. EGFR mutations in lung cancer: correlation with clinical response to gefitinib therapy. Science 2004;304(5676):1497–500.
17. Endoh H, Tomida S, Yatabe Y, et al. Prognostic model of pulmonary adenocarcinoma by expression profiling of eight genes as determined by quantitative real-time reverse transcriptase polymerase chain reaction. J Clin Oncol 2004;22(5): 811–9.
18. Gordon GJ, Richards WG, Sugarbaker DJ, et al. A prognostic test for adenocarcinoma of the lung from gene expression profiling data. Cancer Epidemiol Biomarkers Prev 2003;12(9):905–10.
19. Hayes DN, Monti S, Parmigiani G, et al. Gene expression profiling reveals reproducible human lung adenocarcinoma subtypes in multiple independent patient cohorts. J Clin Oncol 2006; 24(31):5079–90.
20. Parmigiani G, Garrett-Mayer ES, Anbazhagan R, et al. A cross-study comparison of gene expression studies for the molecular classification of lung cancer. Clin Cancer Res 2004;10(9):2922–7.
21. Wee P, Wang Z. Epidermal growth factor receptor cell proliferation signaling pathways. Cancers (Basel) 2017;9(5), [pii:E52].
22. Ullrich A, Coussens L, Hayflick JS, et al. Human epidermal growth factor receptor cDNA sequence and aberrant expression of the amplified gene in A431 epidermoid carcinoma cells. Nature 1984; 309(5967):418–25.
23. Kumar A, Petri ET, Halmos B, et al. Structure and clinical relevance of the epidermal growth factor receptor in human cancer. J Clin Oncol 2008;26(10): 1742–51.
24. Lee JC, Vivanco I, Beroukhim R, et al. Epidermal growth factor receptor activation in glioblastoma through novel missense mutations in the extracellular domain. PLoS Med 2006;3(12):e485.
25. Red Brewer M, Yun CH, Lai D, et al. Mechanism for activation of mutated epidermal growth factor receptors in lung cancer. Proc Natl Acad Sci U S A 2013;110(38):E3595–604.
26. Zhang X, Gureasko J, Shen K, et al. An allosteric mechanism for activation of the kinase domain of epidermal growth factor receptor. Cell 2006; 125(6):1137–49.
27. Barber TD, Vogelstein B, Kinzler KW, et al. Somatic mutations of EGFR in colorectal cancers

and glioblastomas. N Engl J Med 2004;351(27): 2883.

28. Gullick WJ, Marsden JJ, Whittle N, et al. Expression of epidermal growth factor receptors on human cervical, ovarian, and vulval carcinomas. Cancer Res 1986;46(1):285–92.

29. Carey KD, Garton AJ, Romero MS, et al. Kinetic analysis of epidermal growth factor receptor somatic mutant proteins shows increased sensitivity to the epidermal growth factor receptor tyrosine kinase inhibitor, erlotinib. Cancer Res 2006;66(16): 8163–71.

30. Fujino S, Enokibori T, Tezuka N, et al. A comparison of epidermal growth factor receptor levels and other prognostic parameters in non-small cell lung cancer. Eur J Cancer 1996;32A(12):2070–4.

31. Pennell NA, Neal JW, Chaft JE, et al. SELECT: a phase II trial of adjuvant erlotinib in patients with resected epidermal growth factor receptor-mutant non-small-cell lung cancer. J Clin Oncol 2019; 37(2):97–104.

32. Oberndorfer F, Mullauer L. Molecular pathology of lung cancer: current status and perspectives. Curr Opin Oncol 2018;30(2):69–76.

33. Piotrowska Z, Isozaki H, Lennerz JK, et al. Landscape of acquired resistance to osimertinib in EGFR-mutant NSCLC and clinical validation of combined EGFR and RET inhibition with osimertinib and BLU-667 for acquired RET fusion. Cancer Discov 2018;8(12):1529–39.

34. Thress KS, Paweletz CP, Felip E, et al. Acquired EGFR C797S mutation mediates resistance to AZD9291 in non-small cell lung cancer harboring EGFR T790M. Nat Med 2015;21(6):560–2.

35. Niederst MJ, Hu H, Mulvey HE, et al. The allelic context of the C797S mutation acquired upon treatment with third-generation EGFR inhibitors impacts sensitivity to subsequent treatment strategies. Clin Cancer Res 2015;21(17):3924–33.

36. Borczuk AC. Keeping up with testing guidelines in lung cancer. Arch Pathol Lab Med 2018;142(7): 783–4.

37. Lindeman NI, Cagle PT, Aisner DL, et al. Updated molecular testing guideline for the selection of lung cancer patients for treatment with targeted tyrosine kinase inhibitors: guideline from the College of American Pathologists, the International Association for the Study of Lung Cancer, and the Association for Molecular Pathology. Arch Pathol Lab Med 2018;142(3):321–46.

38. Bayliss R, Choi J, Fennell DA, et al. Molecular mechanisms that underpin EML4-ALK driven cancers and their response to targeted drugs. Cell Mol Life Sci 2016;73(6):1209–24.

39. Pan Y, Zhang Y, Li Y, et al. ALK, ROS1 and RET fusions in 1139 lung adenocarcinomas: a comprehensive study of common and fusion pattern-

specific clinicopathologic, histologic and cytologic features. Lung Cancer 2014;84(2):121–6.

40. Rosenbaum JN, Bloom R, Forys JT, et al. Genomic heterogeneity of ALK fusion breakpoints in non-small-cell lung cancer. Mod Pathol 2018;31(5): 791–808.

41. Stumpfova M, Janne PA. Zeroing in on ROS1 rearrangements in non-small cell lung cancer. Clin Cancer Res 2012;18(16):4222–4.

42. Drilon A, Ou SI, Cho BC, et al. Repotrectinib (TPX-0005) is a next-generation ROS1/TRK/ALK inhibitor that potently inhibits ROS1/TRK/ALK solvent-front mutations. Cancer Discov 2018;8(10):1227–36.

43. Sheikine Y, Pavlick D, Klempner SJ, et al. BRAF in lung cancers: analysis of patient cases reveals recurrent BRAF mutations, fusions, kinase duplications, and concurrent alterations. JCO Precis Oncol 2018;2:1–5.

44. Suh JH, Johnson A, Albacker L, et al. Comprehensive genomic profiling facilitates implementation of the national comprehensive cancer network guidelines for lung cancer biomarker testing and identifies patients who may benefit from enrollment in mechanism-driven clinical trials. Oncologist 2016; 21(6):684–91.

45. Chen D, Zhang LQ, Huang JF, et al. BRAF mutations in patients with non-small cell lung cancer: a systematic review and meta-analysis. PLoS One 2014;9(6):e101354.

46. Schmid T, Buess M. Overcoming resistance in a BRAF V600E-mutant adenocarcinoma of the lung. Curr Oncol 2018;25(3):e217–9.

47. Khunger A, Khunger M, Velcheti V. Dabrafenib in combination with trametinib in the treatment of patients with BRAF V600-positive advanced or metastatic non-small cell lung cancer: clinical evidence and experience. Ther Adv Respir Dis 2018;12, 1753466618767611.

48. Piva S, Ganzinelli M, Garassino MC, et al. Across the universe of K-RAS mutations in non-small-cell-lung cancer. Curr Pharm Des 2014;20(24): 3933–43.

49. Ferrer I, Zugazagoitia J, Herbertz S, et al. KRAS-Mutant non-small cell lung cancer: from biology to therapy. Lung Cancer 2018;124:53–64.

50. Matikas A, Mistriotis D, Georgoulias V, et al. Targeting KRAS mutated non-small cell lung cancer: a history of failures and a future of hope for a diverse entity. Crit Rev Oncol Hematol 2017;110:1–12.

51. Riely GJ, Kris MG, Rosenbaum D, et al. Frequency and distinctive spectrum of KRAS mutations in never smokers with lung adenocarcinoma. Clin Cancer Res 2008;14(18):5731–4.

52. Mao C, Qiu LX, Liao RY, et al. KRAS mutations and resistance to EGFR-TKIs treatment in patients with non-small cell lung cancer: a meta-analysis of 22 studies. Lung Cancer 2010;69(3):272–8.

53. Herbst RS, Heymach JV, Lippman SM. Lung cancer. N Engl J Med 2008;359(13):1367–80.

54. Dong ZY, Zhong WZ, Zhang XC, et al. Potential predictive value of TP53 and KRAS mutation status for response to PD-1 blockade immunotherapy in lung adenocarcinoma. Clin Cancer Res 2017;23(12):3012–24.

55. Govindan R, Fakih MG, Price TJ, et al. Phase I study of safety, tolerability, PK and efficacy of AMG 510, a novel KRAS G12C inhibitor, evaluated in NSCLC. IASLC 2019 World Conference on Lung Cancer. Barcelona, Spain, September 7–10, 2019.

56. Lu X, Peled N, Greer J, et al. MET exon 14 mutation encodes an actionable therapeutic target in lung adenocarcinoma. Cancer Res 2017;77(16):4498–505.

57. Lee GD, Lee SE, Oh DY, et al. MET exon 14 skipping mutations in lung adenocarcinoma: clinicopathologic implications and prognostic values. J Thorac Oncol 2017;12(8):1233–46.

58. Zeng L, Xia C, Zhang Y, et al. Identification of a novel MET exon 14 skipping variant coexistent with EGFR mutation in lung adenocarcinoma sensitive to combined treatment with afatinib and crizotinib. J Thorac Oncol 2019;14(4):e70–2.

59. Kim S, Kim TM, Kim DW, et al. Acquired resistance of MET-amplified non-small cell lung cancer cells to the MET inhibitor capmatinib. Cancer Res Treat 2019;51(3):951–62.

60. Li A, Yang JJ, Zhang XC, et al. Acquired MET Y1248H and D1246N mutations mediate resistance to MET inhibitors in non-small cell lung cancer. Clin Cancer Res 2017;23(16):4929–37.

61. Gainor JF, Shaw AT. Novel targets in non-small cell lung cancer: ROS1 and RET fusions. Oncologist 2013;18(7):865–75.

62. Gainor JF, Shaw AT. The new kid on the block: RET in lung cancer. Cancer Discov 2013;3(6):604–6.

63. Saito M, Ishigame T, Tsuta K, et al. A mouse model of KIF5B-RET fusion-dependent lung tumorigenesis. Carcinogenesis 2014;35(11):2452–6.

64. Wang R, Hu H, Pan Y, et al. RET fusions define a unique molecular and clinicopathologic subtype of non-small-cell lung cancer. J Clin Oncol 2012;30(35):4352–9.

65. Gainor JF, Lee DH, Curigliano G, et al. Clinical activity and tolerability of BLU-667, a highly potent and selective RET inhibitor, in patients with advanced RET-fusion+ non-small cell lung cancer (NSCLC). 2019 American Society of Clinical Oncology Annual Meeting. Chicago, IL, May 31–June 4, 2019.

66. Drilon A, Oxnard G, Wirth L, et al. Registrational results of LIBRETTO-001: A phase 1/2 trial of LOXO-292 in patients with RET fusion-positive lung cancers. IASLC 2019 World Conference on Lung Cancer. Barcelona, Spain, September 7–10, 2019.

67. Nelson-Taylor SK, Le AT, Yoo M, et al. Resistance to RET-inhibition in RET-rearranged NSCLC is mediated by reactivation of RAS/MAPK signaling. Mol Cancer Ther 2017;16(8):1623–33.

68. Arcila ME, Chaft JE, Nafa K, et al. Prevalence, clinicopathologic associations, and molecular spectrum of ERBB2 (HER2) tyrosine kinase mutations in lung adenocarcinomas. Clin Cancer Res 2012;18(18):4910–8.

69. Cappuzzo F, Varella-Garcia M, Shigematsu H, et al. Increased HER2 gene copy number is associated with response to gefitinib therapy in epidermal growth factor receptor-positive non-small-cell lung cancer patients. J Clin Oncol 2005;23(22):5007–18.

70. Shigematsu H, Takahashi T, Nomura M, et al. Somatic mutations of the HER2 kinase domain in lung adenocarcinomas. Cancer Res 2005;65(5):1642–6.

71. Peters S, Stahel R, Bubendorf L, et al. Trastuzumab emtansine (T-DM1) in patients with previously treated HER2-Overexpressing metastatic non-small cell lung cancer: efficacy, safety, and biomarkers. Clin Cancer Res 2019;25(1):64–72.

72. Li BT, Shen R, Buonocore D, et al. Ado-Trastuzumab emtansine for patients with HER2-mutant lung cancers: results from a phase II basket trial. J Clin Oncol 2018;36(24):2532–7.

73. Farago AF, Taylor MS, Doebele RC, et al. Clinicopathologic features of non-small-cell lung cancer harboring an NTRK gene fusion. JCO Precis Oncol 2018;2018:1–14.

74. Friedlaender A, Banna G, Malapelle U, et al. Next generation sequencing and genetic alterations in squamous cell lung carcinoma: where are we today? Front Oncol 2019;9:166.

75. Pennell NA, Mutebi A, Zhou ZY, et al. Economic impact of next-generation sequencing versus single-gene testing to detect genomic alterations in metastatic non–small-cell lung cancer using a decision analytic model. JCO Precis Oncol 2019;3:1–9.

76. Cancer Genome Atlas Research Network. Comprehensive genomic characterization of squamous cell lung cancers. Nature 2012;489(7417):519–25.

77. Chan AW, Chau SL, Tong JH, et al. The landscape of actionable molecular alterations in immunomarker-defined large-cell carcinoma of the lung. J Thorac Oncol 2019;14(7):1213–22.

78. Pelosi G, Fabbri A, Papotti M, et al. Dissecting pulmonary large-cell carcinoma by targeted next generation sequencing of several cancer genes pushes genotypic-phenotypic correlations to emerge. J Thorac Oncol 2015;10(11):1560–9.

79. Barnard W. The nature of the 'oat-celled sarcoma' of the mediastinum. J Pathol 1926;29:241–4.

80. Karachaliou N, Pilotto S, Lazzari C, et al. Cellular and molecular biology of small cell lung cancer: an overview. Transl Lung Cancer Res 2016;5(1):2–15.

81. Park KS, Liang MC, Raiser DM, et al. Characterization of the cell of origin for small cell lung cancer. Cell Cycle 2011;10(16):2806–15.

82. Reynolds SD, Giangreco A, Power JH, et al. Neuroepithelial bodies of pulmonary airways serve as a reservoir of progenitor cells capable of epithelial regeneration. Am J Pathol 2000;156(1):269–78.

83. Bunn PA Jr, Minna JD, Augustyn A, et al. Small cell lung cancer: can recent advances in biology and molecular biology be translated into improved outcomes? J Thorac Oncol 2016;11(4):453–74.

84. George J, Lim JS, Jang SJ, et al. Comprehensive genomic profiles of small cell lung cancer. Nature 2015;524(7563):47–53.

85. Saunders LR, Bankovich AJ, Anderson WC, et al. A DLL3-targeted antibody-drug conjugate eradicates high-grade pulmonary neuroendocrine tumor-initiating cells in vivo. Sci Transl Med 2015; 7(302):302ra136.

86. Rudin CM, Pietanza MC, Bauer TM, et al. Rovalpituzumab tesirine, a DLL3-targeted antibody-drug conjugate, in recurrent small-cell lung cancer: a first-in-human, first-in-class, open-label, phase 1 study. Lancet Oncol 2017;18(1):42–51.

87. Paz-Ares LG, Perez JMG, Besse B, et al. Efficacy and safety profile of lurbinectedin in second-line SCLC patients: results from a phase II single-agent trial. J Clin Oncol 2019;37(15_suppl):8506.

88. Borghaei H, Paz-Ares L, Horn L, et al. Nivolumab versus docetaxel in advanced nonsquamous non-small-cell lung cancer. N Engl J Med 2015; 373(17):1627–39.

89. Brahmer J, Reckamp KL, Baas P, et al. Nivolumab versus docetaxel in advanced squamous-cell non-small-cell lung cancer. N Engl J Med 2015;373(2): 123–35.

90. Reck M, Rodriguez-Abreu D, Robinson AG, et al. Pembrolizumab versus chemotherapy for PD-L1-positive non-small-cell lung cancer. N Engl J Med 2016;375(19):1823–33.

91. Seebacher NA, Stacy AE, Porter GM, et al. Clinical development of targeted and immune based anti-cancer therapies. J Exp Clin Cancer Res 2019; 38(1):156.

92. Haslam A, Prasad V. Estimation of the percentage of US patients with cancer who are eligible for and respond to checkpoint inhibitor immunotherapy drugs. JAMA Netw Open 2019;2(5): e192535.

93. Sozzi G, Conte D, Mariani L, et al. Analysis of circulating tumor DNA in plasma at diagnosis and during follow-up of lung cancer patients. Cancer Res 2001;61(12):4675–8.

94. Wei Z, Shah N, Deng C, et al. Circulating DNA addresses cancer monitoring in non small cell lung cancer patients for detection and capturing the dynamic changes of the disease. Springerplus 2016; 5:531.

95. Wu TH, Hsiue EH, Yang JC. Opportunities of circulating tumor DNA in lung cancer. Cancer Treat Rev 2019;78:31–41.

96. Alexander M, Galeas J, Cheng H. Tumor mutation burden in lung cancer: a new predictive biomarker for immunotherapy or too soon to tell? J Thorac Dis 2018;10(Suppl 33):S3994–8.

97. Lam VK, Zhang J. Blood-based tumor mutation burden: continued progress toward personalizing immunotherapy in non-small cell lung cancer. J Thorac Dis 2019;11(6):2208–11.

98. Chong CR, Janne PA. The quest to overcome resistance to EGFR-targeted therapies in cancer. Nat Med 2013;19(11):1389–400.

99. Wakelee H, Kelly K, Edelman MJ. 50 years of progress in the systemic therapy of non-small cell lung cancer. Am Soc Clin Oncol Educ Book 2014;34: 177–89.

100. Cerami E, Gao J, Dogrusoz U, et al. The cBio cancer genomics portal: an open platform for exploring multidimensional cancer genomics data. Cancer Discov 2012;2(5):401–4.

101. Gao J, Aksoy BA, Dogrusoz U, et al. Integrative analysis of complex cancer genomics and clinical profiles using the cBioPortal. Sci Signal 2013; 6(269):pl1.

Pulmonary Neuroendocrine Tumors

Alain C. Borczuk, MD

KEYWORDS

- Carcinoid • Neuroendocrine • Small-cell carcinoma • Large-cell neuroendocrine • Atypical

Key points

- Carcinoid tumors are graded based on necrosis and mitotic rate, with typical carcinoids as low grade and atypical carcinoids as intermediate grade. The use of a Ki-67–based classification is emerging but still not established.
- Large-cell neuroendocrine carcinoma is an uncommon tumor type, with one subset that molecularly resembles small-cell carcinoma and one that resembles adenocarcinoma.
- Small-cell carcinoma is a relatively common lung tumor that represents a clinically relevant category of high-grade neuroendocrine carcinoma.

ABSTRACT

Pulmonary neuroendocrine tumors represent a morphologic spectrum of tumors from the well-differentiated typical carcinoid tumor, to the intermediate-grade atypical carcinoid tumor, to the high-grade neuroendocrine carcinomas composed of small-cell carcinoma and large-cell neuroendocrine carcinoma. The addition of immunohistochemistry in diagnostics is helpful and often essential, especially in the classification of large-cell neuroendocrine carcinoma. The importance of the intermediate-grade atypical carcinoid group is underscored by the impact of this diagnosis on therapy. The distinction of pulmonary small-cell carcinoma from large-cell neuroendocrine carcinoma, despite both being in the high-grade group, is of relevance to the therapeutic approach to these tumor types.

be challenging, due to several pitfalls that are partially resolvable at the current time. The distinction of typical carcinoid from atypical carcinoid, which affects therapy and in some scenarios supersedes tumor stage, often requires examination of the resected tumor for accurate assessment. Refinement of small sample diagnosis using biomarkers such as Ki-67 appears promising but is not yet fully realized. In contrast, the distinction of small-cell carcinoma from large-cell neuroendocrine carcinoma in small samples is often desired clinically, but is met with the significant challenges of morphologic and biomarker overlap in these 2 entities. Emerging data indicate overlap between solid pattern adenocarcinoma and large-cell neuroendocrine carcinoma. A combination of clinical presentation, staging, and pathologic parameters can help define treatment strategies in these challenging scenarios.

OVERVIEW

The classification of pulmonary neuroendocrine tumors is critical to the assignment of correct treatment regimens. However, although the definitions have been established in several versions of the World Health Organization classification, applying those definitions to individual cases can

CARCINOID TUMORS (TYPICAL AND ATYPICAL)

This group of tumors in the lung are considered together, as they have similar precursor lesions, clinical presentation, and molecular characteristics.

Department of Pathology, Weill Cornell Medicine, 1300 York Avenue, ST10-1000A, New York, NY 10065, USA
E-mail address: alb9003@med.cornell.edu

Surgical Pathology 13 (2020) 35–55
https://doi.org/10.1016/j.path.2019.10.002
1875-9181/20/© 2019 Elsevier Inc. All rights reserved.

surgpath.theclinics.com

PRECURSOR LESIONS

Neuroendocrine cell hyperplasia (NCH), in some instances, is thought to be a precursor of carcinoid tumors. It is defined as a proliferation of neuroendocrine cells confined to the bronchial or bronchiolar epithelium; when generalized, it is termed diffuse idiopathic pulmonary neuroendocrine cell hyperplasia (DIPNECH).[1] This NCH is manifested by an increased number of neuroendocrine cells in the small airways of the lung, usually with rows or clusters of such cells. Morphologically, this can be identified by a prominence of a basally oriented layer of uniform cells that lift up the normal respiratory epithelium (**Fig. 1**A). Whether truly exophytic or the product of dyscohesion caused by these cells, strips of epithelium projecting or sloughed into the airway lumen, with associated NCH, can be a feature that draws attention to this diagnosis (**Fig. 1**B). These proliferations can be highlighted by immunohistochemistry for neuroendocrine markers, such as synaptophysin or chromogranin. When proliferations extend out of the airway epithelium into adjacent peribronchiolar stroma, they are termed carcinoid tumorlets. These tumorlets are nodules of neuroendocrine cells adjacent to the airways, but measure smaller than 0.5 cm to distinguish them from carcinoid tumors (**Fig. 1**C). Tumorlets can be an incidental finding, are frequently seen in association with NCH, and help define the radiologic features of DIPNECH.

DIPNECH is the diffuse form of NCH. Although rare, increasing recognition of these diffuse forms radiologically by airway-based findings of thickening and dilatation, and parenchymal findings such as mosaic attenuation on computed tomography (CT) scan with presence of small nodules, have increased detection of DIPNECH.[2,3] The gross appearance of this lesion can be subtle, and the target nodule can distract from these other findings of small nodules and airway thickening (**Fig. 1**D, E). Although the exact minimum definition of the extent of NCH and tumorlets needed to establish DIPNECH as a diagnosis remains unclear,[4] the correlation of histology and imaging appears to be critical. In addition, associated findings, such as obstructive lung disease due to constrictive bronchiolitis, add an important reason to correctly identify and diagnose this condition.[5] However, NCH as a secondary airway finding in chronic obstructive pulmonary disease and granulomatous disease, and carcinoid tumorlets as incidental findings in lung resections, create a situation in which the histopathologic diagnosis of NCH and tumorlets is best established by the

pathologist, whereas the clinical syndrome of DIPNECH is established through multidisciplinary clinico-pathologic correlation.

Overall, the main evidence of NCH or DIPNECH as precursor lesions of carcinoids is limited to the frequent finding of these lesions in patients with carcinoid tumors.[6] In a series of patients with DIPNECH, a large proportion have stable disease, whereas others develop worsening pulmonary function, so that the nature of DIPNECH as an obligate or nonobligate precursor is not fully established.[7]

NEUROENDOCRINE CELL HYPERPLASIA

- Uniform cells in rows and nests
- Sloughed epithelium
- Associated with tumorlets

CARCINOIDS

Pulmonary carcinoids are defined as malignant neuroendocrine neoplasms measuring larger than 5.0 mm, with typical carcinoids having fewer than 2 mitoses per 2 mm^2 (10 high-powered fields [HPF]) and lacking necrosis. There may be observed an increase in incidence, with a rate of 1.4 to 2.0 per 100,000 in more recent analyses.[8] Pulmonary carcinoid tumors as a group are not associated with cigarette smoking,[9] have a relatively equal male/female incidence[10] (although some series report a female predominance), and occur in younger patients than higher-grade neuroendocrine tumors, such as small-cell carcinoma.[11]

Carcinoid tumors of the lung are often centrally located, in relation to a large airway, although as many as 30% are found in peripheral locations (**Fig. 2**A, B). Carcinoids are usually solitary lesions (approximately 95% of cases),[12] although tumorlets can be found in many cases.

These tumors are known for the histologic diversity of their growth patterns, and include solid nests with intervening stroma (organoid), trabecular or ribbonlike (**Fig. 3**A), oncocytic (**Fig. 3**B), rosette (**Fig. 3**C), paragangliomalike, and spindle cell (**Fig. 3**D). Although these patterns can be helpful in recognizing carcinoid tumors, they do not by themselves predict biological behavior.

The most consistent histologic finding is the cytologic uniformity of the cell nucleus with little cell-to-cell variation. In addition, the chromatin in most cells is described as salt and pepper, with a stippling of chromatin without intranuclear vesicular chromatin or prominent nucleoli. It is important to realize that this is most cells, so that

Fig. 1. Pulmonary neuroendocrine cell hyperplasia (NCH). (*A*) In NCH, neuroendocrine cells form a uniform confluent basally placed proliferation with some small clusters. The proliferation lifts up normal epithelium. (hematoxylin-eosin [H&E], original magnification ×100). (*B*) In addition to basally placed cells, strips of epithelium project into the airway lumen and are seen sloughed into the space. In addition, neighboring alveolar spaces are lined by neuroendocrine cells (H&E, original magnification ×100). (*C*) A carcinoid tumorlet is seen next to a bronchus, and associated with NCH. A strip of epithelium with NCH is seen sloughed into the airway lumen (H&E, original magnification ×25).

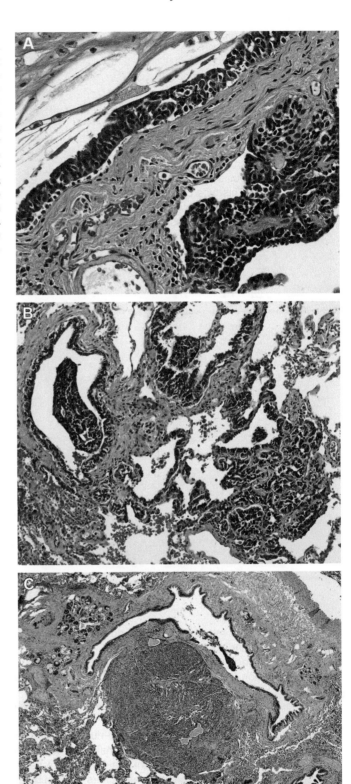

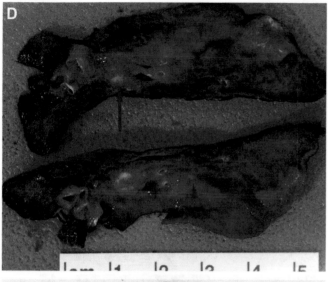

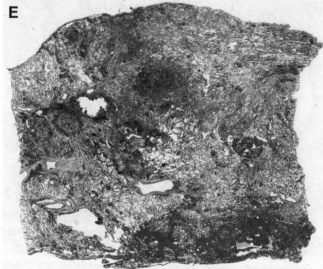

Fig. 1. (*continued*). (*D*) A gross image from a case of DIPNECH. In addition to the index lesion, which is a carcinoid tumor (*arrow*), tumorlets are seen in the adjacent lung (*arrowheads*). (*E*) A lower-power view shows airway-based NCH and tumorlets in 1 section, demonstrating the extent of proliferation in DIPNECH (H&E, original magnification ×1).

exceptions within a microscopic field do not negate the overall finding.

Other features encountered in carcinoid tumors include calcification (see **Fig. 3**D), stromal hyalinization (**Fig. 3**E), and stromal amyloid. In fact, calcification has been described as a CT imaging feature suggestive of the diagnosis.[13]

Because of the cellular uniformity and the nuclear features, carcinoid tumors are often considered by morphologic assessment alone. However, there are several carcinoid mimickers that can result in a differential diagnosis requiring ancillary studies to resolve. In some cases, low-grade tumors, such as mucoepidermoid carcinoma, can have morphologic similarity and can occur endobronchially in an overlapping age group. The presence of mucous-producing cells can be helpful, but the uniformity of the nuclei can be a pitfall when these tumors have a predominance of intermediate cells. Nuclear chromatin pattern is crucial in these instances. On frozen section, the nuclear features of plasma cells can resemble the nuclei of carcinoid tumors, and the characteristic perinuclear Golgi zone of plasma cells can be inapparent. Cytologic preparations are helpful in this setting. Spindle cell carcinoids can be mistaken for benign spindle cell neoplasms of smooth muscle or meningothelial origin. Some metastatic carcinomas can grow in solid patterns and can have deceptively bland nuclei. Paragangliomas, although rare in the lung, are difficult to resolve from carcinoid tumors with

Fig. 2. Carcinoid tumor: gross features. (*A*) A well-circumscribed yellow, tan, and red mass without central umbilication is seen in this wedge resection of a peripheral carcinoid. (*B*) A more centrally located tan-yellow–circumscribed carcinoid tumor fills the bronchial lumen and invades into adjacent lung tissue.

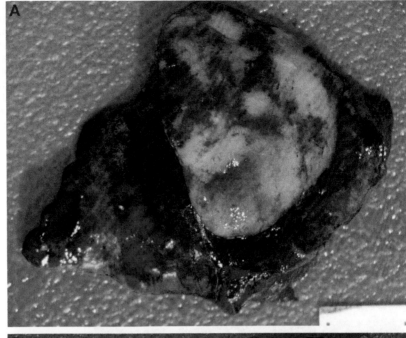

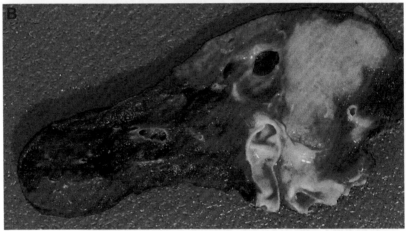

paragangliomalike pattern by morphology alone. The occasional presence of pigment in carcinoid tumors can raise concern for malignant melanoma.

Immunohistochemistry is a useful adjunct to morphologic assessment. Cytokeratin immunoreactivity is present in carcinoid tumors; however, it is important to recognize that as many as 10% of carcinoids are negative for cytokeratin AE1:AE3 and require a low molecular weight cytokeratin such as CAM5.2 to demonstrate cytokeratin reactivity. Neuroendocrine markers are often performed as well, including synaptophysin, chromogranin, and CD56. Because carcinoids are relatively well differentiated, these markers are relatively sensitive in this setting, with

chromogranin as the most specific. There is an emerging marker, insulinoma-associated-1 (INSM1), that may be useful in this setting, with higher sensitivity and specificity than the other individual markers.[14] It is a transcriptional regulator, and localizes to the nucleus, providing a nuclear immunohistochemistry pattern. It may be most useful in the higher-grade setting, however, when compared with the other markers.

Another use of immunohistochemistry in carcinoid tumors may be considered when the tumor is of unknown primary site, in disseminated disease. In this setting, thyroid transcription factor 1 (TTF1), CDX2, and PAX8 may be used to help guide primary site determination, with TTF1 indicative of lung origin,[15] CDX2 of gastrointestinal tract

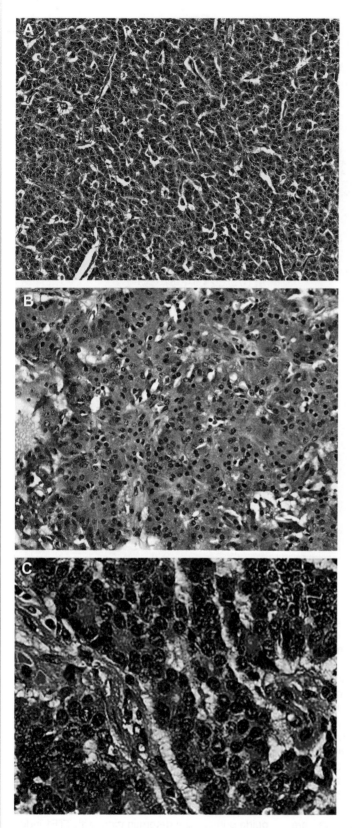

Fig. 3. Histologic patterns of carcinoid tumors. (*A*) Tumor cells growing in rows or ribbonlike pattern (trabecular) (H&E, original magnification ×100). (*B*) Abundant cytoplasm from eosinophilic to lightly basophilic (oncocytic) (H&E, original magnification ×100). (*C*) Tumor cells forming small clusters around a central space, with nuclei peripherally located (rosette) (H&E, original magnification ×150).

Fig. 3. (continued). (*D*) Elongated spindle-shaped cells in vague bundles (spindle). Calcifications are present (H&E, original magnification ×100). (*E*) Dense hyalinized stroma is seen in some cases (H&E, original magnification ×100).

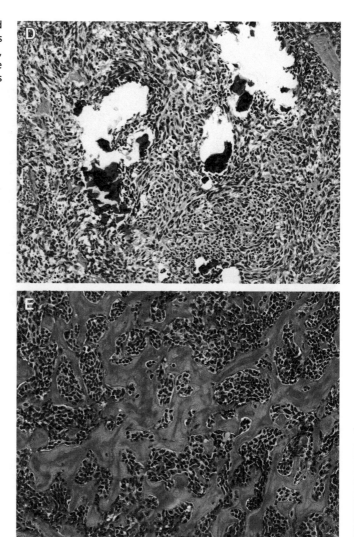

origin,[16] and PAX8 of pancreatic (vs ileal and pulmonary)[17] or thymic origin.[18] Although potentially useful, it is unclear whether treatment regimens differ in the metastatic setting based on primary site of origin, but can help identify an organ source for the tumor.

Once it is determined that a tumor is in the carcinoid group, the decision between typical and atypical carcinoid needs to be made. This decision is based on 2 features: necrosis and mitotic activity.[19] In small samples, it may not be possible to detect either of these features, as necrosis may not have been sampled, and mitotic activity may not reflect the highest rate in the tumor. In this setting, the diagnosis of carcinoid tumor can be rendered, but the precise characterization deferred to the resection. Although the use of Ki-67 is discussed further later in this article, the precise cutoff on cytology cell block or small biopsy for prediction of atypical carcinoid at resection has not as yet been established.

At resection, extensive or entire sampling of a tumor may be needed to detect areas of necrosis, after careful gross examination (**Fig. 4**A). Necrosis is generally represented by focal patches of tumoral necrosis rather than large central tumoral necrosis with cavitation (**Fig. 4**B). One pitfall is the presence of focal necrosis or granulation tissue due to prior biopsy. The location and distribution of necrosis and association with granulation tissue may be important in the decision that it is biopsy related. Some investigators have emphasized the presence of comedolike necrosis in this setting, with patients showing this feature having increased tumor recurrence and mortality.[20]

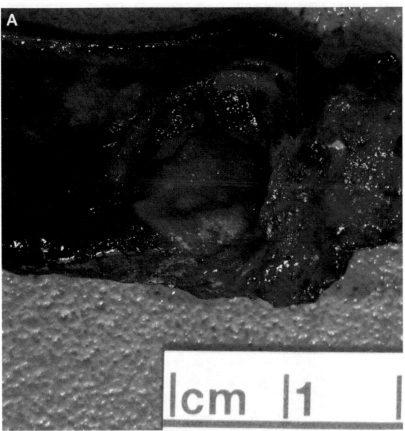

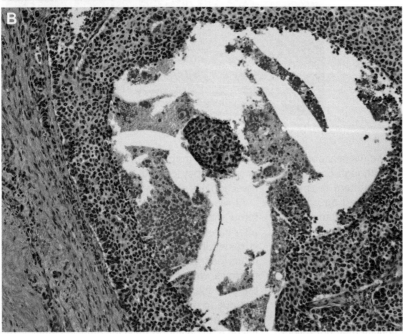

Fig. 4. Atypical carcinoid. (*A*) The gross image reveals a circumscribed tan tumor with an area of central softening with yellow discoloration and a red rim. This area should be sampled to identify necrosis. (*B*) A tumor nest shows central comedolike tumor necrosis (H&E, original magnification ×50).

Fig. 4. (continued). (*C*) The organoid pattern and uniform nuclei with fine stippled chromatin ("salt and pepper pattern") are characteristic of a carcinoid, but with increased mitotic activity (3 mitoses on this field) (H&E, original magnification ×100). (*D*) In this example, mitotic rate warranted a typical carcinoid designation, but Ki-67 was higher than 5% (diaminobenzidine [DAB] IHC, ×50).

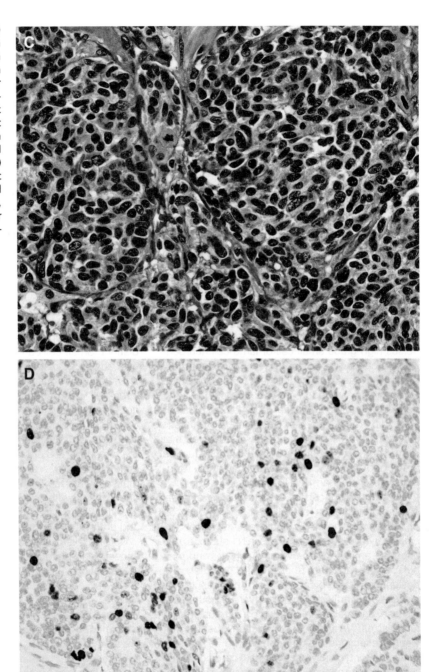

Mitotic activity in a carcinoid tumor needs to be carefully assessed. Two to 9 mitoses in 10 HPFs (2 mm²) is the established definition for atypical carcinoid (**Fig. 4**C). Although in the past this was the strict definition, it was modified in the last World Health Organization classification to account for borderline cases.[20] In cases that are near the cutoff, a total of 30 fields need to be counted, and the total averaged to be 2 or above. Although this clarification encourages more rigorous counting, it does not fully clarify what to do if one set of fields reaches 4 in 2 mm², but suggests that 6 (or >5) total in 3 sets of 2 mm² (or 30 HPFs) is needed. It is acknowledged that in most instances this resolves the lower end of the range, and that the upper end of the range (vs large-cell neuroendocrine carcinoma) is less commonly a problem, as these carcinomas often are highly mitotic.

The use of Ki-67 could help in this tumor type, and it has been implemented in neuroendocrine tumors of other organs. In fact, in small biopsies, the use of Ki-67, especially in limited samples or samples with suboptimal morphology, can help distinguish low-grade from high-grade neuroendocrine tumors; that is, very low values (<5%) versus high values (>50%).[21] From a practical point of view, Ki-67 in a small sample that shows greater than 5% cell staining may be used to suggest an increased possibility of a tumor of at least intermediate grade.[22] Whether this information is useful in an organ localized tumor before resection is not clear, so a general recommendation cannot be made. In one series, correlation of biopsy and resection was good, although a cutoff of 20% was used to divide high grade from low and intermediate grade.[23]

More controversial is its use in classification of typical carcinoid and atypical carcinoids at resection. Although at the extremes it is no doubt helpful (very low <5% vs 15%–20%) the best cutoff values remain elusive and at this point do not supersede the mitotic count (**Fig. 4D**).[24,25] In addition, the upper end of the range of Ki-67 index of atypical carcinoid versus high-grade small-cell or large-cell neuroendocrine carcinoma has not been fully established, again with very high counts (eg, >50%) reserved for the higher-grade tumors. In 2 studies, the addition of Ki-67 to the traditional morphologic parameters did not provide additional prognostic information.[26,27] It may be the case, however, that a small number of relatively high Ki-67 index tumors are of poorer prognosis.[22,27] This may apply to tumors with more than 10% Ki-67 index.

Once the diagnosis of typical versus atypical carcinoid has been established, the impact on prognosis and therapy is significant. In typical carcinoids, lymph node metastasis in N1 stations may not have an impact on overall survival[10] and may not require adjuvant therapy. In contrast, the designation of atypical carcinoid may result in a discussion of adjuvant therapy even without nodal disease, and may be influenced by T status (mainly tumor size).[28] In addition, completion lobectomy in wedge resections may be considered.[29] The survival data for typical versus atypical carcinoid supports this approach. Five-year survival for typical carcinoids exceeds 90%,[30] whereas that of atypical carcinoids is closer to 60%,[31] with even greater separation at 10 years, greater than 80% and 40%, respectively.[32]

SMALL-CELL CARCINOMA AND LARGE-CELL NEUROENDOCRINE CARCINOMA

The distinction between these 2 tumor types is very challenging, and due to sampling, may not always be achievable. This is compounded by the fact that small-cell carcinomas frequently have large-cell neuroendocrine carcinoma components as part of the tumor, and that such combinations are overall designated as combined small-cell carcinoma.[33] The finding of any small-cell component should drive classification toward small-cell carcinoma, albeit as a combined small-cell carcinoma when the large-cell neuroendocrine carcinoma exceeds 10% of the total tumor.[34] This classification has clinical impact for lung cancer treatment, as small-cell carcinoma remains an important histologic subtype with well-defined, generally nonsurgical therapeutic approaches,[35] whereas large-cell neuroendocrine carcinoma is uncommon with a greater propensity toward primary surgical approaches followed by less established nonsurgical approaches.[36]

CLINICAL ASPECTS

Despite these histologic challenges in classification, it does appear that these 2 entities are distinct. Small-cell carcinomas most often present with advanced disease, and are relatively rarer as a single lung nodule (approximately 5%), whereas large-cell neuroendocrine carcinomas (LCNEC) are of early stage in as many as 50% of cases.[37] Small-cell carcinomas are associated with a variety of paraneoplastic syndromes,[38] whereas these are rare in LCNEC.[39] LCNECs are typically peripheral, lobulated, and sometimes spiculated masses, whereas small-cell carcinomas are more often central with bulky disease. Both tumors are smoking associated, high grade, PET positive, and anticipate a poor prognosis.

Careful histopathologic analysis is needed, especially in tumors that do not follow the classic presentation. Although uncommon, lung localized small-cell carcinomas do occur, perhaps at as high a rate as 5% of small-cell carcinoma. Because these are often encountered in resection specimens, some features, such as crush artifact, are less prominent. In addition, in a series of 100 such resected small-cell carcinomas, 40% had at least a focus of large-cell neuroendocrine carcinoma.[33] Therefore, the histopathologic aspects need to be carefully synthesized to draw the correct diagnostic conclusion.

PATHOLOGIC ASPECTS

The main distinction in small-cell and LCNECs is cell size and nuclear features. The cells of small-cell carcinoma have high nuclear-to-cytoplasmic ratio with scant cytoplasm. This leads to nuclear molding. Small-cell carcinoma cells are fragile, leading to frequent crush artifact (**Fig. 5A**).

Fig. 5. Small-cell carcinoma versus LCNEC. (*A*) Small-cell carcinoma histology with nuclear molding, crush artifact, and frequent apoptotic debris (H&E, original magnification ×150). (*B*) Small-cell carcinoma with necrosis, scant cytoplasm, and fine chromatin pattern (H&E, original magnification ×150).

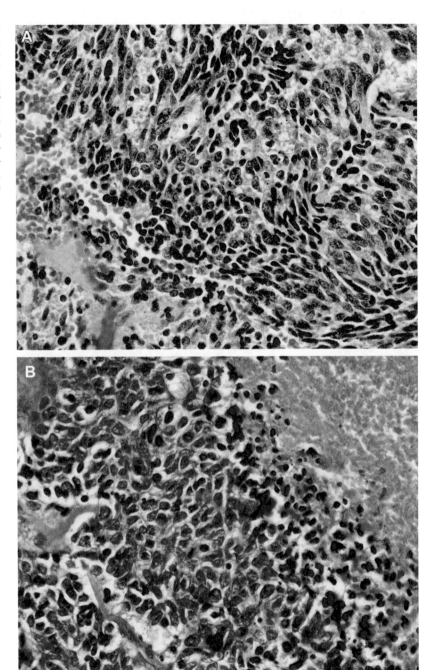

Apoptotic debris is frequent in both types of high-grade neuroendocrine carcinoma. Small-cell carcinoma nuclei have classic salt and pepper chromatin with fine chromatin without nucleoli (**Fig. 5**B). Necrosis can be seen in both small-cell and LCNECs. In contrast, LCNECs have large cells with more visible cytoplasm (although usually not abundant) and identifiable nucleoli that are not macronucleoli.[40] This chromatin is therefore coarser than that of small-cell carcinoma

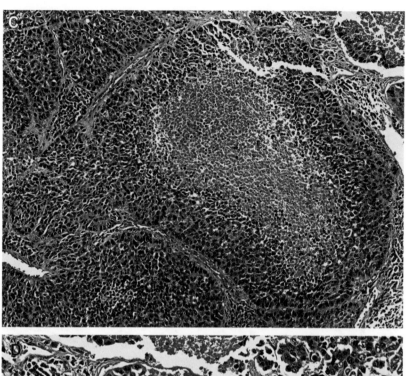

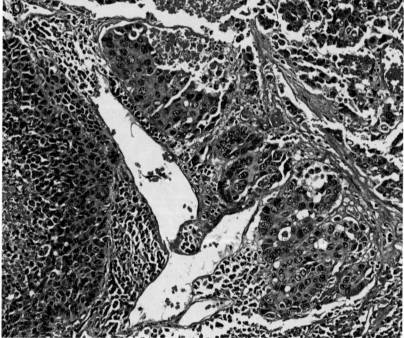

Fig. 5. (continued). (C) LCNEC with comedolike necrosis and peripheral palisading of cells (H&E, original magnification ×50). (D) The cells of LCNEC have more visible cytoplasm, polygonal irregular nuclei, and coarse chromatin with small nucleoli (H&E, original magnification ×100).

(Fig. 5C, D). Perhaps because of the cytoplasm in these cells, palisading and rosette formation may be easier to recognize in LCNEC. As noted, similar to both tumors is frequent apoptosis, mitotic activity, and necrosis. Of note, although in small and crushed samples mitoses can be hard to appreciate, apoptosis is usually easily identified and its absence should lead to questions as to the accuracy of the small-cell (or LCNEC) diagnosis representing an opportunity for the use of Ki-67, as previously discussed.

Unfortunately, immunohistochemistry does not resolve this problem. Although TTF1 is positive at a high rate in small-cell carcinoma, the rate of immunoreactivity in LCNEC is also relatively high.[41] While neuroendocrine markers are not required for the diagnosis of small-cell carcinoma, if they are performed, the pattern will be the same in both tumors. Ki-67 is high (over 50%) in both tumor types. Immunohistochemistry for cytokeratin and synaptophysin is often dotlike in small-cell, while either membranous for cytokeratin or diffusely cytoplasmic for LCNEC. While this can highlight a dual cell population in a combined tumor (supporting the presence of 2 histologic patterns) the finding is not sufficiently consistent a diagnostic tool in morphologically difficult cases.

There are some circumstances in which immunohistochemistry may be of use in cases of high grade neuroendocrine carcinoma. In nonsmokers or patients under the age of 40, the diagnosis of primary pulmonary small-cell carcinoma warrants additional examination. In this setting, confirmation of neuroendocrine differentiation by immunohistochemistry is strongly suggested, as well as cytokeratin staining. The high rate of TTF1 immunoreactivity in small-cell carcinoma can be exploited. Therefore, an approach to rule out other tumors such as primitive neuroectodermal tumor, lymphoma, synovial sarcoma, desmoplastic small round cell tumor, mesenchymal chondrosarcoma, and small-cell osteosarcoma, among other tumors, is recommended. Finally, immunohistochemistry will not eliminate extrapulmonary small-cell carcinoma, with the exception of Merkel cell carcinoma, which is uniquely CK20 positive and negative for TTF1 and CK7.

For LCNEC, in addition to small-cell carcinoma, the differential diagnosis includes nonkeratinizing squamous cell carcinomas, basaloid carcinoma, and solid pattern adenocarcinoma (see more in next section). Cytokeratin and neuroendocrine markers are needed to confirm LCNEC, and use of p40 will help eliminate squamous carcinomas. It has been suggested that staining for more than one neuroendocrine marker is more specific for LCNEC,[42] with the caveat that it is critical that an immunohistochemistry approach be reserved for tumors with neuroendocrine morphology, as it is known that squamous and adenocarcinomas can be positive for neuroendocrine markers, a problem of using immunohistochemistry (IHC) for neuroendocrine classification. The use of INSM1 may provide more sensitivity and specificity in this setting than other markers (**Fig. 6A–C**).

In summary, after ruling out morphologic mimickers and confirming neuroendocrine morphology with IHC in the case of LCNEC, the differential diagnosis of small-cell versus LCNECs remains largely morphologic. Especially in small samples

from extrapulmonary metastatic sites, the focus should be to identify any small-cell component as a small-cell or combined small-cell carcinoma is more likely in that setting and the treatment of high-stage small-cell carcinoma is better established. Morphologic features are summarized in **Table 1**.

LARGE-CELL NEUROENDOCRINE CARCINOMA VERSUS SOLID-TYPE ADENOCARCINOMA

Although at first glance this does not seem like a difficult problem, in practice, the overlap between the organoid pattern of a neuroendocrine tumor and the solid pattern of adenocarcinoma can be challenging. In addition, distinction of a cribriform pattern of adenocarcinoma from pseudorosettes and rosettes is also quite subjective. As a result, this problem has led to overlapping classification, which has been partially unearthed with molecular testing.

Both tumor types can be a lobulated or spiculated peripheral mass lesion in the lung, and both are associated with cigarette smoking. Although there are architectural similarities in growth pattern histologically in some cases, LCNEC nests are more likely to have central necrosis (comedolike) than adenocarcinoma. Beyond that, however, the differences become focused on cellular features. In adenocarcinoma, nuclei have vesicular chromatin with macronucleoli, whereas LCNECs have coarse chromatin with visible nucleoli, but not macronucleoli. In addition, although LCNECs have visible cytoplasm when compared with small-cell carcinomas, adenocarcinoma cells often have more abundant cytoplasm than LCNECs. Although mitotic rates are high in both tumor types, adenocarcinomas generally have a lower mitotic rate than LCNECs and also a lower Ki-67 index.[43] However, cutoff values have not been established for this distinction (**Fig. 7A–E**).

Beyond morphology, IHC should be a useful adjunct. The requirement of neuroendocrine immunohistochemistry in the differential of LCNEC when compared with adenocarcinoma should resolve negative cases as adenocarcinoma, but positive cases do not automatically lead to an LCNEC conclusion. It is known that non–small-cell lung cancer can be positive for synaptophysin or CD56 and this tumor type, that of neuroendocrine differentiation by IHC alone, raises a problem in this analysis when such tumors have overlapping morphologic features with neuroendocrine tumors.[44] This specificity problem is greatest for CD56 and synaptophysin

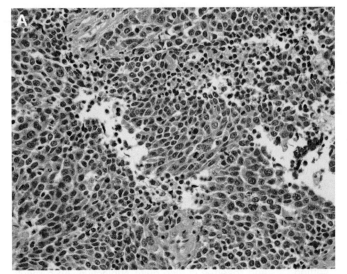

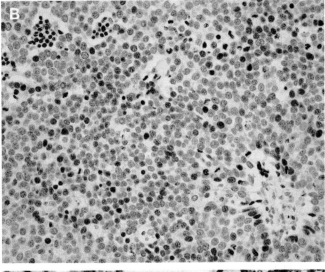

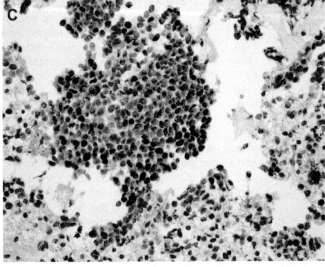

Fig. 6. IHC for INSM1. (*A*) A tumor with a solid growth pattern and cells with visible cytoplasm and high mitotic rate. The nuclei show salt and pepper chromatin. Neuroendocrine morphology is suggested but immunohistochemistry negative for synaptophysin, chromogranin, and CD56 (H&E, original magnification ×100). (*B*) INSM1 is variably but consistently positive in the tumor cells in (*A*) (DAB, original magnification ×100). (*C*) INSM1 is also useful in cytology cell blocks (DAB, original magnification ×100).

Table 1
Pathologic features of low-grade and high-grade neuroendocrine carcinomas

Feature	Typical Carcinoid	Atypical Carcinoid	SCLC	LCNEC
Gross	>5.0 mm Circumscribed Lung localized	>5.0 mm Circumscribed Lung localized	Bulky Extrapulmonary	Peripheral lung mass Necrosis
Histology	Uniform cells Fine chromatin Cytoplasm visible No necrosis Rare apoptosis	Uniform cells Fine chromatin Cytoplasm visible Necrosis can be present Some apoptosis	Nuclear molding Crush artifact Fine chromatin Scant cytoplasm Necrosis Apoptosis	Irregular nuclei Larger cells Coarse chromatin Small nucleoli Visible cytoplasm Palisading/rosettes Necrosis
Mitoses	<2 in 2 mm^2 (10 HPF) <6 in 3 sets of 2 mm^2 fields (30 HPF)	$\geq$2–9 in 2 mm^2 (10 HPF) $\geq$6 in 3 sets of 2 mm^2 fields (30 HPF)	$\geq$10 in 2 mm^2 (10 HPF)	$\geq$10 in 2 mm^2 (10 HPF)
Ki-67[a]	Usually <5%	>5%, <20%	Usually >50%	Usually >50%

Abbreviations: HPF, high-power field; LCNEC, large-cell neuroendocrine carcinoma; SCLS, small-cell lung cancer.
[a] Cutoff not established.

and lowest for chromogranin. However, chromogranin is also the least sensitive in high-grade neuroendocrine carcinomas overall. It has been proposed that 2 markers positive would favor LCNEC. In addition, it appears that INSM1 may be more sensitive than chromogranin but equally specific in this arena,[45] and may combine the sensitivity of CD56 and the specificity of chromogranin.

Given that the primary therapy is surgical for either LCNEC or adenocarcinoma, this problem may be most problematic in the decision for chemotherapy or targeted therapies. As a result, molecular data also may play a role in the decision-making process; however, such analyses have rendered interesting results in terms of refinement of classification. In one series using napsin A, p40, CD56, synaptophysin, and chromogranin to resolve morphologically difficult cases, 47 cases of LCNEC studied showed no KRAS mutation–positive tumors, an alteration seen in 20% to 30% of lung adenocarcinomas.[46] In contrast, a series of 45 LCNECs showed 18 cases with TP53 and RB1 alterations ("small-cell–like") whereas 20 cases harbored either KRAS and/or STK11 mutations without RB1 alterations ("adenocarcinomalike"). Interestingly, this subset of tumors was more likely napsin A positive and Ki-67 intermediate than their small-cell–like counterparts.[43] It is suggested that napsin A and intermediate Ki-67 index (see **Fig. 7**E) indicate an adenocarcinoma with IHC determined neuroendocrine differentiation, giving a potential role for these markers in this distinction. It is unclear how INSM1 would impact this decision, as neither study explored this marker.

In another molecular analysis of LCNEC,[47] 2 subtypes were also reported, with some overlap with other studies. Interestingly, the profile of LCNEC that was "adenocarcinomalike" had STK11/KEAP1 alterations and were achaete-scute family BHLH transcription factor 1 (ASCL1) high and DLL3 high, and NOTCH low, whereas the LCNEC "small-cell–like" group, although similar to the small-cell group with TP53 and RB1 mutation, had low ASCL1 and DLL3, with high NOTCH, whereas small-cell had ASCL1 high and DLL3 high, NOTCH low. This study included combined small-cell carcinomas, which seemed to group with small-cell carcinomas.

These studies underscore the complexity that remains in the diagnosis of LCNEC and the resultant molecular heterogeneity of that group (**Table 2**). It may be that this uncommon tumor is composed of 2 or 3 subtypes; it is also possible that one subset belongs with small-cell carcinoma, whereas the other as a variant of adenocarcinoma. It also highlights that neuroendocrine markers as currently performed are imperfect, and that they should not be performed when tumors are not neuroendocrine by morphology. In addition, focal staining, especially for CD56 and synaptophysin should not be the sole determinant of tumor class in a morphologically difficult case. It remains unclear whether the distinct clinicopathologic and therapeutic features of LCNEC are the consequence of the inclusion of tumors that are in fact molecular adenocarcinoma.

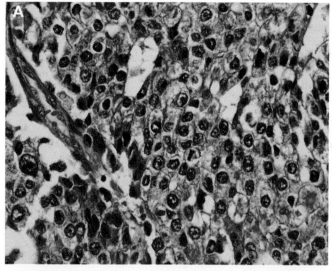

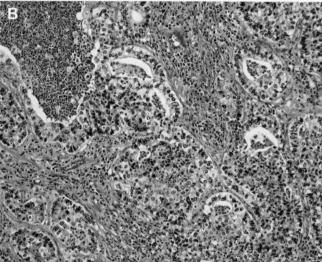

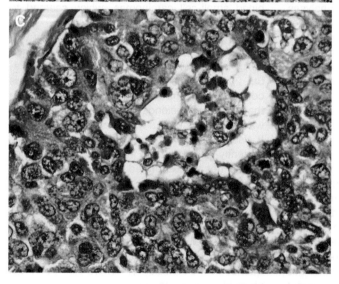

Fig. 7. LCNEC and solid pattern adenocarcinoma. (*A*) A solid pattern histology with cells having moderate to abundant cytoplasm, vesicular chromatic, and nucleoli. Neuroendocrine morphology was considered, and IHC was positive for synaptophysin (H&E, original magnification ×150). (*B*) Some areas of the tumor in (*A*) show gland formation and were napsin A positive. A diagnosis of combined adenocarcinoma and LCNEC was rendered (H&E, original magnification ×100). (*C*) A solid pattern histology with cells having visible cytoplasm, irregular nuclei, vesicular chromatin, and prominent nucleoli. Neuroendocrine morphology was considered and IHC was positive for synaptophysin (H&E, original magnification ×150).

Fig. 7. (*continued*). (*D*) Areas of the tumor in (*C*) were mucicarmine positive and molecular testing showed a KRAS-positive tumor ("adenocarcinomalike"). Is this tumor a variant of adenocarcinoma rather than LCNEC? (Mucicarmine, original magnification ×150). (*E*) Ki-67 in the tumor from (*C*) is approximately 30%, which is lower than most LCNECs (DAB, original magnification ×100).

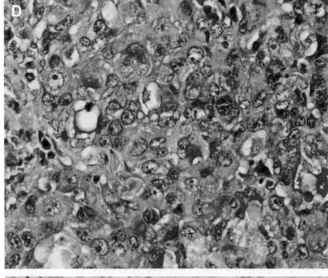

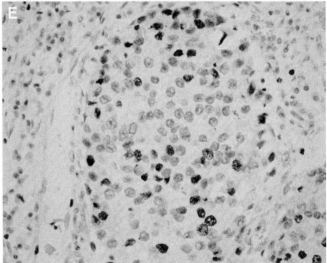

MIMICKERS OF HIGH-GRADE NEUROENDOCRINE CARCINOMAS

Many of the tumors mentioned in the differential diagnosis of small-cell carcinoma are encountered in clinical circumstances that largely do not overlap with small-cell carcinoma. As a result, one pitfall of these mimickers is that they are not considered in thoracic tumors in older patients with smoking history. In addition, the frequent presentation of small-cell carcinoma at metastatic sites also may reduce the suspicion for alternative diagnoses; these other entities are often rarer tumors than small-cell carcinoma. This is compounded by the use of small samples in the diagnosis of high-stage tumors, which may not allow for as extensive a panel of ancillary tests.

Review of clinical features as well as tumor location is critical. Younger patients with never-smoking or light-smoking histories should raise concern for a misdiagnosis of small-cell carcinoma. The tumor distribution is also important: tumors that are more chest wall associated than lung associated should raise consideration for an expanded differential diagnosis.[48]

The use of IHC for cytokeratin and CD56 in this setting can be especially misleading (**Table 3**). Cytokeratin reactivity in synovial sarcoma, primitive neuroectodermal tumor, and desmoplastic small round cell tumor are either typical or sufficiently common

Table 2
Features of large-cell neuroendocrine subtypes

LCNEC: Adenocarcinomalike	LCNEC: Small-Cell–Like
Napsin A positive	Napsin A negative
Ki-67 intermediate	Ki-67 high
KRAS/STK11/KEAP1 mutations	TP53 mutation RB1 loss
ASCL1/DLL3 high, NOTCH low	ASCL1/DLL3 low, NOTCH high

Abbreviations: ASCL1, achaete-scute family BHLH transcription factor 1; DLL3, deltalike 3 (*Drosophila*); LCNEC, large-cell neuroendocrine carcinoma.

that this result needs to be considered as part of a panel of stains. In addition, the sole immunoreactivity for CD56 as the basis for a neuroendocrine tumor diagnosis needs to be interpreted with extreme caution. CD56 is seen in a variety of tumor types; some neuroendocrine, some not neuroendocrine. In fact, a wide variety of carcinomas, sarcomas, and hematologic tumors can be CD56 positive at a high rate.[49] As a result, a panel approach, in this setting to include TTF1 to support small-cell carcinoma, markers such as WT1, desmin, and actin and potentially judicious use of molecular testing and fluorescence in situ hybridization are recommended to avoid misclassification.

OTHER CONSIDERATIONS IN NEUROENDOCRINE TUMORS

DELTALIKE 3 (*DROSOPHILA*) IN SMALL-CELL CARCINOMA

ASCL1 expression, a transcription factor important for neuronal cell lineage commitment and differentiation, is critical to the generation of neuroendocrine cells.[50] Although ASCL1 may be useful in determining cells that are destined to be neuroendocrine, its role in diagnosis remains uncertain.[51] There is an important interaction between ASCL1 and Deltalike 3 (*Drosophila*) (DLL3), and the interaction of DLL3 with Notch promotes proliferation and cell survival.[52] This interaction can be inhibited and this has been exploited as a potential therapy in small-cell carcinoma. One agent, rovalpituzumab tesirine, showed promise in a Phase 1 study,[53] and there is continued research to determine the feasibility of this treatment approach.

PROGRAMMED DEATH LIGAND 1 IN NEUROENDOCRINE TUMORS

There have been a few studies of programmed death ligand 1 (PD-L1) expression in neuroendocrine tumors. The rate in small-cell carcinoma is low, and ranges from 0% to 5.8% in 2 studies.[54,55] It is also reported as absent in carcinoid tumors.[55] The LCNEC subgroup again appears to be distinct from small-cell carcinoma. PD-L1 expression was 11% in one series of LCNEC,[55] and there is a suggestion that checkpoint inhibitor therapy may be active in this tumor type[56] when associated with high tumor mutation burden. It may be that PD-L1 expression in the inflammatory stroma is more relevant to survival prediction than tumoral expression,[57] and that CD8 infiltration in LCNEC may also have prognostic significance.[58]

DISCLOSURE

The author has nothing to disclose.

Table 3
Tumors positive for CD56 by immunohistochemistry

Neuroendocrine Tumors	Non-neuroendocrine Tumors Commonly (>50%)	Non-neuroendocrine Tumors Less Commonly (25%)
Merkel cell carcinoma	Wilms tumor	Papillary thyroid carcinoma
Medullary thyroid carcinoma	Rhabdomyosarcoma	Mesothelioma
Small-cell carcinoma	Desmoplastic round cell tumor	
Paraganglioma	Synovial sarcoma	
Primitive neuroectodermal tumor (20%)	Ovarian/endometrial stromal	
	Mesenchymal chondrosarcoma	
	Natural killer cell tumors	
	Acute myeloid leukemia	
	Multiple myeloma	
	Granular cell tumor	
	Solid pseudopapillary	

REFERENCES

1. Brambilla E, Beasley MB, Austin JHM, et al. Neuroendocrine tumors. Lyon (France): International Agency for Research on Cancer; 2015.

2. Brown MJ, English J, Muller NL. Bronchiolitis obliterans due to neuroendocrine hyperplasia: high-resolution CT–pathologic correlation. AJR Am J Roentgenol 1997;168(6):1561–2.

3. Lee JS, Brown KK, Cool C, et al. Diffuse pulmonary neuroendocrine cell hyperplasia: radiologic and clinical features. J Comput Assist Tomogr 2002;26(2): 180–4.

4. Marchevsky AM, Wirtschafter E, Walts AE. The spectrum of changes in adults with multifocal pulmonary neuroendocrine proliferations: what is the minimum set of pathologic criteria to diagnose DIPNECH? Hum Pathol 2015;46(2):176–81.

5. Davies SJ, Gosney JR, Hansell DM, et al. Diffuse idiopathic pulmonary neuroendocrine cell hyperplasia: an under-recognised spectrum of disease. Thorax 2007;62(3):248–52.

6. Rizvi SM, Goodwill J, Lim E, et al. The frequency of neuroendocrine cell hyperplasia in patients with pulmonary neuroendocrine tumours and non-neuroendocrine cell carcinomas. Histopathology 2009;55(3):332–7.

7. Gorshtein A, Gross DJ, Barak D, et al. Diffuse idiopathic pulmonary neuroendocrine cell hyperplasia and the associated lung neuroendocrine tumors: clinical experience with a rare entity. Cancer 2012; 118(3):612–9.

8. Yao JC, Hassan M, Phan A, et al. One hundred years after "carcinoid": epidemiology of and prognostic factors for neuroendocrine tumors in 35,825 cases in the United States. J Clin Oncol 2008;26(18): 3063–72.

9. Hemminki K, Li X. Incidence trends and risk factors of carcinoid tumors: a nationwide epidemiologic study from Sweden. Cancer 2001;92(8):2204–10.

10. Crocetti E, Paci E. Malignant carcinoids in the USA, SEER 1992-1999. An epidemiological study with 6830 cases. Eur J Cancer Prev 2003;12(3):191–4.

11. Caplin ME, Baudin E, Ferolla P, et al. Pulmonary neuroendocrine (carcinoid) tumors: European Neuroendocrine Tumor Society expert consensus and recommendations for best practice for typical and atypical pulmonary carcinoids. Ann Oncol 2015;26(8):1604–20.

12. Ferolla P, Daddi N, Urbani M, et al. Tumorlets, multicentric carcinoids, lymph-nodal metastases, and long-term behavior in bronchial carcinoids. J Thorac Oncol 2009;4(3):383–7.

13. Meisinger QC, Klein JS, Butnor KJ, et al. CT features of peripheral pulmonary carcinoid tumors. AJR Am J Roentgenol 2011;197(5):1073–80.

14. Rooper LM, Sharma R, Li QK, et al. INSM1 demonstrates superior performance to the individual and combined use of synaptophysin, chromogranin and CD56 for diagnosing neuroendocrine tumors of the thoracic cavity. Am J Surg Pathol 2017; 41(11):1561–9.

15. Oliveira AM, Tazelaar HD, Myers JL, et al. Thyroid transcription factor-1 distinguishes metastatic pulmonary from well-differentiated neuroendocrine tumors of other sites. Am J Surg Pathol 2001;25(6): 815–9.

16. Yang Z, Klimstra DS, Hruban RH, et al. Immunohistochemical characterization of the origins of metastatic well-differentiated neuroendocrine tumors to the liver. Am J Surg Pathol 2017;41(7):915–22.

17. Long KB, Srivastava A, Hirsch MS, et al. PAX8 Expression in well-differentiated pancreatic endocrine tumors: correlation with clinicopathologic features and comparison with gastrointestinal and pulmonary carcinoid tumors. Am J Surg Pathol 2010;34(5):723–9.

18. Weissferdt A, Tang X, Wistuba II, et al. Comparative immunohistochemical analysis of pulmonary and thymic neuroendocrine carcinomas using PAX8 and TTF-1. Mod Pathol 2013;26(12):1554–60.

19. Travis WD, Rush W, Flieder DB, et al. Survival analysis of 200 pulmonary neuroendocrine tumors with clarification of criteria for atypical carcinoid and its separation from typical carcinoid. Am J Surg Pathol 1998;22(8):934–44.

20. Tsuta K, Raso MG, Kalhor N, et al. Histologic features of low- and intermediate-grade neuroendocrine carcinoma (typical and atypical carcinoid tumors) of the lung. Lung Cancer 2011;71(1):34–41.

21. Aslan DL, Gulbahce HE, Pambuccian SE, et al. Ki-67 immunoreactivity in the differential diagnosis of pulmonary neuroendocrine neoplasms in specimens with extensive crush artifact. Am J Clin Pathol 2005; 123(6):874–8.

22. Marchio C, Gatti G, Massa F, et al. Distinctive pathological and clinical features of lung carcinoids with high proliferation index. Virchows Arch 2017;471(6): 713–20.

23. Fabbri A, Cossa M, Sonzogni A, et al. Ki-67 labeling index of neuroendocrine tumors of the lung has a high level of correspondence between biopsy samples and surgical specimens when strict counting guidelines are applied. Virchows Arch 2017;470(2):153–64.

24. Pelosi G, Rindi G, Travis WD, et al. Ki-67 antigen in lung neuroendocrine tumors: unraveling a role in clinical practice. J Thorac Oncol 2014;9(3):273–84.

25. Rindi G, Klersy C, Inzani F, et al. Grading the neuroendocrine tumors of the lung: an evidence-based proposal. Endocr Relat Cancer 2014;21(1):1–16.

26. Swarts DR, Rudelius M, Claessen SM, et al. Limited additive value of the Ki-67 proliferative index on

patient survival in World Health Organization-classified pulmonary carcinoids. Histopathology 2017;70(3):412–22.

27. Walts AE, Ines D, Marchevsky AM. Limited role of Ki-67 proliferative index in predicting overall short-term survival in patients with typical and atypical pulmonary carcinoid tumors. Mod Pathol 2012;25(9):1258–64.

28. Herde RF, Kokeny KE, Reddy CB, et al. Primary pulmonary carcinoid tumor: a long-term single institution experience. Am J Clin Oncol 2015;41(1):24–9.

29. Canizares MA, Matilla JM, Cueto A, et al. Atypical carcinoid tumours of the lung: prognostic factors and patterns of recurrence. Thorax 2014;69(7):648–53.

30. Pusceddu S, Catena L, Valente M, et al. Long-term follow up of patients affected by pulmonary carcinoid at the Istituto Nazionale Tumori of Milan: a retrospective analysis. J Thorac Dis 2010;2(1):16–20.

31. Asamura H, Kameya T, Matsuno Y, et al. Neuroendocrine neoplasms of the lung: a prognostic spectrum. J Clin Oncol 2006;24(1):70–6.

32. Aydin E, Yazici U, Gulgosteren M, et al. Long-term outcomes and prognostic factors of patients with surgically treated pulmonary carcinoid: our institutional experience with 104 patients. Eur J Cardiothorac Surg 2011;39(4):549–54.

33. Nicholson SA, Beasley MB, Brambilla E, et al. Small cell lung carcinoma (SCLC): a clinicopathologic study of 100 cases with surgical specimens. Am J Surg Pathol 2002;26(9):1184–97.

34. Kinoshita T, Yoshida J, Ishii G, et al. The differences of biological behavior based on the clinicopathological data between resectable large-cell neuroendocrine carcinoma and small-cell lung carcinoma. Clin Lung Cancer 2013;14(5):535–40.

35. Hanna N, Bunn PA Jr, Langer C, et al. Randomized phase III trial comparing irinotecan/cisplatin with etoposide/cisplatin in patients with previously untreated extensive-stage disease small-cell lung cancer. J Clin Oncol 2006;24(13):2038–43.

36. Eichhorn F, Dienemann H, Muley T, et al. Predictors of survival after operation among patients with large cell neuroendocrine carcinoma of the lung. Ann Thorac Surg 2015;99(3):983–9.

37. Takei H, Asamura H, Maeshima A, et al. Large cell neuroendocrine carcinoma of the lung: a clinicopathologic study of eighty-seven cases. J Thorac Cardiovasc Surg 2002;124(2):285–92.

38. Luiz JE, Lee AG, Keltner JL, et al. Paraneoplastic optic neuropathy and autoantibody production in small-cell carcinoma of the lung. J Neuroophthalmol 1998;18(3):178–81.

39. Nakamura T, Fujisaka Y, Tamura Y, et al. Large cell neuroendocrine carcinoma of the lung with cancer-associated retinopathy. Case Rep Oncol 2015;8(1):153–8.

40. Hoshi R, Furuta N, Horai T, et al. Discriminant model for cytologic distinction of large cell neuroendocrine carcinoma from small cell carcinoma of the lung. J Thorac Oncol 2010;5(4):472–8.

41. Sturm N, Rossi G, Lantuejoul S, et al. Expression of thyroid transcription factor-1 in the spectrum of neuroendocrine cell lung proliferations with special interest in carcinoids. Hum Pathol 2002;33(2):175–82.

42. Rossi G, Cavazza A, Marchioni A, et al. Role of chemotherapy and the receptor tyrosine kinases KIT, PDGFRalpha, PDGFRbeta, and Met in large-cell neuroendocrine carcinoma of the lung. J Clin Oncol 2005;23(34):8774–85.

43. Rekhtman N, Pietanza MC, Hellmann MD, et al. Next-generation sequencing of pulmonary large cell neuroendocrine carcinoma reveals small cell carcinoma-like and non-small cell carcinoma-like subsets. Clin Cancer Res 2016;22(14):3618–29.

44. Visscher DW, Zarbo RJ, Trojanowski JQ, et al. Neuroendocrine differentiation in poorly differentiated lung carcinomas: a light microscopic and immunohistologic study. Mod Pathol 1990;3(4):508–12.

45. Mukhopadhyay S, Dermawan JK, Lanigan CP, et al. Insulinoma-associated protein 1 (INSM1) is a sensitive and highly specific marker of neuroendocrine differentiation in primary lung neoplasms: an immunohistochemical study of 345 cases, including 292 whole-tissue sections. Mod Pathol 2019;32(1):100–9.

46. Rossi G, Mengoli MC, Cavazza A, et al. Large cell carcinoma of the lung: clinically oriented classification integrating immunohistochemistry and molecular biology. Virchows Arch 2014;464(1):61–8.

47. George J, Walter V, Peifer M, et al. Integrative genomic profiling of large-cell neuroendocrine carcinomas reveals distinct subtypes of high-grade neuroendocrine lung tumors. Nat Commun 2018;9(1):1048.

48. Mikami Y, Nakajima M, Hashimoto H, et al. Primary pulmonary primitive neuroectodermal tumor (PNET). A case report. Pathol Res Pract 2001;197(2):113–9, [discussion: 121–2].

49. Bahrami A, Truong LD, Ro JY. Undifferentiated tumor: true identity by immunohistochemistry. Arch Pathol Lab Med 2008;132(3):326–48.

50. Linnoila RI, Sahu A, Miki M, et al. Morphometric analysis of CC10-hASH1 transgenic mouse lung: a model for bronchiolization of alveoli and neuroendocrine carcinoma. Exp Lung Res 2000;26(8):595–615.

51. Miki M, Ball DW, Linnoila RI. Insights into the achaete-scute homolog-1 gene (hASH1) in normal and neoplastic human lung. Lung Cancer 2012;75(1):58–65.

52. Sabari JK, Lok BH, Laird JH, et al. Unravelling the biology of SCLC: implications for therapy. Nat Rev Clin Oncol 2017;14(9):549–61.

53. Rudin CM, Pietanza MC, Bauer TM, et al. Rovalpituzumab tesirine, a DLL3-targeted antibody-drug

conjugate, in recurrent small-cell lung cancer: a first-in-human, first-in-class, open-label, phase 1 study. Lancet Oncol 2017;18(1):42–51.

54. Schultheis AM, Scheel AH, Ozretic L, et al. PD-L1 expression in small cell neuroendocrine carcinomas. Eur J Cancer 2015;51(3):421–6.

55. Tsuruoka K, Horinouchi H, Goto Y, et al. PD-L1 expression in neuroendocrine tumors of the lung. Lung Cancer 2017;108:115–20.

56. Wang VE, Urisman A, Albacker L, et al. Checkpoint inhibitor is active against large cell neuroendocrine carcinoma with high tumor mutation burden. J Immunother Cancer 2017;5(1):75.

57. Kasajima A, Ishikawa Y, Iwata A, et al. Inflammation and PD-L1 expression in pulmonary neuroendocrine tumors. Endocr Relat Cancer 2018;25(3): 339–50.

58. Hermans BCM, Derks JL, Thunnissen E, et al. Prevalence and prognostic value of PD-L1 expression in molecular subtypes of metastatic large cell neuroendocrine carcinoma (LCNEC). Lung Cancer 2019; 130:179–86.

Lung Cancer Staging

Leila Kutob, MD, Frank Schneider, MD*

KEYWORDS

• Lung cancer • Staging • TNM • AJCC • Subtyping • Multiple nodules

---

Key points

- Only the size of the invasive component is used to assign T stage in adenocarcinomas with lepidic component.
- Comprehensive histology subtyping together with molecular testing results is helpful in staging synchronous lung adenocarcinomas.
- Spread through air spaces, now considered a form of invasion, is associated with higher rate of recurrence in limited resections.
- Effective targeted molecular and immunotherapies as first-line treatment increase the importance of standardized assessment of treatment response.

ABSTRACT

Lung cancer staging is a foundation of patient care, informing management decisions and prognosis. This comprehensive overview of the current 8th edition American Joint Committee on Cancer Cancer Staging Manual addresses common difficulties in staging, such as measuring the invasive component of adenocarcinomas and staging multiple lung nodules.

OVERVIEW

Tumor staging is a critical aspect of patient care because it allows for the classification of disease extent as well as informing management decisions and prognostication.[1] It also provides a system that facilitates consistent communication among clinicians, researchers, and patients. The Union for International Cancer Control TNM classification is the internationally accepted standard for cancer staging. The T category defines the size and/or extent of the primary tumor; the N category defines involvement of regional lymph nodes, and the M category defines presence of distant metastases. The TNM system is developed and periodically reviewed in collaboration with the American Joint Committee on Cancer (AJCC).[1] The AJCC formally defines staging as "the severity of an individual's cancer based on the magnitude of the original (primary) tumor as well as on the extent cancer has spread in the body." Staging is broadly divided into clinical staging and pathologic staging. Clinical staging is presurgical and based on clinical examination and imaging as well as diagnostic sampling of tumors, lymph nodes, or metastases. Pathologic staging is based on clinical stage information that is supplemented or modified based on the surgical resection of the tumor, lymph nodes, or metastases. As opposed to some other organ systems, lung cancer staging in the TNM scheme does not incorporate any nonanatomic factors. This review seeks to highlight common problems encountered in lung cancer staging.

EIGHTH EDITION AMERICAN JOINT COMMITTEE ON CANCER CANCER STAGING MANUAL

Changes in the current TNM classification of lung cancer include a different T descriptor for every centimeter of tumor less than 5 cm ("every centimeter counts"), introduction of adenocarcinoma in situ (AIS) and minimally invasive

---

Department of Pathology and Laboratory Medicine, Emory University School of Medicine, Emory University Hospital, 1364 Clifton Road Northeast, Atlanta, GA 30322, USA
* Corresponding author.
E-mail address: frank.schneider@emory.edu

Surgical Pathology 13 (2020) 57–71
https://doi.org/10.1016/j.path.2019.10.003

adenocarcinoma (MIA), reclassification of endo-bronchial tumors located less than 2 cm from the carina as T2, designating total atelectasis/pneumonitis as a T2 based on prognosis, classification of diaphragmatic invasion as T4, and removing mediastinal pleura invasion as T descriptor (**Table 1**).[2,3] The N component descriptors remain the same, but the number of involved lymph node stations has prognostic impact. Although the intrathoracic metastases descriptor (M1a) remained unchanged, extrathoracic metastases are currently divided into a single extrathoracic metastasis (M1b) and multiple extrathoracic metastases in a single organ or multiple organs (M1c). Pathologists should only report an M stage if present (the term MX is obsolete and should not be used).[1] Prognostic stage groups are typically not reported by pathologists. They are not included in the synoptic cancer reporting protocols of the College of American Pathologists.[4]

SIZE AND CONTIGUOUS EXTENSION OF THE PRIMARY TUMOR (T STAGE)

The T stage of lung cancers is based on tumor size. Proper grossing and measurement techniques are critical to assign the correct T category. Formalin fixation can change tumor size by 5%.[5] Most tumors shrink, but some also increase in size. In about 3% of tumors, measurement after fixation leads to a different T stage than measuring the fresh specimen. Radiologic ground glass and subsolid nodules are mostly affected by this change. Although measuring tumor size after fixation may underestimate true tumor size, it is fair to assume that the more than 70,000 lung cancers in the International Association for the Study of Lung Cancer (IASLC) International Staging Project database (which forms the basis for the T stage groupings) were not all measured before the specimen was formalin fixed.

It is of great importance to correlate any gross measurement of the tumor with the microscopic examination. First, tumors are not infrequently associated with organizing lung injury, solid post-obstructive changes, or parenchymal scarring that can lead to overestimating tumor size at the time of gross examination. Second, microscopic examination is often necessary to differentiate invasive components of tumor from noninvasive components.

INVASIVE COMPONENT DETERMINES T CATEGORY

With the publication of a new lung adenocarcinoma classification in 2011, the terminology of "mixed adenocarcinoma" and "bronchioloalveolar carcinoma" became obsolete, whereas the concepts of comprehensive histologic subtyping, lepidic growth pattern, MIA, and AIS were introduced (**Fig. 1**).[6] The AJCC requires that for invasive adenocarcinomas with lepidic component only the invasive component be used to assign the T category.[7] Invasion in adenocarcinoma is defined by the World Health Organization (WHO) as any histologic subtype other than a lepidic pattern, tumor cells infiltrating myofibroblastic stroma, or tumor cells spreading through air spaces or invading pleura or vasculature.[8] Other histologic types of lung cancer are not subject to this measurement rule. Proper staging in partially invasive tumors is complicated by the following. First, distinguishing lepidic adenocarcinoma from invasive patterns shows good reproducibility in straightforward cases and among pulmonary pathologists, but only poor to fair reproducibility in difficult cases and among nonexpert pathologists (**Fig. 2**).[9] Second, in some cases the invasive component does not form a single measurable focus. In this scenario, it is recommended to calculate invasive tumor size by estimating the percentage of the invasive component and multiply it by the total tumor size (**Fig. 3**).[10] Third, lepidic components of adenocarcinomas are difficult or impossible to see grossly. It is prudent to review the preoperative chest computed tomography (CT) and confirm that the surgically resected tumor is adequately represented on the slide (**Fig. 4**). Omitting this step could lead to understaging or overstaging of partial ground glass/solid nodules, for example, by not appreciating that a large ground glass component on the CT was not seen grossly or microscopically, by classifying a tumor as minimally invasive while not recognizing that its ground glass component is larger than 3 cm, or by underestimating the invasive component of a cancer by not submitting the entire solid component of the tumor. When the pathologist finds that gross measurement and tumor size by imaging are discrepant even after adequate histologic sampling, reportable maximum tumor size of the lepidic (ground glass) and invasive (solid) components may be best obtained from the CT (and such course of action should be documented in the surgical pathology report).[7]

IN SITU CARCINOMA

Outcome studies have found that size of invasion in nonmucinous lung adenocarcinomas is an independent predictor of outcome. Tumors lacking invasion (now referred to as adenocarcinoma in situ)

Table 1
T, N, and M descriptors for the eighth edition of the TNM classification for lung cancer

T: Primary tumor		
TX	Primary tumor cannot be assessed or tumor proven by presence of malignant cells in sputum or bronchial washings but not visualized by imaging or bronchoscopy	
T0	No evidence of primary tumor	
Tis	Carcinoma in situ	
T1	Tumor ≤3 cm in greatest dimension surrounded by lung or visceral pleura without bronchoscopic evidence of invasion more proximal than the lobar bronchus (ie, not in the main bronchus)[a]	
T1mi	Minimally invasive adenocarcinoma[b]	
T1a	Tumor ≤1 cm in greatest dimension[a]	
T1b	Tumor >1 cm but ≤2 cm in greatest dimension[a]	
T1c	Tumor >2 cm but ≤3 cm in greatest dimension[a]	
T2	Tumor >3 cm but ≤5 cm or tumor with any of the following features[c]: Involving main bronchus regardless of distance from the carina but without involvement of the carina; invading visceral pleura; associated with atelectasis or obstructive pneumonitis that extends to the hilar region, involving part or all of the lung	
T2a	Tumor >3 cm but ≤4 cm in greatest dimension	
T2b	Tumor >4 cm but ≤5 cm in greatest dimension	
T3	Tumor >5 cm but ≤7 cm in greatest dimension or associated with separate tumor nodule(s) in the same lobe as the primary tumor or directly invades any of the following structures: chest wall (including the parietal pleura and superior sulcus tumors), phrenic nerve, parietal pericardium	
T4	Tumor >7 cm in greatest dimension or associated with separate tumor nodule(s) in a different ipsilateral lobe than that of the primary tumor or invades any of the following structures: diaphragm, mediastinum, heart, great vessels, trachea, recurrent laryngeal nerve, esophagus, vertebral body, and carina	
N: Regional lymph node involvement		
NX	Regional lymph nodes cannot be assessed	
N0	No regional lymph node metastasis	
N1	Metastasis in ipsilateral peribronchial and/or ipsilateral hilar lymph nodes and intrapulmonary nodes, including involvement by direct extension	
N2	Metastasis in ipsilateral mediastinal and/or subcarinal lymph node(s)	
N3	Metastasis in contralateral mediastinal, contralateral hilar, ipsilateral or contralateral scalene, or supraclavicular lymph node(s)	
M: Distant metastasis		
M0	No distant metastasis	
M1	Distant metastasis present	
M1a	Separate tumor nodule(s) in a contralateral lobe; tumor with pleural or pericardial nodule(s) or malignant pleural or pericardial effusion[d]	
M1b	Single extrathoracic metastasis[e]	
M1c	Multiple extrathoracic metastases in 1 or more organs	

[a] The uncommon superficial spreading tumor of any size with its invasive component limited to the bronchial wall, which may extend proximal to the main bronchus, is also classified as T1a.
[b] Solitary adenocarcinoma, ≤3 cm with a predominately lepidic pattern and ≤5 mm invasion in any 1 focus.
[c] T2 tumors with these features are classified as T2a if ≤4 cm in greatest dimension or if size cannot be determined, and T2b if >4 cm but ≤5 cm in greatest dimension.
[d] Most pleural (pericardial) effusions with lung cancer are due to tumor. In a few patients, however, multiple microscopic examinations of pleural (pericardial) fluid are negative for tumor and the fluid is nonbloody and not an exudate. When these elements and clinical judgment dictate that the effusion is not related to the tumor, the effusion should be excluded as a staging descriptor.
[e] This includes involvement of a single distant (nonregional) lymph node.
Adapted from Goldstraw et al.[3] (with permission).

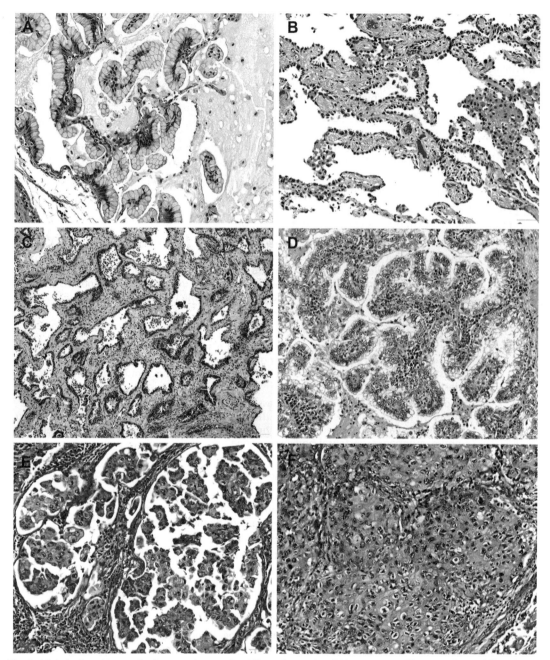

Fig. 1. Histologic patterns of adenocarcinoma. Lepidic patterns should be separated into mucinous (*A*) and non-mucinous (*B*). Purely lepidic mucinous tumors are uncommon; with adequate sampling the vast majority of mucinous adenocarcinomas can be shown to have invasive areas. (*B*) Lepidic adenocarcinoma with retained lung architecture and tumor cells growing along variably thickened alveolar septa. Tumors up to 3 cm showing this pattern exclusively, lacking stromal, vascular, and pleural invasion and without tumor cells in air spaces, can be classified as AIS. (*C*) Acinar adenocarcinoma is characterized by glands or glandlike spaces. Glands in which the central lumen fills up with tumor cells as well as cribriform patterns are considered patterns of acinar adenocarcinoma. (*D*) Papillary adenocarcinoma shows papillae with fibrovascular cores that typically occupy air spaces (as opposed to tangentially sectioned alveolar septa in the lepidic growth pattern). (*E*) Micropapillary adenocarcinoma is characterized by tufts of tumor cells lacking fibrovascular cores that appear to float in air spaces. This pattern is often accompanied by STAS. (*F*) Solid adenocarcinoma shows sheets of tumor cells that cannot be placed into any of the above patterns. When no other pattern is present, confirming this pattern with immunohistochemical stains (eg, thyroid transcription factor 1 (TTF1)) or by demonstrating intracellular mucin in least 5 tumor cells in each of 2 high-power fields is recommended (hematoxylin-eosin, original magnification × 100 (C) and × 200 (A, B, D–F)).[6]

Fig. 2. Transition of lepidic growth pattern (*left*) into acinar growth pattern (*right*) adenocarcinoma. Measuring the size of the invasive component is important because it determines the T stage. Solid, papillary, and micropapillary patterns as well as STAS are by definition considered invasive (hematoxylin-eosin, original magnification × 100).

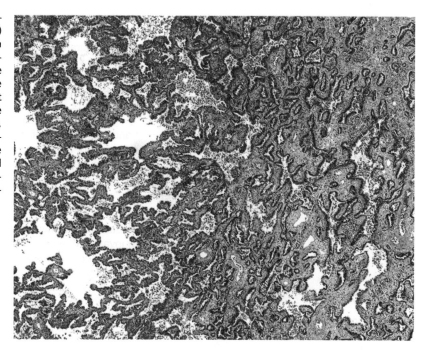

or showing 5 mm or less invasion (now referred to as minimally invasive adenocarcinoma) show essentially 100% 5-year survival.[6,11] The 8th edition AJCC staging manual introduced stage pTis for AIS and pTmi for MIA. To qualify for a diagnosis of pT1mi adenocarcinoma, the tumor must be solitary, less than 3 cm, predominantly lepidic, and lack tumor necrosis, spread through air spaces (STAS), invasion into lymphatics, blood vessels, and pleura. Such tumors need to be entirely submitted for microscopic examination to ascertain all of the above criteria are met. In situ adenocarcinomas (stage pTis) must meet the above criteria

except that they are purely lepidic with no invasion.

SPREAD THROUGH AIR SPACES

STAS is defined as micropapillary clusters, solid nests, or single cells of tumor extending beyond the edge of the tumor into the air spaces of surrounding lung parenchyma (**Fig. 5**). STAS has been associated with increased incidence of recurrence in tumors that have undergone only limited resection and with lower survival.[12,13] The concept of STAS has been included in the 2015

Fig. 3. Multiple invasive areas in adenocarcinoma. In this 2.7-cm tumor (keeping in mind sometimes fair interobserver variability), 30% could be interpreted as invasive (*circled areas*), resulting in a 0.81-cm (= 2.2 × 0.3) invasive component that is staged pT1a (as opposed to pT1c if T staging were based on the size of the entire lesion) (hematoxylin-eosin, original magnification × 40).

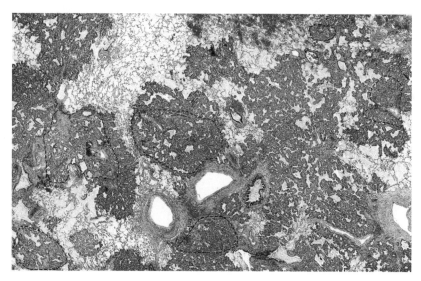

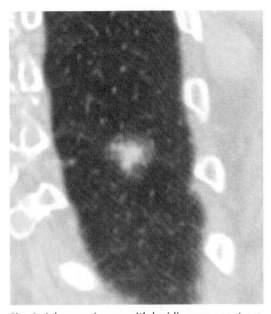

Fig. 4. Adenocarcinoma with lepidic component presenting as ground glass, part-solid nodule: The gross measurement of the tumor and the slide measurement of the invasive component correlated with the size of the ground glass and solid components, respectively.

WHO classification as a form of invasion. There is ongoing controversy whether STAS is truly a biological characteristic of the tumor or an artifact caused by tissue handling and processing.[14] Although STAS is by definition a pattern of invasion, it is not to be considered in determining tumor size or size of the invasive component. There is currently no guidance on how one should handle a tumor that is invasive based solely on the presence of STAS yet has no measurable invasion because the tumor is otherwise purely lepidic.

VISCERAL PLEURAL INVASION

Visceral pleural invasion, invasion across a fissure, or invasion directly into an adjacent ipsilateral lobe with an incomplete fissure upstages tumors less than 3 cm to pT2a. Pleural invasion is present when tumor cells are present on the pleural side of the outermost (external) elastic layer of the pleura (**Fig. 6**). Surgical pathologists should use special stains (eg, elastic-Van Gieson [EVG]) liberally because they can aid in (not only difficult) questions of pleural invasion. Penetration beyond the external elastic and presence of tumor on the visceral pleural surface behave similarly, and distinguishing those has no impact on staging.[15] Direct invasion of the parietal pleura or chest wall

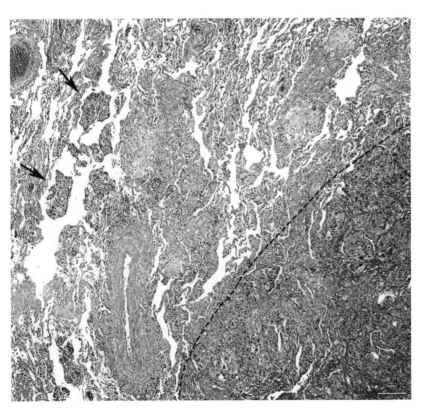

Fig. 5. STAS, defined by WHO as "spread of micropapillary clusters, solid nests, or single cancer cells into air spaces in the lung parenchyma (*arrows*) beyond the edge of the main tumor (*right of dotted line*) (hematoxylin-eosin, original magnification × 100)."[8]

Fig. 6. Pleural invasion can more easily and reliably be identified using elastic fiber stains (EVG stain). To qualify as pleural invasion, tumor cells must breach not only the internal (*stars*) but also through the external elastic lamina (*arrows*) of the visceral pleura (Elastic-van Gieson, original magnification × 400).

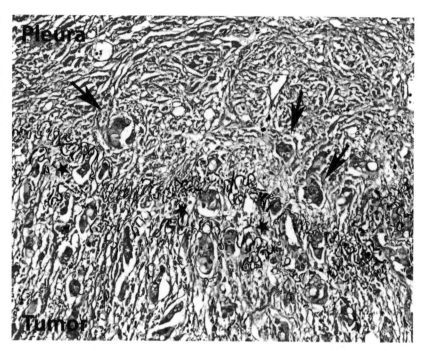

receives a designation of pT3. Parietal pleural invasion can be difficult to assess in the presence of pleural adhesions or inflammatory changes unless the tumor is intimately associated with chest wall components such skeletal muscle. The presence of fat is not specific for chest wall because fat can be seen in the peripheral lung beneath the visceral pleura. Tumors that adhere to the parietal pleura but in which the parietal pleural elastic layer is not recognizable even on EVG stains show outcomes similar to pT3 tumors and may be best managed similar to tumors with confirmed parietal pleural invasion.[16]

INVASION OF THE BRONCHUS

Invasion of the bronchus less than 2 cm from the carina is identified as an independent prognostic factor that requires upstaging a small tumor such as pT2. Pathologists are occasionally puzzled by this criterion and wonder if a tumor at hand meets it. When in doubt, distance of a tumor from the carina may be most easily assessed by pathologists using the coronal reconstruction of the preoperative chest CT. In general, the bronchial margin of any lobectomy will always be more than 2 cm from the carina. When faced with more proximal tumors near a pneumonectomy bronchial margin or involving a sleeve resection of a main bronchus, pathologists best course of action is to discuss the issue with the surgeon if distance cannot be readily obtained from imaging studies.

ANGIOLYMPHATIC INVASION

Invasion of tumor cells into blood or lymphatic vessels has been associated with poor outcome in several retrospective studies and metaanalyses.[17,18] Not only the presence but also the frequency of invasion may be important for prognosis.[19] At this point, no prospective clinical trials have used vascular invasion to stratify probands, and its evaluation does not determine the TNM stage of a tumor.

STAGING OF MULTIPLE LUNG TUMORS

The presence of more than 1 lung cancer poses a common dilemma for pathologists. Up to one-fifth of lung cancers detected by CT screening are multifocal.[20] The criteria of Martini and Melamed[21] for this situation, although nowadays supplemented by comprehensive histology subtyping and molecular studies, remain the cornerstone of the pathologist's initial light microscopic assessment whether 2 lung cancers are independent synchronous primaries. When the histologic types of 2 tumors are different (eg, 1 squamous cell carcinoma and 1 adenocarcinoma), they can be interpreted and staged as independent primary lung cancers with separate TNM designations. When tumors were histologically similar but in different segments or lobes of the lung, interpretation as separate primaries was recommended when (a) both tumors arose from in situ carcinoma, (b) no tumor was seen in lymphatics that were common to both tumors, and (c) no extrapulmonary metastases were present.[21]

MULTIPLE ADENOCARCINOMAS

Once metastatic disease of an extrapulmonary cancer is excluded, most cancers presenting with multiple lung nodule are either adenocarcinoma or squamous cell carcinomas.[22,23] In the setting of multifocal adenocarcinoma, pathologists should use comprehensive histologic subtyping, immunophenotype, and results of molecular studies to distinguish synchronous (and metachronous) primary tumors from intrapulmonary metastases. The current 8th edition of the AJCC staging manual places patients with multiple lung adenocarcinomas into 1 of 4 categories (Table 2).[1]

Table 2
Disease patterns of multifocal lung cancers recognized by the eighth edition of the American Joint Committee on Cancer staging manual

Histologic Finding	Disease Pattern Relationship of the Tumors	Imaging Findings	TNM Classification
Histologically different (eg, 1 squamous, 1 adenocarcinoma) or different by comprehensive histologic subtyping (eg, 1 lepidic-predominant, 1 solid adenocarcinoma)	*Independent primary cancers* Clonally unrelated May have different driver mutations	Two or more distinct masses, each typical for primary lung cancer	Separate T, N, and M for each tumor (separate synoptic report for each tumor)
Same histologic type or subtype	*Intrapulmonary metastases* Related nodules of same cancer	Typical lung cancer (solid, spiculated) with separate solid nodule	T3 if in the same lobe T4 if ipsilateral lobe M1a if contralateral lobe Single N and M (1 synoptic report)
Adenocarcinomas with lepidic growth pattern (including AIS, MIA, LPA)	*Multifocal ground glass/ lepidic adenocarcinoma* Conflicting data whether clonally related (ie, intrapulmonary metastasis) or not (many cases appear to represent multiple primary tumors), prognosis favorable	Multiple ground glass or part-solid nodules	T based on highest T lesion with (m) for multiplicity (or a number, if countable) Single N and M (1 synoptic report)
Tumor with uniform histology (often invasive mucinous adenocarcinoma) involving (sometimes seemingly patchy) expanses of the lobe (or more than 1 lobe)	*Pneumonic-type adenocarcinoma* Conflicting data whether clonally related (some show different clonality in different lobes), prognosis worse than multifocal ground glass/ lepidic adenocarcinoma, but typically without nodal or systemic metastases	Patchy areas of ground glass and consolidation	Areas of involvement determine T stage: T3 if confined to 1 lobe, T4 if involving different lobes in 1 lung, and M1a if involving both lungs (1 synoptic report)

Abbreviation: LPA, lepidic-predominant adenocarcinoma.
  Adapted from AJCC Cancer Staging Manual. 8th ed. New York: Springer; 2017; and Detterbeck FC, Franklin WA, Nicholson AG, et al. The IASLC Lung Cancer Staging Project: Background Data and Proposed Criteria to Distinguish Separate Primary Lung Cancers from Metastatic Foci in Patients with Two Lung Tumors in the Forthcoming Eighth Edition of the TNM Classification for Lung Cancer. J Thorac Oncol. 2016;11(5):651-665.

Each tumor should first undergo comprehensive histology subtyping and evaluation of the cytologic and stromal features (and each tumor be assigned the percentage of each subtype: lepidic, acinar, papillary, solid, and micropapillary). Pathologists should then follow the algorithm proposed by Girard and colleagues[24] to determine whether the tumors are best interpreted as separate primaries or intrapulmonary metastases (**Fig. 7**). This procedure should result in the best possible staging of multiple solid lung nodules. Limitations of this method include accuracy of subtyping in small biopsies and aggressive subtypes being overrepresented in metastatic foci. The AJCC staging manual considers morphologic similarities or difference a relative argument in favor or against clonality, respectively.

The only evidence accepted by the AJCC staging manual to prove that 2 tumors are clonal (ie, intrapulmonary metastasis) is exactly matching breakpoints identified by comparative genomic hybridization (CGH).[25] However, CGH is not available to most surgical pathologists and, in clinical practice, has been largely replaced in routine clinical practice by next-generation DNA sequencing (NGS) because the latter requires less DNA and provides more information on clinically actionable mutations.

The AJCC staging manual considers a similar biomarker pattern (usually genomic alterations) a relative argument in favor of 2 tumors representing intrapulmonary metastases. Because molecular testing for oncogenic mutations has become standard of care for lung cancer, finding the same genomic alteration in a separate tumor can be used to support a clonal origin.[26–28] Several studies have shown a high concordance rate for driver mutations between primary lung tumors and matched metastases.[29] Such information is not accepted as unequivocal proof, however, because (a) the same mutation may be incidentally present in separate tumors (and has been found in morphologically different tumors), (b) driver mutations can occur in normal appearing lung tissue, (c) germline mutations (eg, EGFR) may be misleading, and (d) tumors may show genomic heterogeneity with discordance rate up to 45% between primary tumor and metastasis.[30–33] According to the 2013 Molecular Testing Guideline, each tumor in a patient with multiple, apparently separate, primary lung adenocarcinomas may be tested for genomic aberrations.[26,34] The decision

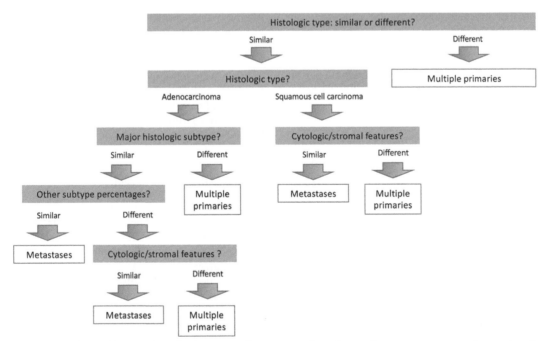

Fig. 7. Algorithm to distinguish multiple primary lung cancers from intrapulmonary metastases. Comprehensive histologic assessment includes evaluation of the percentages of histologic subtypes, cytologic features, and stromal characteristics, such as collagen, inflammation, lymphoid hyperplasia, and necrosis. Tumors exhibiting similar histologic features can be considered metastases, and those showing different histologic features can be considered multiple primaries. (*Adapted from* Girard N, Deshpande C, Lau C, et al. Comprehensive histologic assessment helps to differentiate multiple lung primary nonsmall cell carcinomas from metastases. *Am J Surg Pathol.* 2009;33(12):1752-1764; with permission.)

whether to test each tumor should always be made based on the clinical context. In some cases, it may be informative for staging; in some cases, it may be unnecessary for clinical decision making. Notably, there is no need to test multiple different areas within a single tumor.[26,34]

In some situations, multiple tumors cannot be staged unequivocally even after the best possible pathologic examination and clinical and radiographic correlation. In such cases, it may be best to give the patient the benefit of the doubt and stage tumors as independent primaries with a comment on the difficulty of proper staging. There is no evidence-based recommendation to which tumor one should assign lymph node metastases, but most pathologists would probably associate them with the tumor with the most resemblance in histologic and cytologic features.

MULTIPLE SQUAMOUS CELL CARCINOMAS

Squamous cell carcinomas are currently classified as keratinizing, nonkeratinizing, or basaloid.[8] Assessing keratinization, basaloid, or sarcomatoid features, clear cell change, necrosis, and background stroma (desmoplasia, inflammation, myxoid change hyalinization) may help distinguish multiple primary squamous cell carcinomas. Some of these features can be assessed with good interobserver variability.[35]

Molecular profiling of squamous cell carcinoma is not routinely performed in most institutions. Limited gene panels failed to demonstrate significant improvement in staging of multifocal squamous cell carcinoma.[28]

MULTIPLE NEUROENDOCRINE TUMORS

Patients with multiple carcinoid tumors in the same, an ipsilateral, or even contralateral lobe have excellent prognosis. The staging of multiple carcinoid tumors may require different staging than non–small cell lung cancer, but there are too few data points at present to address this properly.[36]

MULTIPLE GROUND GLASS/PART SOLID NODULES

The third category of multiple lung tumors in Table 2 is those that radiologically present as multiple ground glass opacities or part solid nodules. Histologically, these tumors are typically adenocarcinomas with variable lepidic component. This situation is addressed separately in the staging scheme because of the good outcome (5-year survival between 64% and 100%) and low frequency

of N2 lymph node metastases in these tumors, even when multifocal.[37,38] The genomic alterations of multiple ground glass nodules are not well studied yet. Studies so far suggest that molecular profiles are different, yet some mutations (including EGFR and KRAS) are shared between lesions in the same patient.[39] One hypothesis is that although tumors in the same patient are different, they may either arise from a common precursor or develop in a suitable genomic background ("field effect") characterized by the shared mutation (which may even be present before tumors start forming). For now, tumors in this category are thought of as biologically separate tumors, albeit with some similarities.[38] The T-category designation for multiple ground glass nodules is based on the T category of the lesion with the largest T, followed by the suffix "m" to indicate multiplicity (or a discrete number corresponding to number of tumors). Lymph node (N) stage is assigned for all tumors collectively. If the highest T stage is in situ or MIAs, pTis or pTmi should be used, respectively (eg, pTmi(4)N0).[38]

Mucinous tumors with lepidic growth pattern comprise a special category of ground glass opacity. Mucinous in situ adenocarcinoma is uncommon because one can usually find areas of invasion if the tumor is sampled extensively. Although one should consider separate foci of pure mucinous in situ carcinoma biologically separate tumors (just as other in situ adenocarcinomas), most mucinous adenocarcinomas present with intrapulmonary spread. Therefore, multiple mucinous tumors are typically best considered to represent metastatic foci, a notion supported by multiple mucinous tumors having worse outcome than their nonmucinous counterparts.[8,40]

"PNEUMONIC-TYPE" ADENOCARCINOMA

The fourth category of tumors in Table 2 comprises tumor with radiologic manifestation as diffuse consolidation. These "pneumonic-type" lung cancers are most frequently, but not exclusively, invasive mucinous adenocarcinomas (Fig. 8). The hallmark feature of this designation is a diffuse growth pattern as opposed to formation of discrete nodules. As a result, pneumonic-type adenocarcinomas often pose a challenge in measurement/size determination. The T-category designation essentially follows that for intrapulmonary metastases: pT3 when the adenocarcinoma is limited to a single lobe, pT4 with involvement of a second ipsilateral lobe, and M1a when there is contralateral lung involvement. Although these tumors show slow

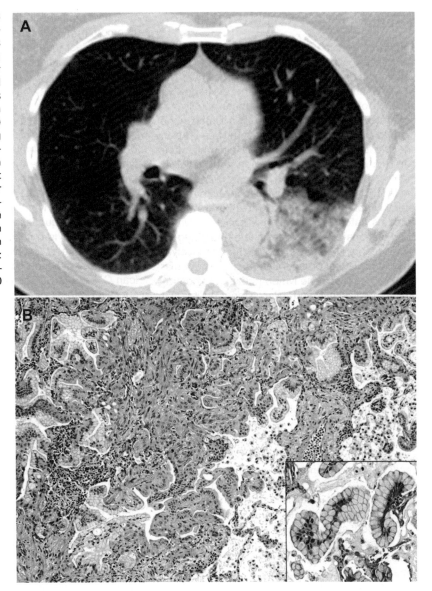

Fig. 8. Invasive mucinous adenocarcinoma radiologically presenting as "pneumonic-type" lung cancer. (*A*) The left lower lobe is diffusely involved by ground glass opacities and consolidation with air bronchograms. (*B*) Most tumors presenting this way are mucinous adenocarcinomas. Although they often show lepidic growth with columnar mucinous cells lining alveolar septa (*inset*), invasion can typically be found in these tumors when adequately sampled (B: hematoxylin-eosin, original magnification × 200 and × 400 (inset)).

progression, their prognosis is worse than that of multifocal ground glass nodules. For pathologists encountering a mucinous tumor involving large areas of the lung parenchyma in a patchy fashion, it would be prudent to review the chest CT to see if the tumor forms a diffuse consolidation rather than a focal lesion with some spread in its periphery.

METACHRONOUS TUMORS

Metachronous tumors are those that arise in patients with a history of lung cancer with a newly diagnosed tumor. To be considered a new primary lung cancer, the new tumor must either be

of a different histologic type or be the same as the previous histologic type with a ≥4-year interval and no evidence of systemic metastases.[41] Occasionally, the question arises whether a histologically similar tumor arising more than 4 years after the first could represent a recurrence or metastasis because recurrence after more than 5 years is known to occur in about 5% of patients with lung cancer.[42] No guidance exists on how to interpret a new tumor as late recurrence. Using the criteria set forth by Martini and Melamed with comprehensive histologic subtyping and consideration of molecular testing results appears to be an acceptable method in this situation.

LYMPH NODE INVOLVEMENT (N STAGE)

The N category is used to designate lymph node metastases, a poor prognostic indicator. The N category is divided into 5 subcategories (NX, N0, N1, N2, and N3) based on the presence or absence of lymph node involvement and lymph node station. The IASLC created a lymph node map to eliminate discrepancies between Asian and Western lymph node maps, allowing standardized documentation of lymph node involvement in patients with lung cancer.[43] Based on the IASLC lymph node classification system, ipsilateral lymph node stations 10 to 14+ are designated as category N1, whereas ipsilateral lymph node stations 2 to 9 are designated as category N2. Category N3 is given to lymph node involvement in ipsilateral or contralateral supraclavicular (station 1) and scalene lymph nodes, and contralateral mediastinal and hilar lymph nodes. Of note, direct extension of a primary tumor into a lymph node is considered lymph node involvement (pN1). At present, extranodal extension does not change the N category. Reporting of extranodal extension may be included in a future edition of the staging manual since metaanalysis has found its presence to be associated with significantly increased risk of mortality.[44]

Both AJCC and IASLC recommend that for accurate staging at least 6 lymph node stations are sampled during surgical resection of a lung cancer: 3 N1 stations and 3 N2 stations for accurate staging. Pathologists should assign an N stage upon microscopic examination of lymph nodes, even if fewer than the recommended number of lymph node stations have been sampled.[1] Of note, fine needle aspirations and core needle biopsies both satisfy the requirement that a lymph node has been examined microscopically.[1] There is no consensus yet whether limited sampling should be classified as pN0 or pN0(un) to acknowledge uncertainty.

Staging information from procedures before a cancer resection should be incorporated. Endobronchial ultrasound-guided lymph node aspirates especially have become a common preoperative staging procedure with prospective trials showing their usefulness compared with mediastinoscopy.[45,46]

The distinction between N1 and N2 lymph node involvement is a clinical break point for treatment decisions. Briefly, the National Comprehensive Cancer Network recommends surgical resection with consideration for neoadjuvant therapy for patients with N0-N1 disease.[47] However, patients with N2 disease are typically considered for definitive concurrent chemoradiation or induction chemotherapy, because randomized controlled trials suggest that surgery does not increase survival in these patients.[47]

LYMPH NODE REPORTING

Lymph node sampling (especially by mediastinoscopy or video-assisted thoracoscopic surgery) often results in submission of fragmentation of lymph nodes to the pathology department. It is impossible to determine whether fragments of lymph nodes originate from a single lymph node or from multiple lymph nodes. Therefore, lymph nodes are best quantified only if the actual number is known. If it is not known, it is acceptable to report the site of involvement without specifying the number of lymph node fragments. The American College of Surgeons Commission of Cancer surveils patterns of care by capturing whether at least 10 regional lymph nodes were removed for low-stage cancers. Pathologists may not be able to provide documentation for such external quality-of-care measures without an understanding of which tissue samples represent individual lymph nodes.

METASTASES (M STAGE)

The M category is based on the presence of distant metastases and is split into 3 subcategories (M1a, M1b, and M1c). Note that the AJCC defines pathologic (p) stage by timing (ie, at the time of surgical resection) and not by the professional performing the staging. Therefore, a 6-cm lung cancer with involved N2 lymph nodes in a patient who, by clinical stage, also has a brain metastasis, should be staged as pT3N2M1b even if the brain metastasis is not biopsied or resected. If a pathologist feels unprepared to incorporate clinical stage into the pathologic stage of their report because a metastasis is not available for microscopic examination, it is acceptable to omit reporting of the M category in the pathology report of a lung cancer resection and pass that responsibility back to the treating physician. Note, that the treating physician also incorporates other pathology reports into the clinical stage that are not formally staged by pathologists, for example, mediastinal lymph node sampling by fine needle aspiration.

Extrathoracic metastases are now classified as single (M1b, in 1 organ) or multiple (M1c, usually in more than 1 organ). Although the survival difference between M1a (pleural/pericardial dissemination) and M1b is minimal, the committee favored documenting oligometastatic disease separately because patients with oligometastatic disease nowadays receive more aggressive local therapy in addition to their systemic treatment.[3]

STAGING FOLLOWING PREOPERATIVE THERAPY

Neoadjuvant chemotherapy improves overall survival, time to distant recurrence, and recurrence-free survival in resectable non–small lung cancer.[48] The histologic features seen in treated tumors after neoadjuvant chemotherapy include necrosis, fibrosis, inflammation, and variable amounts of viable tumor. Immunotherapy induces similar histologic changes, possibly with fewer viable tumor cells and more fibrosis.[49] The amount of viable tumor appears to be the most important histologic predictor of outcome.[50,51] Of note, tumor necrosis (including cavitation), fibrosis, and inflammation can also be seen in resected tumors that have not undergone prior therapy. Stromal fibrosis by itself has been associated with poor prognosis in previously untreated resection specimens.[52,53]

Major pathologic response to neoadjuvant therapy has been defined as 10% or less of viable tumor, although recent data suggest that a higher percentage of viable tumors may still portend a favorable prognosis in adenocarcinoma.[50,54–56] Complete pathologic response requires the absence of residual viable tumor at the primary site as well as regional lymph nodes. Such specimens should be staged as ypT0N0.

Currently, there is no universally accepted guidance on how to assess the pathologic response of lung cancer to preoperative therapy (including chemotherapy, radiation, immunotherapy, or molecular targeted therapy). Recommendations on this subject by the IASLC are expected to be published by early 2020. Until then, estimating the percentage of viable tumor on each slide (assessed on the routine hematoxylin and eosin stains) and averaging over all sections of the tumor bed is an appropriate method to determine the amount of residual viable tumor.[51]

SUMMARY

Lung cancer staging is important to plan treatment and predict prognosis. The most important features for pathologists to assess include tumor size, pleural invasion, and lymph node involvement. In nonmucinous adenocarcinomas with lepidic component, only the invasive component determines T stage. In patients with multiple lung nodules, careful histopathologic examination is necessary to distinguish separate primary lung cancers (each of which should be staged separately) from intrapulmonary metastases. With increased aggressive systemic treatment, including preoperative chemotherapy, immunotherapy, and targeted therapy, assessing treatment response in resection specimen will become more important.

DISCLOSURE

The authors have nothing to disclose.

REFERENCES

1. Amin MB, Edge SB, Greene FL, et al, editors. AJCC cancer staging manual. 8th edition. New York: Springer; 2017.
2. Rami-Porta R, Asamura H, Travis WD, et al. Lung cancer–major changes in the American Joint Committee on Cancer eighth edition cancer staging manual. CA Cancer J Clin 2017;67(2):138–55.
3. Goldstraw P, Chansky K, Crowley J, et al. The IASLC Lung Cancer Staging Project: proposals for revision of the TNM Stage Groupings in the Forthcoming (Eighth) Edition of the TNM Classification for Lung Cancer. J Thorac Oncol 2016;11(1):39–51.
4. Protocol for the examination of resection specimens from patients with primary non-small cell carcinoma, small cell carcinoma, or carcinoid tumor of the lung. 2019. Available at: https://www.cap.org/protocols-and-guidelines/cancer-reporting-tools/cancer-protocol-templates.
5. Park HS, Lee S, Haam S, et al. Effect of formalin fixation and tumour size in small-sized non-small-cell lung cancer: a prospective, single-centre study. Histopathology 2017;71(3):437–45.
6. Travis WD, Brambilla E, Noguchi M, et al. International Association for the Study of Lung Cancer/American Thoracic Society/European Respiratory Society International Multidisciplinary Classification of lung adenocarcinoma. J Thorac Oncol 2011; 6(2):244–85.
7. Travis WD, Asamura H, Bankier AA, et al. The IASLC Lung Cancer Staging Project: proposals for coding T categories for subsolid nodules and assessment of tumor size in part-solid tumors in the forthcoming eighth edition of the TNM classification of lung cancer. J Thorac Oncol 2016;11(8):1204–23.
8. Travis WD, Brambilla E, Burke AP, et al. World Health Organization classification of tumours. Lyon (France): International Agency for Research on Cancer; 2015.
9. Thunnissen E, Beasley MB, Borczuk AC, et al. Reproducibility of histopathological subtypes and invasion in pulmonary adenocarcinoma. An international interobserver study. Mod Pathol 2012;25(12): 1574–83.

10. Yoshizawa A, Motoi N, Riely GJ, et al. Impact of proposed IASLC/ATS/ERS classification of lung adenocarcinoma: prognostic subgroups and implications for further revision of staging based on analysis of 514 stage I cases. Mod Pathol 2011; 24(5):653–64.

11. Borczuk AC, Qian F, Kazeros A, et al. Invasive size is an independent predictor of survival in pulmonary adenocarcinoma. Am J Surg Pathol 2009;33(3): 462–9.

12. Masai K, Sakurai H, Sukeda A, et al. Prognostic impact of margin distance and tumor spread through air spaces in limited resection for primary lung cancer. J Thorac Oncol 2017;12(12):1788–97.

13. Uruga H, Fujii T, Fujimori S, et al. Semiquantitative assessment of tumor spread through air spaces (STAS) in early-stage lung adenocarcinomas. J Thorac Oncol 2017;12(7):1046–51.

14. Blaauwgeers H, Russell PA, Jones KD, et al. Pulmonary loose tumor tissue fragments and spread through air spaces (STAS): invasive pattern or artifact? A critical review. Lung Cancer 2018;123: 107–11.

15. Shimizu K, Yoshida J, Nagai K, et al. Visceral pleural invasion classification in non-small cell lung cancer: a proposal on the basis of outcome assessment. J Thorac Cardiovasc Surg 2004;127(6):1574–8.

16. Mikubo M, Nakashima H, Naito M, et al. Prognostic impact of uncertain parietal pleural invasion at adhesion sites in non-small cell lung cancer patients. Lung Cancer 2017;108:103–8.

17. Wang J, Chen J, Chen X, et al. Blood vessel invasion as a strong independent prognostic indicator in non-small cell lung cancer: a systematic review and meta-analysis. PLoS One 2011;6(12):e28844.

18. Mollberg NM, Bennette C, Howell E, et al. Lymphovascular invasion as a prognostic indicator in stage I non-small cell lung cancer: a systematic review and meta-analysis. Ann Thorac Surg 2014;97(3): 965–71.

19. Okada S, Mizuguchi S, Izumi N, et al. Prognostic value of the frequency of vascular invasion in stage I non-small cell lung cancer. Gen Thorac Cardiovasc Surg 2017;65(1):32–9.

20. Vazquez M, Carter D, Brambilla E, et al. Solitary and multiple resected adenocarcinomas after CT screening for lung cancer: histopathologic features and their prognostic implications. Lung Cancer 2009;64(2):148–54.

21. Martini N, Melamed MR. Multiple primary lung cancers. J Thorac Cardiovasc Surg 1975;70(4):606–12.

22. Rosengart TK, Martini N, Ghosn P, et al. Multiple primary lung carcinomas: prognosis and treatment. Ann Thorac Surg 1991;52(4):773–8, [discussion: 778–9].

23. Martini N, Bains MS, Burt ME, et al. Incidence of local recurrence and second primary tumors in resected stage I lung cancer. J Thorac Cardiovasc Surg 1995;109(1):120–9.

24. Girard N, Deshpande C, Lau C, et al. Comprehensive histologic assessment helps to differentiate multiple lung primary nonsmall cell carcinomas from metastases. Am J Surg Pathol 2009;33(12): 1752–64.

25. Detterbeck FC, Franklin WA, Nicholson AG, et al. The IASLC Lung Cancer Staging Project: background data and proposed criteria to distinguish separate primary lung cancers from metastatic foci in patients with two lung tumors in the forthcoming eighth edition of the TNM classification for lung cancer. J Thorac Oncol 2016;11(5):651–65.

26. Lindeman NI, Cagle PT, Aisner DL, et al. Updated molecular testing guideline for the selection of lung cancer patients for treatment with targeted tyrosine kinase inhibitors: guideline from the College of American Pathologists, the International Association for the Study of Lung Cancer, and the Association for Molecular Pathology. Arch Pathol Lab Med 2018;142(3):321–46.

27. Warth A, Macher-Goeppinger S, Muley T, et al. Clonality of multifocal nonsmall cell lung cancer: implications for staging and therapy. Eur Respir J 2012; 39(6):1437–42.

28. Schneider F, Derrick V, Davison JM, et al. Morphological and molecular approach to synchronous non-small cell lung carcinomas: impact on staging. Mod Pathol 2016;29(7):735–42.

29. Vignot S, Frampton GM, Soria JC, et al. Next-generation sequencing reveals high concordance of recurrent somatic alterations between primary tumor and metastases from patients with non-small-cell lung cancer. J Clin Oncol 2013;31(17):2167–72.

30. Tang X, Shigematsu H, Bekele BN, et al. EGFR tyrosine kinase domain mutations are detected in histologically normal respiratory epithelium in lung cancer patients. Cancer Res 2005;65(17):7568–72.

31. Gazdar A, Robinson L, Oliver D, et al. Hereditary lung cancer syndrome targets never smokers with germline EGFR gene T790M mutations. J Thorac Oncol 2014;9(4):456–63.

32. Bozzetti C, Tiseo M, Lagrasta C, et al. Comparison between epidermal growth factor receptor (EGFR) gene expression in primary non-small cell lung cancer (NSCLC) and in fine-needle aspirates from distant metastatic sites. J Thorac Oncol 2008;3(1): 18–22.

33. Schmid K, Oehl N, Wrba F, et al. EGFR/KRAS/BRAF mutations in primary lung adenocarcinomas and corresponding locoregional lymph node metastases. Clin Cancer Res 2009;15(14):4554–60.

34. Lindeman NI, Cagle PT, Beasley MB, et al. Molecular testing guideline for selection of lung cancer patients for EGFR and ALK tyrosine kinase inhibitors: guideline from the College of American Pathologists,

International Association for the Study of Lung Cancer, and Association for Molecular Pathology. J Thorac Oncol 2013;8(7):823–59.

35. Thunnissen E, Noguchi M, Aisner S, et al. Reproducibility of histopathological diagnosis in poorly differentiated NSCLC: an international multiobserver study. J Thorac Oncol 2014;9(9):1354–62.

36. Travis WD, Giroux DJ, Chansky K, et al. The IASLC Lung Cancer Staging Project: proposals for the inclusion of broncho-pulmonary carcinoid tumors in the forthcoming (seventh) edition of the TNM Classification for Lung Cancer. J Thorac Oncol 2008;3(11): 1213–23.

37. Kadota K, Villena-Vargas J, Yoshizawa A, et al. Prognostic significance of adenocarcinoma in situ, minimally invasive adenocarcinoma, and nonmucinous lepidic predominant invasive adenocarcinoma of the lung in patients with stage I disease. Am J Surg Pathol 2014;38(4):448–60.

38. Detterbeck FC, Marom EM, Arenberg DA, et al. The IASLC Lung Cancer Staging Project: background data and proposals for the application of TNM staging rules to lung cancer presenting as multiple nodules with ground glass or lepidic features or a pneumonic type of involvement in the forthcoming eighth edition of the TNM classification. J Thorac Oncol 2016;11(5):666–80.

39. Park E, Ahn S, Kim H, et al. Targeted sequencing analysis of pulmonary adenocarcinoma with multiple synchronous ground-glass/lepidic nodules. J Thorac Oncol 2018;13(11):1776–83.

40. Shim HS, Kenudson M, Zheng Z, et al. Unique genetic and survival characteristics of invasive mucinous adenocarcinoma of the lung. J Thorac Oncol 2015;10(8):1156–62.

41. Kozower BD, Larner JM, Detterbeck FC, et al. Special treatment issues in non-small cell lung cancer: diagnosis and management of lung cancer, 3rd ed: American College of Chest Physicians evidence-based clinical practice guidelines. Chest 2013;143(5 Suppl):e369S–399S.

42. Maeda R, Yoshida J, Ishii G, et al. Long-term outcome and late recurrence in patients with completely resected stage IA non-small cell lung cancer. J Thorac Oncol 2010;5(8):1246–50.

43. Rusch VW, Asamura H, Watanabe H, et al. The IASLC lung cancer staging project: a proposal for a new international lymph node map in the forthcoming seventh edition of the TNM classification for lung cancer. J Thorac Oncol 2009;4(5): 568–77.

44. Luchini C, Veronese N, Nottegar A, et al. Extranodal extension of nodal metastases is a poor prognostic moderator in non-small cell lung cancer: a meta-analysis. Virchows Arch 2018;472(6):939–47.

45. Yasufuku K, Pierre A, Darling G, et al. A prospective controlled trial of endobronchial ultrasound-guided transbronchial needle aspiration compared with mediastinoscopy for mediastinal lymph node staging of lung cancer. J Thorac Cardiovasc Surg 2011;142(6): 1393–400.e1.

46. Navani N, Nankivell M, Lawrence DR, et al. Lung cancer diagnosis and staging with endobronchial ultrasound-guided transbronchial needle aspiration compared with conventional approaches: an open-label, pragmatic, randomised controlled trial. Lancet Respir Med 2015;3(4):282–9.

47. Network NCC. Non-small cell lung cancer (Version 7.2019). Available at: https://www.nccn.org/professionals/physician_gls/pdf/nscl.pdf.

48. NSCLC Meta-analysis Collaborative Group. Preoperative chemotherapy for non-small-cell lung cancer: a systematic review and meta-analysis of individual participant data. Lancet 2014;383(9928): 1561–71.

49. Weissferdt A, Sepesi B, Pataer A, et al. Pathologic assessment following neoadjuvant immunotherapy or chemotherapy demonstrates similar patterns in non-small cell lung cancer (NSCLC). Ann Oncol 2018;29(suppl_8):viii670–82.

50. Hellmann MD, Chaft JE, William WN Jr, et al. Pathological response after neoadjuvant chemotherapy in resectable non-small-cell lung cancers: proposal for the use of major pathological response as a surrogate endpoint. Lancet Oncol 2014;15(1):e42–50.

51. Pataer A, Kalhor N, Correa AM, et al. Histopathologic response criteria predict survival of patients with resected lung cancer after neoadjuvant chemotherapy. J Thorac Oncol 2012;7(5):825–32.

52. Suzuki K, Yokose T, Yoshida J, et al. Prognostic significance of the size of central fibrosis in peripheral adenocarcinoma of the lung. Ann Thorac Surg 2000;69(3):893–7.

53. Takahashi Y, Ishii G, Taira T, et al. Fibrous stroma is associated with poorer prognosis in lung squamous cell carcinoma patients. J Thorac Oncol 2011;6(9): 1460–7.

54. Junker K, Langner K, Klinke F, et al. Grading of tumor regression in non-small cell lung cancer: morphology and prognosis. Chest 2001;120(5): 1584–91.

55. Junker K, Thomas M, Schulmann K, et al. Tumour regression in non-small-cell lung cancer following neoadjuvant therapy. Histological assessment. J Cancer Res Clin Oncol 1997;123(9):469–77.

56. Qu Y, Emoto K, Eguchi T, et al. Pathologic assessment after neoadjuvant chemotherapy for NSCLC: importance and implications of distinguishing adenocarcinoma from squamous cell carcinoma. J Thorac Oncol 2019;14(3):482–93.

Diagnosis of Mesothelioma

Daffolyn Rachael Fels Elliott, MD, PhD*, Kirk D. Jones, MD

KEYWORDS

• Mesothelioma • Epithelioid • Sarcomatoid • Reactive mesothelial proliferation • Pleural effusion

---

Key points

- Radiographic pitfalls that mimic other diseases include bilateral pleural mesothelioma with lymphadenopathy, anterior mediastinal mesothelioma, localized pleural mesothelioma (solitary nodule), and diaphragmatic invasion with liver involvement.

- The three basic patterns of mesothelioma (epithelioid, biphasic, sarcomatoid) each show wide variation in morphology and invoke a broad differential diagnosis.

- A panel of immunohistochemical markers is recommended for the diagnosis of mesothelioma and should include two mesothelial markers and two markers specific for adenocarcinoma or other entity in the differential diagnosis.

- Advances in markers of malignancy include loss of BAP-1 and p16/CDKN2A deletion (with surrogate marker MTAP).

ABSTRACT

Mesothelioma is a rare neoplasm that arises from mesothelial cells lining body cavities including the pleura, pericardium, peritoneum, and tunica vaginalis. Most malignant mesotheliomas occur in the chest and are frequently associated with a history of asbestos exposure. The diagnosis of malignant mesothelioma is challenging and fraught with pitfalls, particularly in small biopsies. This article highlights what the pathologist needs to know regarding the clinical and radiographic presentation of mesothelioma, histologic features including subtypes and variants, and recent advances in immunohistochemical markers and molecular testing.

OVERVIEW

Mesothelioma is a rare neoplasm that arises from mesothelial cells lining body cavities including the pleura, pericardium, peritoneum, and tunica vaginalis.[1] Most malignant mesotheliomas (70%–90%) occur in the chest and are frequently associated with a history of asbestos exposure.[2,3] The diagnosis of malignant mesothelioma is challenging, particularly in small biopsies, with diagnostic difficulties, such as differentiating between atypical mesothelial hyperplasia (AMH) versus epithelioid mesothelioma and fibrous pleuritis versus sarcomatoid mesothelioma. This article outlines a framework for diagnosis of mesothelioma using the constellation of clinical presentation, radiographic features, microscopic findings, and recent advances in immunohistochemical markers and molecular testing.

INCIDENCE AND ASBESTOS EXPOSURE

The highest incidence rates of mesothelioma have been reported in Australia and Great Britain (approximately 30 cases per million people annually) with large variation between different countries.[4,5] The best established risk factor is asbestos exposure, which causes a spectrum of

---

Department of Pathology, University of California San Francisco, 505 Parnassus Avenue, Room M-545, San Francisco, CA 94143, USA
* Corresponding author.
E-mail address: daffolynrachael.felselliott@ucsf.edu

Surgical Pathology 13 (2020) 73–89
https://doi.org/10.1016/j.path.2019.10.001
1875-9181/20/© 2019 Elsevier Inc. All rights reserved.

thoracic diseases in addition to malignant mesothelioma, including pleural fibrosis and pleural plaques, benign asbestos pleural effusion, asbestosis (parenchymal fibrosis), and small cell and non–small cell lung carcinoma.[6–8] The patient may provide a history of occupational asbestos exposure (eg, construction, shipbuilding, or automotive industries) or reside in a region with known industrial contamination or environmental risk.[9,10] Environmental and/or domestic asbestos exposures are thought to contribute to an increasing proportion of mesothelioma in women.[11–14] The average time from asbestos exposure until development of mesothelioma is long, ranging from 20 to greater than 40 years, and depends on the severity and duration of exposure.[3,4,15,16]

CLINICAL PRESENTATION

The risk of developing mesothelioma increases with age, because of the long latency period following asbestos exposure. Most patients are greater than 50 years old at presentation (median, 63 years)[17] and mean age at death is 70 years.[18,19] There is a male preponderance in keeping with historical patterns of occupational exposure (male/female ratio 3–4:1).[13,18] Presenting symptoms include chest wall pain (unilateral or bilateral), pleurisy, cough, and progressive dyspnea secondary to pleural effusion. Unfortunately, by the time patients develop symptoms they often already have a high burden of disease. Sometimes asymptomatic patients are diagnosed at an earlier stage on chest imaging undertaken for other purposes. Occasionally patients present with distant metastases to liver, spleen, thyroid, or brain.[20,21] An unusual presentation of disease is constrictive pericarditis with symptoms of congestive heart failure, such as in localized pericardial mesothelioma.[22] Rarely pulmonary embolus may precede or coincide with the diagnosis of mesothelioma.[23]

IMAGING PRESENTATION

COMPUTED TOMOGRAPHY SCAN FINDINGS

Computed tomography (CT) with contrast enhancement is the primary modality for radiologic diagnosis and staging of mesothelioma.[24,25] CT scan features of mesothelioma include nodular or diffuse pleural thickening (60%), multifocal nodules studding pleural surfaces (45%–60%), unilateral (may be loculated) pleural effusion (30%–80%), and ipsilateral lung volume loss.[26] Mesothelioma can involve the pulmonary pleura (with possible spread along interlobar fissures), diaphragmatic or pericardial pleural surfaces, and the disease is usually unilateral.[26,27] Smooth thickening or enhancement of the pleura is seen in either neoplastic, reactive, or infectious conditions, whereas nodular, mass-like thickening is more specific for tumor. Rarely mesothelioma presents as a localized pleural or subpleural nodule, which is large in some cases (10–15 cm), and may mimic solitary fibrous tumor radiographically, particularly if pleural effusion is absent.[20,28–30] Mesothelioma can also pose a diagnostic challenge if it presents as a localized anterior mediastinal mass[31] or involving the diaphragmatic pleura with liver invasion.[32]

The presence of concurrent benign asbestos-related findings can provide additional radiographic support for a diagnosis of mesothelioma. On CT scan, pleural plaques are generally less than 1 cm thick, demonstrate regular margins, may contain calcifications, and are a specific sign for asbestos exposure.[27] Benign plaques are usually bilateral involving the pulmonary pleura in most cases and diaphragmatic pleura in about half of cases. Other radiographic features that are somewhat less specific for asbestos exposure include pleural fibrosis (diffuse thickening of the pleura) and round atelectasis of the lower lobes with adjacent pleural thickening.

MRI AND PET/COMPUTED TOMOGRAPHY IMAGING

MRI and PET are complementary to CT scan and can provide greater detail about tumor extension and distant spread.[26,33] High-resolution MRI with contrast enhancement helps delineate relationships between adjacent structures to assess tumor extension/invasion of the chest wall, diaphragm, or mediastinum and aid in surgical planning.[34] Furthermore, targeting areas of enhancement or diffusion restriction on MRI may be helpful to guide biopsies of pleural-based lesions.[34] PET/CT scan is helpful to evaluate for metastatic spread of disease to intrathoracic and extrathoracic lymph nodes and distant sites.[26] Mediastinal lymph nodes appear enlarged in 50% to 66% of patients[27,29] and when prominent raise the differential diagnosis of metastatic carcinoma with pleural involvement.[35] Hall and colleagues[36] observed that metabolic tumor volume and maximum standardized uptake value on PET/CT were significantly associated with overall survival; however, more data are needed to determine whether PET/CT could be of prognostic value in mesothelioma.[37] There is also some evidence to suggest that integrated PET/CT imaging may help differentiate between malignant mesothelioma versus benign asbestosis-related pleural disease[38] and malignant versus benign pleural effusions.[39]

Imaging Key Features

- Malignant mesothelioma most often presents with unilateral pleural disease
  - Diffuse or nodular pleural thickening
  - Multifocal studding of pleural surfaces
  - Pleural effusion in majority
- Benign asbestos-related disease often coexists and is bilateral
- Mesothelioma most commonly involves lung pleura, followed by diaphragm and pericardial pleura
- May see direct invasion into the abdomen at diagnosis
- Mediastinal lymph nodes are involved in at least 50% of cases
- Other sites of metastasis include liver, spleen, thyroid, and brain

Imaging Pitfalls!

! Mesothelioma can mimic metastatic carcinoma of the pleura, particularly if there are prominent subpleural nodules, bilateral disease, and/or mediastinal lymph node involvement

! Localized pleural mesothelioma can mimic solitary fibrous tumor or anterior mediastinal tumor

! Diaphragmatic invasion with liver involvement can mimic primary liver tumor

DIFFERENTIAL DIAGNOSIS BASED ON MICROSCOPIC FINDINGS

According to the 2015 World Health Organization Classification of Tumors of the Pleura, malignant mesothelioma is broadly classified as epithelioid, sarcomatoid, or biphasic types.[40] These basic patterns encompass a wide variety of histologic appearances, and invoke a broad differential diagnosis for the pathologist, as discussed next.

EPITHELIOID MESOTHELIOMA

Epithelioid mesothelioma is the most common subtype (60%–70%) of malignant mesothelioma

and is associated with better prognosis than sarcomatoid mesothelioma.[17,41] Histologically, the tumor cells have ample cytoplasm with well-defined cell borders imparting an epithelioid appearance. The nuclei are often bland and can resemble reactive mesothelial cells with moderate cytologic atypia. Growth patterns include tubulo-papillary, microglandular (adenomatoid), acinar, and solid (**Fig. 1A–D**). Psammoma bodies are seen in areas of tubulopapillary growth. Morphologic variants of epithelioid mesothelioma include clear cell, small cell, deciduoid, adenoid cystic, lymphangiomatoid, and signet ring cell morphology, and these raise additional diagnostic considerations as summarized in **Table 1**. The pleomorphic subtype of epithelioid mesothelioma is characterized by anaplasia and tumor giant cells and is associated with a worse prognosis, similar to sarcomatoid mesothelioma.[42,43] The differential diagnosis for epithelioid mesothelioma includes pulmonary or metastatic adenocarcinoma, particularly when pseudoglandular or pseudoacinar structures are present. Histologic features that may favor adenocarcinoma include eccentric or overlapping nuclei, vesicular chromatin, increased nuclear pleomorphism, and cytoplasmic mucin vacuoles. Correlation with clinical presentation, radiologic features, and immunohistochemistry (**Fig. 1E, F**) is important for this distinction.

ATYPICAL MESOTHELIAL HYPERPLASIA

AMH or florid reactive mesothelial proliferation is in the differential diagnosis for epithelioid and sarcomatoid mesothelioma.[44] Reactive mesothelial cells can show striking cytologic atypia with nuclear enlargement and prominent nucleoli. Mitotic activity may be increased, but no atypical mitoses should be present. AMH can show simple papillary projections, but the overall growth pattern lacks the complexity of epithelioid mesothelioma. Reactive mesothelial cells may become entrapped in the superficial layers of the pleura and mimic invasion; however, AMH should not penetrate into the deep pleura or infiltrate fat (**Fig. 1G, H**).

WELL-DIFFERENTIATED PAPILLARY MESOTHELIOMA

Well-differentiated papillary mesothelioma (WDPM) warrants discussion, although it occurs predominantly in the peritoneum of middle-aged women and only rarely in the pleura.[45,46] The prognosis is generally favorable with rare reports of an aggressive clinical course.[45] WDPM may present incidentally during surgery as a localized nodule or papillary

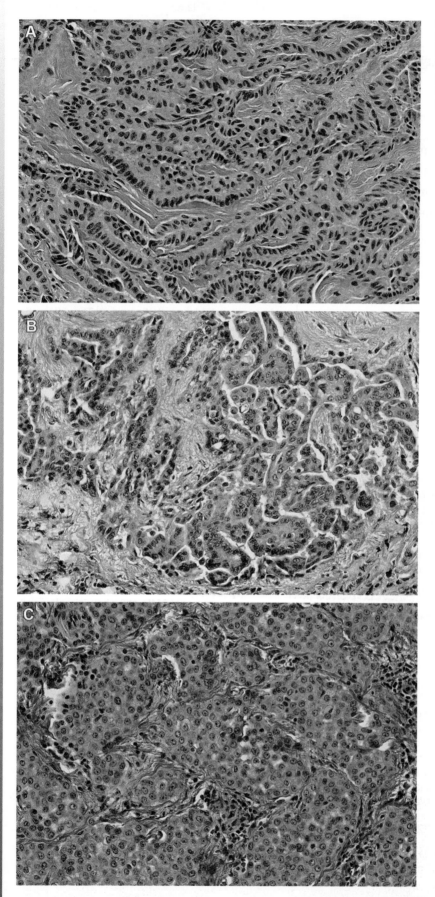

Fig. 1. Epithelioid mesothelioma. (*A*, *B*) Epithelioid mesothelioma with tubulopapillary growth pattern. (*C*) Epithelioid mesothelioma with solid growth pattern.

Fig. 1. (*continued*). (*D*) Epithelioid mesothelioma with myxoid stroma and cytoplasmic vacuoles, mimicking epithelioid hemangioendothelioma. (*E*) Epithelioid mesothelioma infiltrating skeletal muscle, and (*F*) calretinin immunostain showing positive nuclear staining.

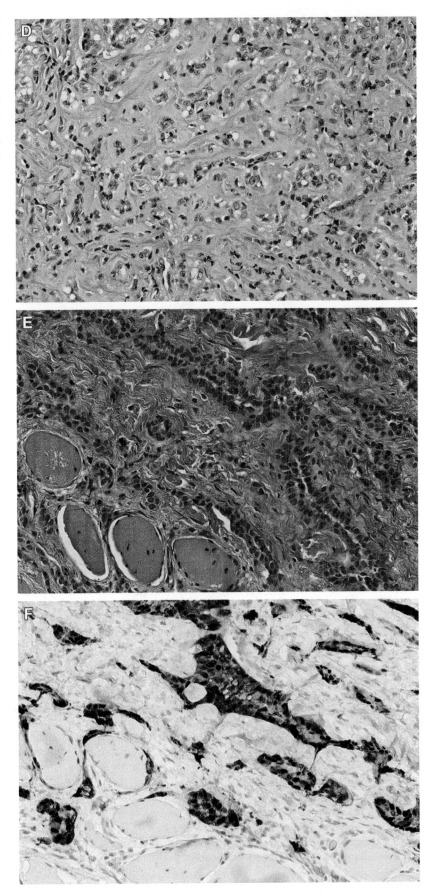

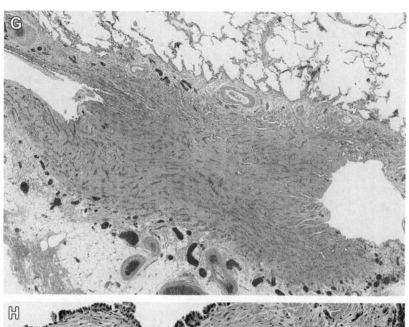

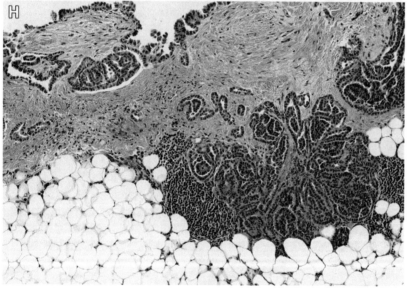

Fig. 1. (*continued*). (*G*) Epithelioid mesothelioma with adhesion between parietal and visceral pleura. (*H*) Infiltration of subpleural fat in early epithelioid mesothelioma.

lesion, and the surgeon may request a frozen section to rule out malignancy. Microscopically, WDPM consists of papillary projections with myxoid fibrovascular cores lined by a single layer of flattened or cuboidal mesothelial cells. There should be minimal nuclear atypia and low mitotic activity. The lesion must be limited to the peritoneal or pleural surface and should not show invasion deeper into soft tissue, which would favor a diagnosis of epithelioid mesothelioma. Recently, a subset of peritoneal WDPM cases were shown to harbor mutually exclusive mutations in TRAF7 and CDC42,[47] supporting a neoplastic process, but these findings have not been validated in the pleura.

SARCOMATOID MESOTHELIOMA

Sarcomatoid mesothelioma is characterized by a proliferation of spindle cells infiltrating dense fibrous stroma with a disorganized growth pattern (**Fig. 2**A, B). The spindle cells are often bland, reminiscent of fibroblasts (**Fig. 2**C), but may show marked nuclear atypia and hyperchromasia (**Fig. 2**D, E). Areas of osseous and cartilaginous differentiation have been reported.[48] Variants of sarcomatoid mesothelioma include desmoplastic and lymphohistiocytic subtypes. Desmoplastic mesothelioma is comprised of dense, hyalinized, collagenous stroma with scant spindle cells in a storiform growth pattern. In the lymphohistiocytic

Table 1
Histologic patterns of mesothelioma and differential diagnosis

Mesothelioma Subtype and Morphologic Variants	Differential Diagnosis	Markers
Epithelioid mesothelioma (tubulopapillary, acinar, adenomatoid, solid)	Adenocarcinoma, epithelioid hemangioendothelioma, benign mesothelial proliferation	MOC-31, Ber-EP4, TTF-1, CD31, BAP-1, CAMTA1
Deciduoid	Squamous cell carcinoma	p40, p63
Clear cell	Metastatic clear cell renal cell carcinoma	PAX8
Small cell	Small cell carcinoma	Synaptophysin, chromogranin A
Lymphangiomatoid	Lymphangioma	Keratin
Pleomorphic	Anaplastic large cell lymphoma	CD30
Biphasic mesothelioma	Synovial sarcoma, pulmonary blastoma, carcinosarcoma	CD99, beta-catenin, X;18 FISH
Sarcomatoid mesothelioma	Fibrous pleuritis, sarcomatoid carcinoma, sarcoma, melanoma	S100, SOX10, keratin (CAM5.2)
Desmoplastic	Fibrous pleuritis	P16/CDKN2A deletion
Lymphohistiocytic	Lymphoma, thymoma	CD20, CD30

variant, mesothelial cells show histiocyte-like morphology within a dense lymphoid stroma.[49] Sarcomatoid mesothelioma is less likely to shed tumor cells into the pleural cavity and thus fluid cytology is often nondiagnostic. The differential diagnosis of sarcomatoid mesothelioma includes fibrous pleuritis, sarcomatoid carcinoma, primary and metastatic sarcomas, and metastatic melanoma. Fibroblasts can stain positively with cytokeratins in fibrous pleuritis, which is a potential pitfall. Features that support mesothelioma include invasion into deep soft tissue, expansile nodules, disorganized or storiform growth patterns, zonation, necrosis, severe nuclear atypia, and atypical mitoses (**Fig. 2F–H**).

BIPHASIC AND "TRANSITIONAL" MESOTHELIOMA SUBTYPES

The 2015 World Health Organization classification defines biphasic mesothelioma as containing greater than 10% of both epithelioid and sarcomatoid components (**Fig. 3**), and suggests that survival may correlate with the amount of sarcomatoid component present within the tumor.[40] This diagnosis is of clinical importance, because selecting patients for surgical intervention is dependent on the absence of a sarcomatoid component and tumor volume and resectability. However, in some cases distinguishing a true sarcomatoid component from florid stromal reaction is challenging; and in other cases the features are

transitional between epithelioid and sarcomatoid mesothelioma. In the former scenario, diagnostic adjuncts, such as BAP-1 immunohistochemistry and fluorescence in situ hybridization (FISH) for CDKN2A (p16) deletion, are helpful and are discussed later in this article (see the section on markers of malignancy). In the latter scenario, Galateau Salle and colleagues[50] advocate that ambiguous cases with transitional features between epithelioid and sarcomatoid mesothelioma should be considered a distinct "transitional" subtype. A panel of 14 pathologists evaluated 42 biopsies of biphasic mesothelioma with moderate agreement (weighted Kappa 0.45), and transitional features (focal or diffuse) were identified in 40% of all diagnoses. The transitional pattern was associated with poorer prognosis (median survival, 6 months) in comparison with biphasic mesothelioma without transitional features (median survival, 12 months; P<.0001). Further validation and reproducibility are needed, but these data are compelling evidence to better define and stratify risk groups within the biphasic mesothelioma subtype.

PROPOSED PATHOLOGIC GRADING SYSTEMS IN MESOTHELIOMA

Pathologic grading schema have been proposed to risk stratify patients with malignant pleural mesothelioma for prognostication, determining therapy options and enrollment into clinical trials, independent of the stage of disease. Although

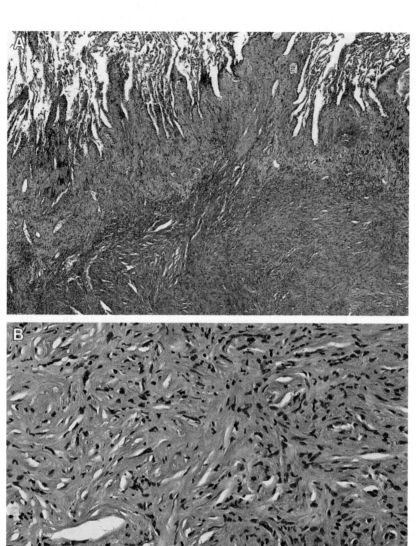

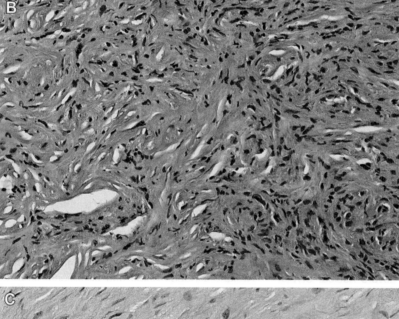

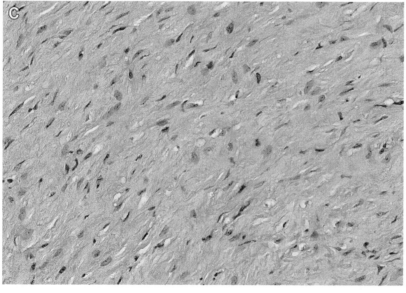

Fig. 2. Sarcomatoid mesothelioma. (*A*) Marked pleural thickening by sarcomatoid mesothelioma with adherent lung. (*B*) Atypical spindle cells infiltrating dense fibrous stroma with a disorganized growth pattern is characteristic of sarcomatoid mesothelioma. (*C*) Bland spindle cells with low cellularity are mistaken for fibroblasts.

Fig. 2. (continued). (*D, E*) Sarcomatoid mesothelioma with high cellularity and nuclear atypia. (*F*) Nodular growth pattern with so-called foci of independent growth, pushing into deep soft tissue.

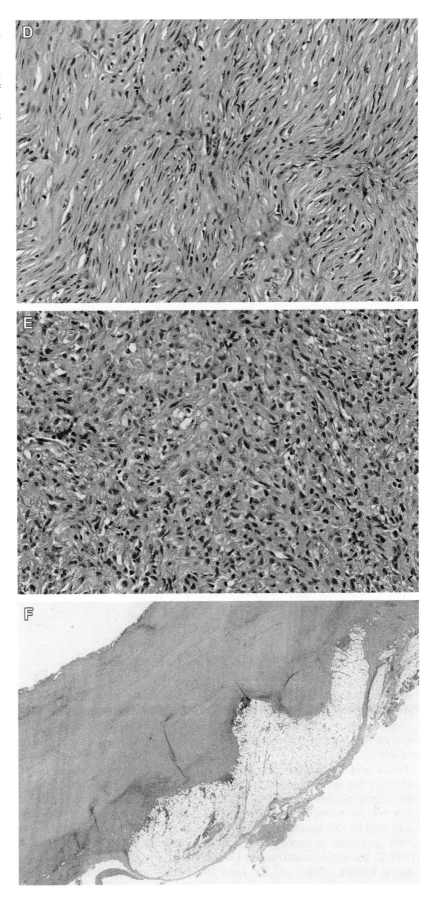

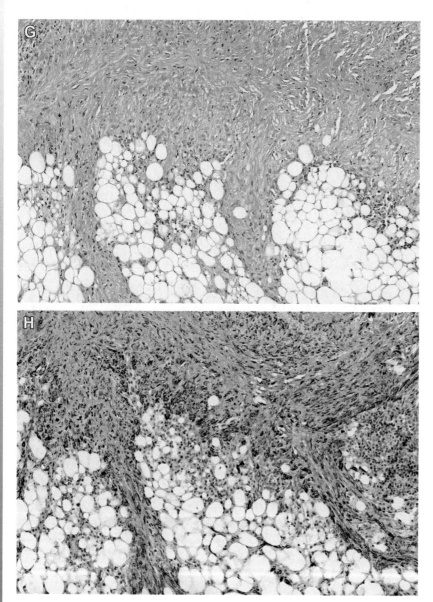

Fig. 2. (continued). (*G*) Sarcomatoid mesothelioma with bland cytology, infiltrating into deep soft tissue, and (*H*) pancytokeratin immunostain.

currently there is no consensus guideline advocating the use of a specific grading system in the evaluation of mesothelioma, in this section we highlight two grading schema with potential clinical utility.

Pelosi and colleagues[51] proposed a points-based grading system to predict survival in malignant pleural mesothelioma based on four factors: (1) histologic subtype, (2) necrosis, (3) mitotic count, and (4) Ki67 proliferation index. The model, which generates a score from 0 to 8 points (**Table 2**), showed a hazard ratio of 1.46 (95% confidence interval, 1.36–1.56) for each one-point increase in score in the training set (n = 328) and 1.28 (95% confidence interval, 1.22–1.34) in the validation cohort (n = 612). The model correlated with decreasing survival from a score of 0 points (median overall survival, 26.3 and 26.9 months, training and validation cohorts) to one to three points (median, 12.8 and 14.4 months) to four to eight points (median, 3.7 and 7.7 months).

Authors at Memorial Sloan-Kettering Cancer Center proposed a nuclear grading system specifically for epithelioid mesothelioma.[52] The study examined seven nuclear features (atypia, nuclear/ cytoplasmic ratio, chromatin pattern, intranuclear

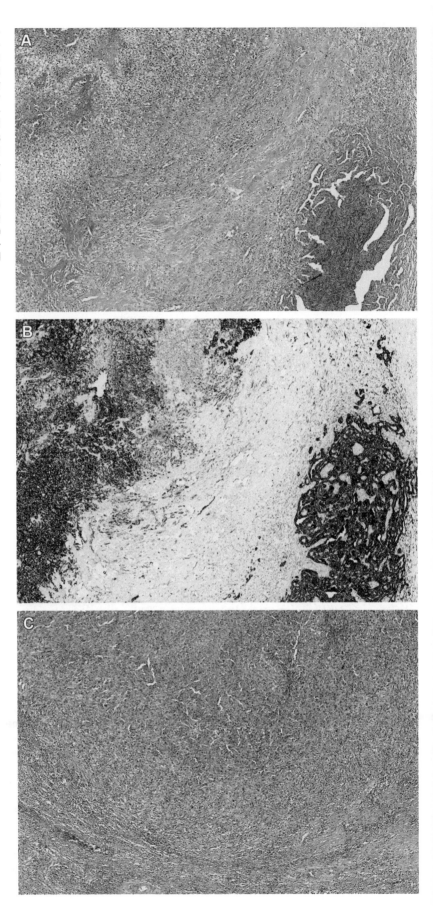

Fig. 3. Biphasic mesothelioma. (*A*) Biphasic mesothelioma with an epithelioid component with tubulopapillary morphology in the lower right, and a solid component with epithelioid and sarcomatoid features in the upper left, and (*B*) pancytokeratin immunostain. (*C*) Sarcomatoid area of the same case, and (*D*) pancytokeratin immunostain. (*E*) Biphasic mesothelioma with intermixed epithelioid and sarcomatoid morphology.

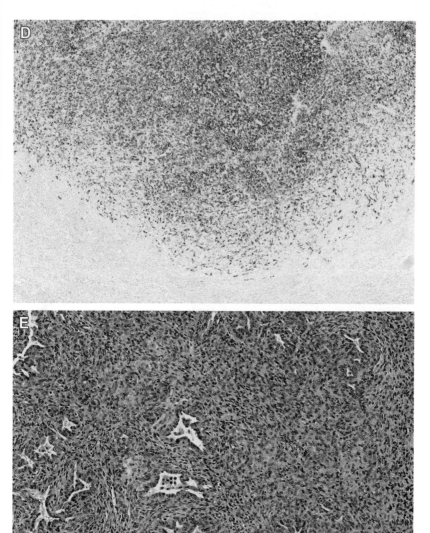

Fig. 3. (continued).

inclusions, prominence of nucleoli, mitotic count, and atypical mitoses) in 232 tumors. By multivariate analysis, nuclear atypia ($P = .012$) and mitotic count ($P<.001$) emerged as independent prognostic factors and were combined into a three-tier score for nuclear grade (Table 3): grade 1 (median overall survival, 28 months), grade 2 (median, 14 months), and grade 3 (median, 5 months). A multi-institutional validation study subsequently confirmed the Memorial Sloan-Kettering Cancer Center nuclear grading system correlated with overall survival ($P<.0001$; n = 776).[53] Adding tumor necrosis to the nuclear grade allowed further

stratification into four prognostic groups: (1) nuclear grade 1 without necrosis (median survival, 29 months), (2) nuclear grade 1 with necrosis and grade 2 without necrosis (16 months), (3) nuclear grade 2 with necrosis (10 months), and (4) nuclear grade 3 with or without necrosis (8 months).

Overall, both grading systems may be effective tools to risk stratify mesothelioma by patient survival times; however, it remains to be determined whether such a system would be of clinical benefit to help inform management decisions (eg, determining eligibility for surgical intervention, systemic therapy, or palliation).

Table 2
Pelosi and colleagues pathologic grading system in malignant pleural mesothelioma

Criteria		Points
Histologic subtype	Epithelioid/biphasic	0
	Sarcomatoid	2
Necrosis	Absent	0
	Present	1
Mitotic count (per square millimeter)	1–2	0
	3–5	1
	6–9	2
	≥10	4
Ki67	<30%	0
	≥30%	1
	Group 1	0
	Group 2	1–3
	Group 3	4–8

Data from Pelosi G, Papotti M, Righi L, Rossi G, Ferrero S, Bosari S, et al. Pathologic grading of malignant pleural mesothelioma: An evidence-based proposal. J Thorac Oncol 2018;13(11):1750-61.

MARKERS OF MESOTHELIAL DIFFERENTIATION

Several immunohistochemical markers for mesothelial cells have been proposed in the literature, including calretinin, WT-1, D2-40 (podoplanin), CK 5/6, HBME-1, thrombomodulin, and mesothelin, but only the first four have sufficient specificity (80% and higher) for routine use in diagnosing mesothelioma.[54,55] The sensitivity and specificity of these markers vary depending on the differential diagnosis in question. For example, calretinin has

high sensitivity to differentiate epithelioid mesothelioma from pulmonary adenocarcinoma (97.5%),[56] but expression can also be seen in other intrathoracic tumors including small cell carcinoma, large cell neuroendocrine carcinoma, pulmonary large cell carcinoma, synovial sarcoma, thymoma/thymic carcinoma; and metastatic tumors, such as ovarian and breast carcinomas, epithelioid sarcoma, and melanoma.[57] WT-1 and mesothelin are expressed in ovarian carcinoma and D2-40 is expressed in most squamous cell carcinomas and lymphatic cells.[57] The addition of thrombomodulin may be helpful in diagnosing the small cell variant of epithelioid mesothelioma, but the marker also shows expression in squamous cell carcinoma, adenocarcinoma, small cell carcinoma, large cell neuroendocrine carcinoma, and sarcomatoid carcinoma, resulting in low specificity.[57,58] Recently, HEG1 (heart development protein with EGF-like domains 1) has been proposed as a new mesothelioma marker with high sensitivity (98.5%) and specificity (82.5%) to differentiate between nonsarcomatoid mesothelioma and lung carcinoma.[59] HEG1 also performed well in biphasic mesothelioma with higher sensitivity than calretinin.

DIFFERENTIAL DIAGNOSIS BASED ON STAINING CHARACTERISTICS

A panel of immunohistochemical markers is recommended for the diagnosis of mesothelioma and should include two mesothelial markers and two markers specific for adenocarcinoma or other entity in the differential diagnosis.[55,60] For example, to differentiate between pulmonary adenocarcinoma and epithelioid mesothelioma, a panel could include calretinin and CK5/6 as mesothelioma markers and MOC-31 and Ber-EP4 as adenocarcinoma markers. Other options for pulmonary adenocarcinoma markers include TTF-1, monoclonal CEA, B72.3, BG8 (Lewis), and claudin 4.[61,62] Although CK5/6 is useful to differentiate between mesothelioma and pulmonary adenocarcinoma, it is strongly expressed in squamous cell carcinoma, which in turn is distinguished by nuclear expression of p63 and p40. In cases where metastatic adenocarcinoma is in the differential diagnosis, using CK7/CK20 is helpful, provided the pathologist is aware that mesothelial cells show positivity for CK7. Incorporating a cytokeratin marker is essential for sarcomatoid mesothelioma (keratin positive) where the differential diagnosis includes sarcoma (keratin negative). Kushitani and colleagues[63] found that CAM5.2 was the most sensitive marker to differentiate

Table 3
Kadota and colleagues nuclear grading system in epithelioid mesothelioma

Criteria		Points
Nuclear atypia	Mild	1
	Moderate	2
	Severe	3
Mitotic count (per 10 high-power field)	Low (0–1)	1
	Intermediate (2–4)	2
	High (≥5)	3
	Nuclear grade 1	2–3
	Nuclear grade 2	4–5
	Nuclear grade 3	6

Data from Kadota K, Suzuki K, Colovos C, Sima CS, Rusch VW, Travis WD, Adusumilli PS. A nuclear grading system is a strong predictor of survival in epithelioid diffuse malignant pleural mesothelioma. Mod Pathol 2012, Feb;25(2):260-71.

sarcomatoid mesothelioma from a sarcoma. A screening panel for sarcomatoid mesothelioma could include CAM5.2, cytokeratin AE1/AE3, and WT-1, with additional markers as needed for classification of sarcoma (eg, desmin, smooth muscle actin, S100, CD34, ALK). Panels of diagnostic markers may vary depending on availability in local laboratories but each marker should have a minimum of 80% specificity to achieve high diagnostic accuracy, which is of particular importance in evaluation of small biopsies and pleural fluids.[60]

MARKERS OF MALIGNANCY

Loss of BRCA1-associated protein 1 (BAP-1) has been described in a subset of epithelioid (~80%) and biphasic (~50%) mesotheliomas[64] and rarely sarcomatoid mesothelioma,[65] and is particularly helpful distinguishing between malignant mesothelioma and reactive mesothelial proliferation in small biopsies.[66] The sensitivity for BAP-1 loss in epithelioid mesothelioma ranges from 55% to 85% and specificity is 98% to 100%.[62] Therefore, when BAP-1 is lost the pathologist can diagnose mesothelioma with confidence, but retained BAP-1 does not exclude the diagnosis.

In cases with retained BAP-1 or sarcomatoid mesothelioma, homozygous deletion of p16/CDKN2A may be detected using FISH and is 70% to 90% sensitive and 100% specific for a diagnosis of mesothelioma.[62] Deletion of p16/CDKN2A has been reported in 90% to 100% of sarcomatoid mesotheliomas and up to 70% of epithelioid and biphasic mesotheliomas.[62,65,67] A few studies have suggested that p16/CDKN2A deletion may be associated with poor survival, but further data are required to determine the clinical significance with respect to prognosis and treatment decisions.[68–71]

Methylthioadenosine phosphorylase (MTAP) immunohistochemistry has been proposed as a reliable surrogate marker for p16/CDKN2A FISH.[72,73] The MTAP gene, which encodes an enzyme involved in purine metabolism, is located at the 9p21 locus near to CDKN2A such that both genes are frequently deleted in tandem. Chapel and colleagues[72] showed that MTAP loss by immunohistochemistry was 96% specific and 78% sensitive for CDKN2A homozygous deletion in a multi-institution cohort of 99 malignant mesotheliomas and 20 benign mesothelial lesions. Another study demonstrated loss of MTAP immunostaining in 13/20 (65%) epithelioid mesotheliomas, whereas no cases (0/17) of reactive mesothelial proliferation showed MTAP loss.[74] Using BAP-1 in combination with MTAP enabled

the authors to distinguish between benign and malignant mesothelioma in 18/20 (90%) cases. Similarly, Kinoshita and colleagues[75] showed that a combination of MTAP and BAP-1 distinguished sarcomatoid (n = 18) and biphasic (n = 12) mesotheliomas from fibrous pleuritis (n = 17) with 90% sensitivity and 100% specificity.

GENOMIC LANDSCAPE OF MALIGNANT MESOTHELIOMA

Comprehensive genomic analysis (exome sequencing, RNA sequencing, methylation, copy-number array) of 74 cases of malignant pleural mesothelioma was performed as part of The Cancer Genome Atlas.[76] This study revealed a low mutational burden (<2 nonsynonymous mutations per megabase) and confirmed known mutations and frequent copy-number loss in tumor suppressor genes BAP1, CDKN2A, and NF2, and identifying recurrent mutations in TP53, LATS2, and SETD2. The mutational signature of smoking was not observed, and no mutational signature specific to asbestos exposure was elucidated. These data support that the pathogenesis of malignant mesothelioma is driven primarily by inactivation of tumor suppressor genes. Integrating data from The Cancer Genome Atlas and the International Cancer Genome Consortium revealed a novel molecular subtype of mesothelioma characterized by genome-wide loss of heterozygosity and near-haploid karyotype (5/154 [3.2%] cases). All five cases showed loss of function mutations in SETDB1, which encodes a gene silencing histone methyltransferase, and four cases had TP53 mutations. Clinically this molecular subtype was associated with younger age and female predominance (female/male = 4:1).

IMMUNOHISTOCHEMICAL AND MOLECULAR MARKERS KEY POINTS

- Use two mesothelial markers: calretinin, WT-1, D2-40, CK 5/6
- Use two epithelial markers: MOC-31, Ber-EP4, monoclonal CEA, B72.3, BG8, claudin 4
- HEG1 is a recently proposed mesothelioma marker that may be helpful in diagnosing epithelioid and biphasic mesothelioma (vs adenocarcinoma)
- Add markers specific for the differential diagnosis as necessary (eg, TTF-1 and Napsin A for pulmonary adenocarcinoma)
- Markers of malignancy in mesothelioma:

- ○ Loss of BAP-1 (useful in epithelioid or biphasic mesothelioma, detect using immunohistochemistry)
- ○ p16/CDKN2A deletion (useful in sarcomatoid mesotheliomas or if BAP-1 is retained, detect using FISH)
- ○ MTAP is a reliable surrogate marker for p16/CDKN2A deletion (useful in combination with BAP-1 to increase sensitivity)

DISCLOSURE

The authors have no disclosures.

REFERENCES

1. Hiriart E, Deepe R, Wessels A. Mesothelium and malignant mesothelioma. J Dev Biol 2019;7(2), [pii:E7].
2. Price B, Ware A. Time trend of mesothelioma incidence in the United States and projection of future cases: an update based on SEER data for 1973 through 2005. Crit Rev Toxicol 2009;39(7):576–88.
3. Neumann V, Löseke S, Nowak D, et al. Malignant pleural mesothelioma: incidence, etiology, diagnosis, treatment, and occupational health. Dtsch Arztebl Int 2013;110(18):319–26.
4. Bianchi C, Bianchi T. Malignant mesothelioma: global incidence and relationship with asbestos. Ind Health 2007;45(3):379–87.
5. Robinson BM. Malignant pleural mesothelioma: an epidemiological perspective. Ann Cardiothorac Surg 2012;1(4):491–6.
6. Wagner JC, Sleggs CA, Marchand P. Diffuse pleural mesothelioma and asbestos exposure in the North Western Cape province. Br J Ind Med 1960;17:260–71.
7. Strauchen JA. Rarity of malignant mesothelioma prior to the widespread commercial introduction of asbestos: the Mount Sinai autopsy experience 1883-1910. Am J Ind Med 2011;54(6):467–9.
8. Solbes E, Harper RW. Biological responses to asbestos inhalation and pathogenesis of asbestos-related benign and malignant disease. J Investig Med 2018;66(4):721–7.
9. Ruffie P, Feld R, Minkin S, et al. Diffuse malignant mesothelioma of the pleura in Ontario and Quebec: a retrospective study of 332 patients. J Clin Oncol 1989;7(8):1157–68.
10. Bianchi C, Brollo A, Ramani L, et al. Asbestos exposure in malignant mesothelioma of the pleura: a survey of 557 cases. Ind Health 2001;39(2):161–7.
11. Marsh GM, Riordan AS, Keeton KA, et al. Non-occupational exposure to asbestos and risk of pleural mesothelioma: review and meta-analysis. Occup Environ Med 2017;74(11):838–46.
12. Xu R, Barg FK, Emmett EA, et al. Association between mesothelioma and non-occupational asbestos exposure: systematic review and meta-analysis. Environ Health 2018;17(1):90.
13. Marinaccio A, Corfiati M, Binazzi A, et al. The epidemiology of malignant mesothelioma in women: gender differences and modalities of asbestos exposure. Occup Environ Med 2018;75(4):254–62.
14. Panou V, Vyberg M, Meristoudis C, et al. Non-occupational exposure to asbestos is the main cause of malignant mesothelioma in women in North Jutland, Denmark. Scand J Work Environ Health 2019;45(1):82–9.
15. Marinaccio A, Binazzi A, Cauzillo G, et al. Analysis of latency time and its determinants in asbestos related malignant mesothelioma cases of the Italian register. Eur J Cancer 2007;43(18):2722–8.
16. Frost G. The latency period of mesothelioma among a cohort of British asbestos workers (1978-2005). Br J Cancer 2013;109(7):1965–73.
17. Rusch VW, Giroux D, Kennedy C, et al. Initial analysis of the International Association for the Study of Lung Cancer mesothelioma database. J Thorac Oncol 2012;7(11):1631–9.
18. Delgermaa V, Takahashi K, Park EK, et al. Global mesothelioma deaths reported to the World Health Organization between 1994 and 2008. Bull World Health Organ 2011;89(10):716–24, 724A–C.
19. Craighead JE. Epidemiology of mesothelioma and historical background. Recent Results Cancer Res 2011;189:13–25.
20. Ertan G, Eren A, Ulus S. Rare presentation of a localised malignant pleural mesothelioma with cranial metastasis. BMJ Case Rep 2016;2016, [pii: bcr2016217348].
21. Finn RS, Brims FJH, Gandhi A, et al. Postmortem findings of malignant pleural mesothelioma: a two-center study of 318 patients. Chest 2012;142(5):1267–73.
22. Edel JP, Balink H. 18F-FDG PET/CT revealing constrictive pericarditis as the only manifestation of malignant mesothelioma. Clin Nucl Med 2019;44(1):55–6.
23. Koksal D, Safak O, Ozcan A, et al. Thromboembolic events in malignant pleural mesothelioma. Clin Appl Thromb Hemost 2016;22(4):390–4.
24. Odisio EG, Marom EM, Shroff GS, et al. Malignant pleural mesothelioma: diagnosis, staging, pitfalls and follow-up. Semin Ultrasound CT MR 2017;38(6):559–70.
25. Zhou H, Tamura T, Kusaka Y, et al. Development of a guideline on reading CT images of malignant pleural mesothelioma and selection of the reference CT films. Eur J Radiol 2012;81(12):4203–10.
26. Nickell LT, Lichtenberger JP, Khorashadi L, et al. Multimodality imaging for characterization, classification, and staging of malignant pleural mesothelioma. Radiographics 2014;34(6):1692–706.
27. Polverosi R, Vigo M, Citton O. Pleural and parenchymal lung diseases from asbestos exposure. CT

diagnosis. Radiol Med 2000;100(5):326–31, [in Italian].

28. Crotty TB, Myers JL, Katzenstein AL, et al. Localized malignant mesothelioma. A clinicopathologic and flow cytometric study. Am J Surg Pathol 1994; 18(4):357–63.

29. Yao W, Yang H, Huang G, et al. Massive localized malignant pleural mesothelioma (LMPM): manifestations on computed tomography in 6 cases. Int J Clin Exp Med 2015;8(10):18367–74.

30. Kim KC, Vo HP. Localized malignant pleural sarcomatoid mesothelioma misdiagnosed as benign localized fibrous tumor. J Thorac Dis 2016;8(6): E379–84.

31. Hino T, Kamitani T, Sagiyama K, et al. Localized malignant pleural mesothelioma mimicking an anterior mediastinal tumor. Eur J Radiol Open 2019;6:72–7.

32. Huang JW, Li ZH, Wang Z, et al. Primary malignant mesothelioma of the diaphragm with liver invasion: a case report and review of literature. Medicine (Baltimore) 2019;98(15):e15147.

33. Carter BW, Betancourt SL, Shroff GS, et al. MR imaging of pleural neoplasms. Top Magn Reson Imaging 2018;27(2):73–82.

34. Raptis CA, McWilliams SR, Ratkowski KL, et al. Mediastinal and pleural MR imaging: practical approach for daily practice. Radiographics 2018; 38(1):37–55.

35. Bakhshayesh Karam M, Karimi S, Mosadegh L, et al. Malignant mesothelioma versus metastatic carcinoma of the pleura: a CT challenge. Iran J Radiol 2016;13(1):e10949.

36. Hall DO, Hooper CE, Searle J, et al. 18F-Fluorodeoxyglucose PET/CT and dynamic contrast-enhanced MRI as imaging biomarkers in malignant pleural mesothelioma. Nucl Med Commun 2018;39(2):161–70.

37. Armato SG, Francis RJ, Katz SI, et al. Imaging in pleural mesothelioma: a review of the 14th International Conference of the International Mesothelioma Interest Group. Lung Cancer 2019;130:108–14.

38. Yildirim H, Metintas M, Entok E, et al. Clinical value of fluorodeoxyglucose-positron emission tomography/computed tomography in differentiation of malignant mesothelioma from asbestos-related benign pleural disease: an observational pilot study. J Thorac Oncol 2009;4(12):1480–4.

39. Sun Y, Yu H, Ma J, et al. The role of 18F-FDG PET/CT integrated imaging in distinguishing malignant from benign pleural effusion. PLoS One 2016;11(8): e0161764.

40. Travis WD, Brambilla E, Burke AP, et al. WHO classification of tumours of the lung, pleura, thymus and heart. Lyon (France): International Agency for Research on Cancer; 2015.

41. Meyerhoff RR, Yang CF, Speicher PJ, et al. Impact of mesothelioma histologic subtype on outcomes in the surveillance, epidemiology, and end results database. J Surg Res 2015;196(1):23–32.

42. Ordóñez NG. Pleomorphic mesothelioma: report of 10 cases. Mod Pathol 2012;25(7):1011–22.

43. Kadota K, Suzuki K, Sima CS, et al. Pleomorphic epithelioid diffuse malignant pleural mesothelioma: a clinicopathological review and conceptual proposal to reclassify as biphasic or sarcomatoid mesothelioma. J Thorac Oncol 2011;6(5):896–904.

44. Cagle PT, Churg A. Differential diagnosis of benign and malignant mesothelial proliferations on pleural biopsies. Arch Pathol Lab Med 2005;129(11): 1421–7.

45. Butnor KJ, Sporn TA, Hammar SP, et al. Well-differentiated papillary mesothelioma. Am J Surg Pathol 2001;25(10):1304–9.

46. Galateau-Sallé F, Vignaud JM, Burke L, et al. Well-differentiated papillary mesothelioma of the pleura: a series of 24 cases. Am J Surg Pathol 2004;28(4): 534–40.

47. Stevers M, Rabban JT, Garg K, et al. Well-differentiated papillary mesothelioma of the peritoneum is genetically defined by mutually exclusive mutations in TRAF7 and CDC42. Mod Pathol 2019;32(1): 88–99.

48. Klebe S, Mahar A, Henderson DW, et al. Malignant mesothelioma with heterologous elements: clinicopathological correlation of 27 cases and literature review. Mod Pathol 2008;21(9):1084–94.

49. Galateau-Sallé F, Attanoos R, Gibbs AR, et al. Lymphohistiocytoid variant of malignant mesothelioma of the pleura: a series of 22 cases. Am J Surg Pathol 2007;31(5):711–6.

50. Galateau Salle F, Le Stang N, Nicholson AG, et al. New insights on diagnostic reproducibility of biphasic mesotheliomas: a multi-institutional evaluation by the International Mesothelioma Panel from the MESOPATH reference center. J Thorac Oncol 2018;13(8):1189–203.

51. Pelosi G, Papotti M, Righi L, et al. Pathologic grading of malignant pleural mesothelioma: an evidence-based proposal. J Thorac Oncol 2018; 13(11):1750–61.

52. Kadota K, Suzuki K, Colovos C, et al. A nuclear grading system is a strong predictor of survival in epithelioid diffuse malignant pleural mesothelioma. Mod Pathol 2012;25(2):260–71.

53. Rosen LE, Karrison T, Ananthanarayanan V, et al. Nuclear grade and necrosis predict prognosis in malignant epithelioid pleural mesothelioma: a multi-institutional study. Mod Pathol 2018;31(4): 598–606.

54. Chapel DB, Churg A, Santoni-Rugiu E, et al. Molecular pathways and diagnosis in malignant mesothelioma: a review of the 14th International Conference of the International Mesothelioma Interest Group. Lung Cancer 2019;127:69–75 ;.

55. Galateau-Salle F, Churg A, Roggli V, et al, World Health Organization Committee for Tumors of the Pleura. The 2015 World Health Organization classification of tumors of the pleura: advances since the 2004 classification. J Thorac Oncol 2016;11(2): 142–54.

56. Kao SC, Griggs K, Lee K, et al. Validation of a minimal panel of antibodies for the diagnosis of malignant pleural mesothelioma. Pathology 2011;43(4): 313–7.

57. Comin CE, Novelli L, Cavazza A, et al. Expression of thrombomodulin, calretinin, cytokeratin 5/6, D2-40 and WT-1 in a series of primary carcinomas of the lung: an immunohistochemical study in comparison with epithelioid pleural mesothelioma. Tumori 2014; 100(5):559–67.

58. Miettinen M, Sarlomo-Rikala M. Expression of calretinin, thrombomodulin, keratin 5, and mesothelin in lung carcinomas of different types: an immunohistochemical analysis of 596 tumors in comparison with epithelioid mesotheliomas of the pleura. Am J Surg Pathol 2003;27(2):150–8.

59. Tsuji S, Washimi K, Kageyama T, et al. HEG1 is a novel mucin-like membrane protein that serves as a diagnostic and therapeutic target for malignant mesothelioma. Sci Rep 2017;7:45768.

60. Husain AN, Colby TV, Ordóñez NG, et al. Guidelines for pathologic diagnosis of malignant mesothelioma 2017 update of the consensus statement from the International Mesothelioma Interest Group. Arch Pathol Lab Med 2018;142(1):89–108.

61. Yaziji H, Battifora H, Barry TS, et al. Evaluation of 12 antibodies for distinguishing epithelioid mesothelioma from adenocarcinoma: identification of a three-antibody immunohistochemical panel with maximal sensitivity and specificity. Mod Pathol 2006;19(4):514–23.

62. Porcel JM. Biomarkers in the diagnosis of pleural diseases: a 2018 update. Ther Adv Respir Dis 2018;12, 1753466618808660.

63. Kushitani K, Takeshima Y, Amatya VJ, et al. Differential diagnosis of sarcomatoid mesothelioma from true sarcoma and sarcomatoid carcinoma using immunohistochemistry. Pathol Int 2008;58(2):75–83.

64. McGregor SM, Dunning R, Hyjek E, et al. BAP1 facilitates diagnostic objectivity, classification, and prognostication in malignant pleural mesothelioma. Hum Pathol 2015;46(11):1670–8.

65. Hwang HC, Pyott S, Rodriguez S, et al. BAP1 immunohistochemistry and p16 FISH in the diagnosis of sarcomatous and desmoplastic mesotheliomas. Am J Surg Pathol 2016;40(5):714–8.

66. Pillappa R, Maleszewski JJ, Sukov WR, et al. Loss of BAP1 expression in atypical mesothelial proliferations helps to predict malignant mesothelioma. Am J Surg Pathol 2018;42(2):256–63.

67. Sheffield BS, Hwang HC, Lee AF, et al. BAP1 immunohistochemistry and p16 FISH to separate benign from malignant mesothelial proliferations. Am J Surg Pathol 2015;39(7):977–82.

68. Dacic S, Kothmaier H, Land S, et al. Prognostic significance of p16/cdkn2a loss in pleural malignant mesotheliomas. Virchows Arch 2008;453(6): 627–35.

69. Kobayashi N, Toyooka S, Yanai H, et al. Frequent p16 inactivation by homozygous deletion or methylation is associated with a poor prognosis in Japanese patients with pleural mesothelioma. Lung Cancer 2008;62(1):120–5.

70. Singhi AD, Krasinskas AM, Choudry HA, et al. The prognostic significance of BAP1, NF2, and CDKN2A in malignant peritoneal mesothelioma. Mod Pathol 2016;29(1):14–24.

71. Chou A, Toon CW, Clarkson A, et al. The epithelioid bap1-negative and p16-positive phenotype predicts prolonged survival in pleural mesothelioma. Histopathology 2018;72(3):509–15.

72. Chapel DB, Schulte JJ, Berg K, et al. MTAP immunohistochemistry is an accurate and reproducible surrogate for CDKN2A fluorescence in situ hybridization in diagnosis of malignant pleural mesothelioma. Mod Pathol 2019, [Epub ahead of print].

73. Hida T, Hamasaki M, Matsumoto S, et al. Immunohistochemical detection of MTAP and BAP1 protein loss for mesothelioma diagnosis: comparison with 9p21 FISH and BAP1 immunohistochemistry. Lung Cancer 2017;104:98–105.

74. Berg KB, Dacic S, Miller C, et al. Utility of methylthioadenosine phosphorylase compared with BAP1 immunohistochemistry, and CDKN2A and NF2 fluorescence in situ hybridization in separating reactive mesothelial proliferations from epithelioid malignant mesotheliomas. Arch Pathol Lab Med 2018; 142(12):1549–53.

75. Kinoshita Y, Hamasaki M, Yoshimura M, et al. A combination of MTAP and BAP1 immunohistochemistry is effective for distinguishing sarcomatoid mesothelioma from fibrous pleuritis. Lung Cancer 2018;125:198–204.

76. Hmeljak J, Sanchez-Vega F, Hoadley KA, et al. Integrative molecular characterization of malignant pleural mesothelioma. Cancer Discov 2018;8(12): 1548–65.

Pathology of Idiopathic Interstitial Pneumonias

Yoshiaki Zaizen, MD[a,b], Junya Fukuoka, MD, PhD[a,c,d],*

KEYWORDS

- Classification • Guideline • Interstitial lung disease • Idiopathic pulmonary fibrosis

---

Key points

1. Summary of basic anatomy and guidance on how to understand pathology of interstitial pneumonias.

2. Sampling methods used by pathologists for interstitial pneumonia include a new technology, cryobiopsy.

3. Most of the idiopathic interstitial pneumonias are discussed with practical diagnostic points.

4. The concept of the usual interstitial pneumonia bucket is introduced, which helps to understand the progressive fibrosing interstitial lung disease phenotype.

SYNOPSIS

This review discusses diagnostic pathology in idiopathic interstitial pneumonias (IIPs). Accurate understanding of basic structure of lung lobules is critical because the location of abnormalities inside the lobule is an important effector of pathology diagnosis. Depending on the method of obtaining tissue, recognition of the location may be difficult or impossible. Cryobiopsy is a new technology and its coverage of lung lobules is limited. This article discusses fundamental anatomy and approach to interstitial pneumonia. In addition, most histologic types of IIPs are covered, but the focus is on diagnosis of usual interstitial pneumonia because of its clinical importance.

OVERVIEW

Interstitial pneumonias are a group of diseases that includes stromal inflammatory and/or fibrotic changes affecting both lungs. Although interstitial pneumonia is rare, its detection has continued to increase with the progress of radiological images and the use of screening by computed tomography (CT). Among nonpulmonary physicians, this group of diseases is often categorized simply as interstitial pneumonia without further specific diagnosis. However, among this group of interstitial pneumonias, idiopathic pulmonary fibrosis (IPF) is one of the most common and lethal diseases, along with lung cancer, with only 2 to 3 years of survival after the diagnosis.[1–5] With growing availability of treatment options for IPF,[6,7] early detection and accurate classification of interstitial pneumonias has become crucial for personalized medicine. Most interstitial pneumonias are classified based on pathology, on which treatments are designed.

Interstitial pneumonias include several conditions, such as connective tissue disease manifesting in the lung, pneumoconioses, idiosyncratic reaction to drugs, and hypersensitivity reactions to inhaled antigens. Some cases of interstitial pneumonias have no identifiable cause, and are

---

[a] Department of Pathology, Nagasaki University Hospital, 1-7-1 Sakamoto, Nagasaki 852-8501, Japan; [b] Division of Respirology, Neurology and Rheumatology, Department of Medicine, Kurume University School of Medicine, 67 Asahi-machi, Kurume, Fukuoka 830-0011, Japan; [c] Department of Pathology, Nagasaki University Graduate School of Biomedical Sciences, 1-7-1, Sakamoto, Nagasaki 852-8501, Japan; [d] Department of Pathology, Kameda Medical Center, 929 Higashi-machi, Kamogawa, Chiba 296-8602, Japan
* Corresponding author.
E-mail address: junfkoka@gmail.com

Surgical Pathology 13 (2020) 91–118
https://doi.org/10.1016/j.path.2019.11.006

diagnosed as idiopathic interstitial pneumonias (IIPs). Therefore, it is not surprising that IIPs can be heterogeneous because they include cases from multiple undetectable causes. This article focuses on pathology of IIPs.

HISTORY OF IDIOPATHIC INTERSTITIAL PNEUMONIA CLASSIFICATION

The classification of interstitial pneumonia was in some disarray until Travis and colleagues organized a committee sponsored by the American Thoracic Society (ATS) and European Respiratory Society (ERS) and released the first consensus classification in 2002.[8] In 2013, the same group updated the classification,[9] in which most histologic patterns described in the 2002 classification were still listed as major IIPs; however, lymphoid interstitial pneumonia (LIP), along with a newly recognized condition, pleuroparenchymal fibroelastosis (PPFE), were included in the rare IIPs category. Unclassifiable interstitial pneumonia was already mentioned in the 2002 classification but referred only to truly unsolvable conditions. In the updated classification, unclassifiable interstitial pneumonia was listed as one of 4 major categories of IIPs. Acute fibrinous and organizing pneumonia

(AFOP) and bronchiolocentric patterns of interstitial pneumonia were added as rare histologic patterns and separated from unclassifiable IIP (UCIP) (Table 1).

GENERAL OVERVIEW OF THE PATHOLOGY OF IDIOPATHIC INTERSTITIAL PNEUMONIAS

THE CONCEPT OF THE INTERSTITIUM

The term interstitial is difficult to understand in the lungs. The counterpart of interstitium inside the lung is airway and airspace, including alveolar pneumocytes. All other components are potentially included the umbrella term of interstitium. The term interstitium also includes the stroma around the bronchovascular bundles, interlobular septa, and subpleural stroma (Figs. 1A, B). Most interstitial stroma is located around the alveolar duct/sac, where three-dimensional view shows the delicate framework of the fibrous stroma composed of scant collagen and elastic fibers and the membranous alveolar sac[10] (Fig. 1C).

THE STRUCTURE OF THE LOBULE

The primary pulmonary lobule is defined as the alveolar tissue distal to a respiratory bronchiole,

Table 1
Classification of idiopathic interstitial pneumonias

Category	Clinical-Radiological-Pathologic Diagnosis	Associated Radiological and/Or Pathologic-Morphologic Patterns
Major IIPs		
Chronic fibrosing Interstitial Pneumonia	IPF	Usual interstitial pneumonia
	Idiopathic nonspecific interstitial pneumonia	Nonspecific interstitial pneumonia
Acute/subacute Interstitial Pneumonia	Cryptogenic organizing pneumonia	Organizing pneumonia
	Acute interstitial pneumonia	Diffuse alveolar damage
Smoking-related Interstitial Pneumonia	Respiratory bronchiolitis-interstitial lung disease	Respiratory bronchiolitis
	Desquamative interstitial pneumonia	Desquamative interstitial pneumonia
Rare IIPs		
	Idiopathic LIP	Lymphocytic interstitial pneumonia
	Idiopathic pleuroparenchymal fibroelastosis	Pleuroparenchymal fibroelastosis
	UCIP	Variable
Rare Histologic Patterns		
	AFOP	
	Bronchiolocentric patterns of interstitial pneuomnia	

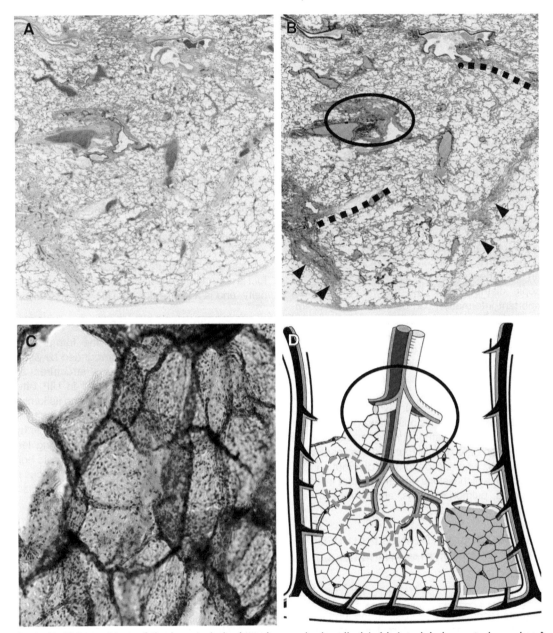

Fig. 1. (*A, B*) Interstitium of the lung includes bronchovascular bundle (*circle*), interlobular septa (*arrowhead*), lymphatic root (*dashed line*), and pleura. (*C*) Three-dimensional view of the lung parenchyma showing fibrovascular framework and membranous alveolar sac. (*D*) Structure of the secondary pulmonary lobule. Red, blue, and orange indicate artery, veins, and lymphatic vessels, respectively. Black circle, green dotted circle, and pink-filled space indicates centrilobular distribution, airway-centered distribution, and area of primary lobule.

and includes a small unit of alveolar ducts and alveolar sacs. The structure of the primary lobule difficult to identify with a microscope in the normal lung, because its boundaries are indistinct. In contrast, the secondary lobule, as defined by Miller,[11] is usually the smallest easily identifiable unit of structure and consists of several primary lobules. The secondary lobule is around 1 to 2 cm in size and is surrounded incompletely by interlobular septa. It often possesses a membranous bronchiole and pulmonary artery in the center of the structure. There are veins and lymphatic vessels running inside the secondary lobule, which usually represent the structure between 2 primary lobules. Areas around terminal airways and respiratory bronchioles are often called centrilobular and centriacinar, respectively. The lung parenchyma directly adjacent to the pleura, large bronchovascular bundle, and pulmonary veins are considered as periphery of the lobule (**Fig. 1D**).

THE DISTRIBUTION OF THE DISEASE

To understand the pathology of IIPs, pathologists must recognize the exact location and distribution of the disease. First, whether lesions occur mainly in the upper parts or the base of the lung, are diffuse or partial, or are centrally or peripherally located within the lung is critical and gives a rough clue to what the disease is. However, such information is often not included with biopsies, and thus data from CT, preferably high-resolution CT (HRCT), should be obtained. Pathologists must be aware that the same microscopic pathology can be seen in completely different settings, which can be differentiated by knowledge of macroscopic distribution of the lesions. In addition, important information can be obtained by examining the disease distribution within the lobule. Pathologists must determine whether the abnormality is distributed diffusely or focally inside the lobule, and whether it is prominent in the centriacinar region, around the airway, or at the periphery of the lobule. Specifically, patchy distribution is a situation in which normal lung abruptly contacts the lesions. Airway-centered or bronchiolocentric distribution is a situation in which lesions are mainly found in the respiratory bronchioles, whereas peripheral distribution is a situation in which lesions directly contact interlobular septa, pulmonary veins, and lymphatic vessels (**Fig. 2**).

BASIC HISTOLOGIC FINDINGS INCLUDED IN IDIOPATHIC INTERSTITIAL PNEUMONIA PATHOLOGY

Fibrosis

Accurate recognition of fibrosis in the lung is critical for the diagnosis of interstitial lung disease (ILD). Fibrosis in the lung includes several different types, and each type represents different biological behavior. The first and most important type is a scarlike dense collagenous fibrosis seen in usual interstitial pneumonia (UIP). Elastica-Van Gieson (EVG) staining is useful in differentiating it from other fibrosis types by highlighting it in red (**Figs. 3A, B**). The second type is a loose fibrosis sometimes seen in nonspecific interstitial pneumonia (NSIP) or smoking-related ILD (SR-ILD), which is a mixture of edema and some increase of collagen fibers. This type of fibrosis often contains small numbers of fibroblasts (**Fig. 3C**). The third type is called fibroelastosis. Fibrosis with

accompanying elastic fibers usually does not occur inside the lung. However, histologic observation gives the impression of fibroelastosis in some cases because of close admixture of elastic and collagenous fibers. The most common example is observed in atelectasis followed by pleuroparenchymal fibroelastosis (PPFE) (**Figs. 3D, E**). The fourth type is young fibroplasia, which is often not called fibrosis, because it is composed of only an increased number of myofibroblasts and edema. It often shows intraluminal osculation and is divided into polypoid, mural, and occluded types by its shape and relationship to the alveolar septum[12] (**Figs. 3F, G**). Masson bodies seen in organizing pneumonia (OP) are the polypoid prototype, and fibroblastic foci are either mural or occluded types. The mixture of chronic dense fibrosis with subacute fibroplasia as fibroblastic foci is commonly referred to as temporal heterogeneity, and is a key feature of UIP[13] (**Fig. 3H**).

Honeycombing and Traction Bronchioloectasis

Honeycombing is defined by the formation of irregularly dilated airspaces surrounded by dense fibrosis, whose underlying lung structures are destroyed.[14] Honeycombing found in UIP often ranges in diameter from 2 to 10 mm and its luminal surface is often coated with bronchial epithelia (**Fig. 4A**). There may be some smooth muscle hyperplasia in the cystic wall. Honeycombing less than 2 mm in diameter is called microscopic honeycombing because it is often filled with mucus or proteinaceous substances and rarely recognized by CT (**Fig. 4B**).

Traction bronchioloectasis is a condition in which the membranous bronchiole is mechanically dilated by contraction of surrounding lung parenchyma by fibrosis.[15] Sometimes the distinction between honeycombing and traction bronchioloectasis is challenging, but traction bronchioloectasis can be identified by the presence of smooth muscle associated with the membranous bronchiole (**Fig. 4C**). Occasional cystic spaces are observed surrounded by dense collagen without an epithelial cell lining. These cysts are called interstitial emphysema, and form when air pressure from the alveolar airspace tears the adjacent interstitial tissues of the lung, resulting in the formation of cystic spaces[16,17] (**Fig. 4D**).

THE ROLE OF PATHOLOGISTS FOR IDIOPATHIC INTERSTITIAL PNEUMONIA DIAGNOSIS

The pathologist's role is to give a specific diagnosis to each patient. However, there are several

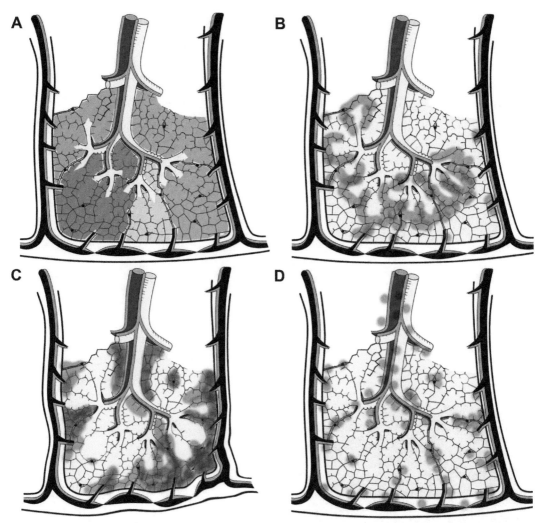

Fig. 2. Distribution of the diseases inside the secondary lobule is important for pathologic diagnosis. (*A*) Diffuse distribution often seen in diffuse alveolar damage and nonspecific interstitial pneumonia. (*B*) Airway-centered distribution is often seen in cases of inhalation-related diseases, such as pneumoconiosis or aspiration pneumonia. (*C*) Peripheral accentuated patchy distribution seen in usual interstitial pneumonia. (*D*) Distribution of lymphatic route. This pattern is often seen in lymphoproliferative disorder and sarcoidosis.

institutional differences that affect pathologists, among which are the choice of sampling method. Although surgical lung biopsy, especially video-associated thoracic surgery (VATS), is the most desirable methodology, if the institute does not have a thoracic surgeon, cryobiopsy or transbronchial lung biopsy (TBLB) may be submitted to pathology. The approach is different for each (**Fig. 5**).

Video-associated Thoracic Surgery Biopsy

The expectation of a VATS biopsy is a specific pathology diagnosis. However, it is difficult on rare occasions, and, for most cases, multidisciplinary discussion (MDD) to give final diagnosis is strongly recommended.[9,18,19] In addition to the histologic

diagnosis, findings suggesting specific diseases, such as connective tissue disease or hypersensitivity pneumonitis, should be reported along with findings that may influence therapeutic options, such as presence or absence of marked inflammatory cell infiltration (**Fig. 6**A). For example, a complex case may show features of UIP pattern based on guidelines,[18] but may also show associated findings, such as marked lymphoid follicles with germinal centers, which suggests association of connective tissue disease[20]; numerous granulomas and/or airway-centered changes, which suggest hypersensitivity pneumonitis[21,22]; or acute exudative inflammation, which suggests exacerbation of UIP.[23,24] Critical points for

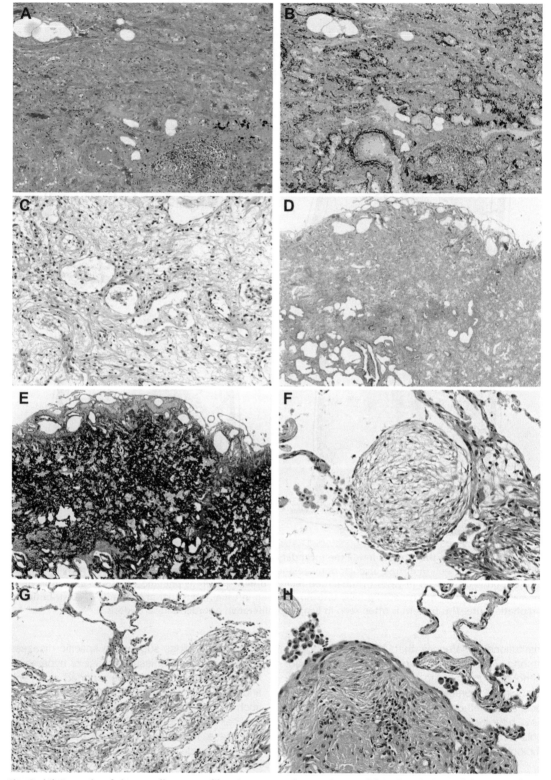

Fig. 3. (*A*) Example of dense collagenous fibrosis, commonly seen in UIP. (*B*) EVG stain is useful in identifying dense collagenous fibrosis. Note the red fibers indicating scarred collagen deposition. (*C*) Loose fibrosis shown by pale color. This type is often seen in nonspecific interstitial pneumonia (NSIP). (*D*) Fibroelastosis is commonly found in collapsed lung. PPFE shows changes mainly seen in the subpleural zone. (*E*) Fibroelastosis is well highlighted by EVG staining. (*F*) Young polypoid-shaped fibroplasia occupying the alveolar space is a typical feature of organizing pneumonia. (*G*) Organizing pneumonia sometimes incorporates into adjacent alveolar septa, called mural or occluded types of organizing pneumonia. (*H*) Fibroblast foci are a key pathologic finding of UIP. Note the dense collagenous fibrosis is located directly adjacent to the pale fibroplasia.

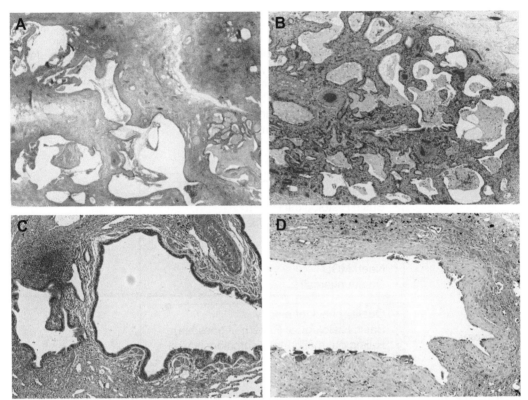

Fig. 4. (*A*) Honeycomb cysts are irregular airspaces of 2 to 10 mm found inside the fibrotic area where alveolar structure is completely distorted. (*B*) In microscopic honeycomb, or small honeycombing unable to be identified by CT, mucus pooling inside the cystic spaces is a common finding. (*C*) Mechanically expanded bronchioles are called traction bronchiolectasis. (*D*) Interstitial emphysema in adults causes cystic spaces surrounded by dense collagen without covering of epithelial cells, but with histiocytes. The spaces arise by the dissection of fibrotic stroma.

diagnosis of IIPs by VATS biopsy are separation between UIP and non-UIP, listing histologic findings suggestive of cause of interstitial pneumonia, detection of components suggestive of diffuse alveolar damage, and indication of findings that may affect the therapeutic protocols, including prominent inflammatory cell infiltration or presence of acute lung injury.

Transbronchial Cryobiopsy

Transbronchial cryobiopsy has been proposed as a less invasive alternative to VATS biopsy in patients with interstitial pneumonia, partly because of the perception that it is a safer procedure.[25] This method uses compressed gas to freeze lung parenchyma at the site of a cryoprobe. Previous reports emphasize the benefits of cryobiopsy for larger specimens and lesser crush artifact compared with TBLB, along with its histologic diagnostic yields of more than 70%.[25–28]

The area included in cryobiopsy is, importantly, not exactly the same as VATS biopsy (**Fig. 6**B). It

often lacks areas around the subpleural zone, and thus observation of the peripheral area inside the secondary lobule is limited to the stroma around the bronchovascular bundle or small venules (**Figs. 6**C, D). EVG staining is strongly recommended because it helps recognition of lung parenchyma of the peripheral lobule (**Fig. 6**E). The diagnostic accuracy in non-UIP cases is currently under investigation, so the method should only be used to determine the presence of UIP pattern or the need for additional VATS biopsy at this point.

Transbronchial Lung Biopsy

The diagnostic yield by TBLB is limited for interstitial pneumonia. Cryptogenic OP may be the only disease that can be diagnosed with TBLB in combination with an MDD.[8] TBLB has limited diagnostic power for UIP, NSIP, desquamative interstitial pneumonia (DIP), LIP, or acute interstitial pneumonia, so it is strongly recommended not to use this method for these diagnoses even

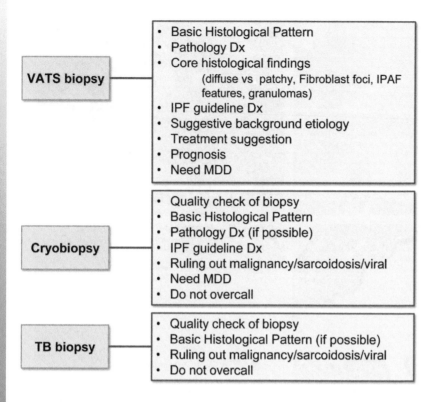

VATS biopsy
- Basic Histological Pattern
- Pathology Dx
- Core histological findings
    (diffuse vs patchy, Fibroblast foci, IPAF features, granulomas)
- IPF guideline Dx
- Suggestive background etiology
- Treatment suggestion
- Prognosis
- Need MDD

Cryobiopsy
- Quality check of biopsy
- Basic Histological Pattern
- Pathology Dx (if possible)
- IPF guideline Dx
- Ruling out malignancy/sarcoidosis/viral
- Need MDD
- Do not overcall

TB biopsy
- Quality check of biopsy
- Basic Histological Pattern (if possible)
- Ruling out malignancy/sarcoidosis/viral
- Do not overcall

Fig. 5. Required tasks for pathologists differ depending on sampling methods. Tips for each method are listed. Dx, diagnosis; TB, transbronchial.

with MDD. The artifactual collapse of the specimen makes pathologic evaluation difficult, and often normal lung can be mistaken for interstitial pneumonia by general pathologists (**Fig. 6F**).

DIAGNOSTIC APPROACH OF IDIOPATHIC INTERSTITIAL PNEUMONIAS

When making a pathologic diagnosis, the clinicians must first determine whether the main abnormality is fibrosis, exudative change, or inflammatory cell infiltration. Then, observation of detailed findings are made, which suggest more specific conditions for each disease, such as levels of architectural destruction; whether it is a loose or dense type of fibrosis; whether fibroblast foci are present or absent; and whether additional features are present, such as granulomas, lymphoid follicles with germinal centers, abnormal smooth muscle, or morphologic changes of pneumocytes or vessels. The detailed histopathology findings for each disease are described here.

FEATURES OF EACH IDIOPATHIC INTERSTITIAL PNEUMONIA

USUAL INTERSTITIAL PNEUMONIA (UIP)

IPF is the most important and common form of chronic interstitial pneumonia, and shows a corresponding condition called UIP. The term UIP was

originally introduced by Carrington and colleagues,[29] who defined it as "chronic lung fibrosis of the common or usual type." The name creates confusions but remains because of great respect to those investigators and long history of its usage.

Clinical Features of Usual Interstitial Pneumonia

IPF is stereotypically observed in older men, usually more than 60 years of age.[30]

Most patients are smokers, but those who have never smoked can also be affected.[31] IPF slowly progresses to irreversible end-stage honeycomb fibrosis with eventual death caused by respiratory failure.[9,32,33] Patients with IPF are at increased risk for developing lung cancer, in which case the prognosis may depend on the cancer behavior.[34,35] From 10% to 20% of patients with IPF experience acute exacerbation and rapidly deteriorate to death.[1] Antifibrotic agents, such as pirfenidone[6] or nintedanib,[7] are the primary choice of treatment, and, importantly, steroid use is contraindicated because it is associated with increased morbidity and mortality.[36,37]

Histopathologic Features of Usual Interstitial Pneumonia

The key histopathologic feature of UIP is its heterogeneous appearance seen at low magnification (**Fig. 7A**). The areas of scarred fibrosis are

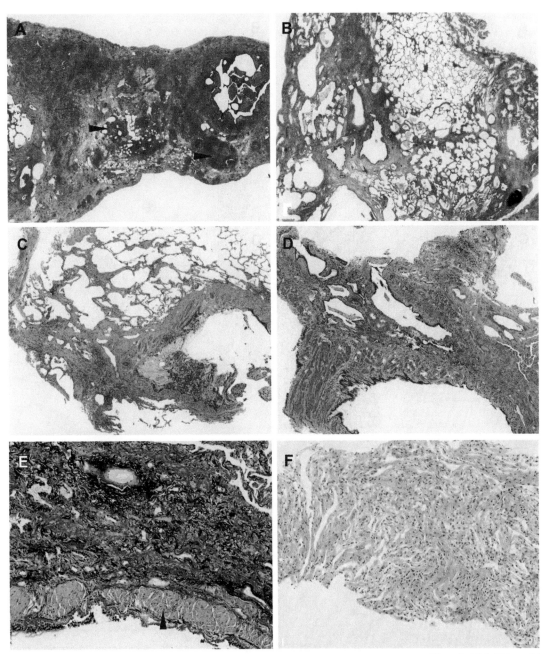

Fig. 6. (*A*) Panoramic view of VATS biopsy. In addition to histologic pattern, presence of lymphoid follicles with germinal centers (*arrowheads*) suggests autoimmune disease as a background condition. (*B*) Dotted line indicates the area sampled by cryobiopsy, mainly including lung parenchyma of 2 to 3 mm surrounding the membranous bronchioles. (*C, D*) UIP seen in cryobiopsy. Parenchyma starting directly from the bronchovascular bundle is the peripheral zone of the pulmonary lobule. Its occupancy by dense and destructive fibrosis is a key finding for UIP diagnosis. (*E*) EVG staining highlights the nature of destructive fibrosis. Note that elastic fibers are irregularly folded with red collagen fibers. The fibrosis begins from the edge of smooth muscle of bronchiole (*arrowhead*). (*F*) Collapsed normal lung seen in transbronchial forceps biopsy. This biopsy was originally reported as cellular interstitial pneumonia because of a misinterpretation of artifactual collapse.

immediately adjacent to normal-looking parenchyma. The dense fibrotic areas are mainly located in the peripheral zones of secondary lobules (**Fig. 7**B).[38] In the transitional areas between chronic dense fibrosis and normal lung, scattered foci of young fibroblastic proliferation, named fibroblast foci, are found[39] (**Fig. 7**C). This coexistence of old and several disconnected foci of

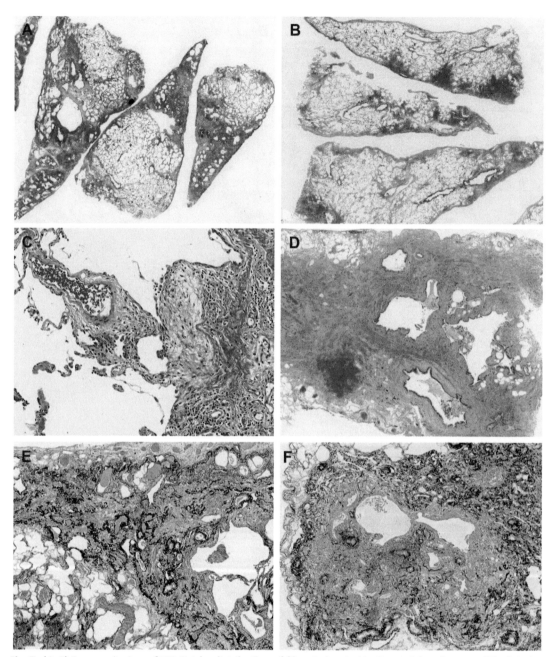

Fig. 7. (*A, B*) Panoramic view of UIP. Patchy distribution of fibrosis, located in the peripheral zones of the lobules, is a key to the diagnosis. (*C*) High magnification of fibroblastic focus. Young fibroplasia is located next to dense collagenous fibrosis. (*D*) Fibrotic lung of a patient with UIP showing complete destruction of normal lung parenchyma. (*E, F*). EVG staining of UIP samples often shows accumulation of elastic fiber in the perilobular zones of lung parenchyma.

young loose fibrosis is referred to as temporal heterogeneity and is one of the most important clues to UIP.[13] This repetitive heterogeneous pattern spreads throughout the lung. In the area of dense fibrosis, normal lung architecture is completely distorted, and an increase in collagenous fibers becomes predominant (**Fig. 7**D). Elastic fibers of the original lung show discontinuity or disappearance at the center of the lobule and accumulate in the perilobular zones (**Figs. 7**E, F). Inflammatory cell infiltration is limited. Disordered proliferation of smooth muscle is a frequent finding as well.[40]

Cystic spaces of various sizes are seen. Some of them are microscopic honeycomb change and others are either traction bronchiolectasis or emphysematous spaces.[14,15]

Diagnosis of Idiopathic Pulmonary fibrosis: An Official American Thoracic Society/European Respiratory Society/Japanese Respiratory Society/Latin American Thoracic Association Clinical Practice Guideline 2018[18]

For cases of suspected IIP, additional description of judgment based on the IPF guideline is also recommended. One important point is that the use of the term UIP in the guideline is limited to only IPF cases and does not include UIP in connective tissue disease or in chronic hypersensitivity pneumonitis (CHP), although such cases are common. These cases are excluded from the guideline. Therefore, cases with known connective tissue disease or with certain other identifiable causes do not require additional notes regarding the guideline. The key findings for UIP diagnosis indicated in the guideline are (1) dense fibrosis with architectural destruction; (2) predominant subpleural and/or paraseptal distribution of fibrosis; (3) patchy involvement of lung parenchyma by fibrosis; (4) fibroblast foci; and (5) absence of features to suggest an alternative diagnosis. Cases with all 5 characteristics are classified as UIP. Depending on the levels of uncertainty, cases are categorized as probable UIP or indeterminate

UIP. The criteria are indicated in **Table 2**. Note that cases with features of other histologic patterns of IIPs in all biopsies or histologic findings indicating other disease are now diagnosed as alternative diagnosis. Pathologists must be aware that this diagnosis has a strong power to exclude the chance of IPF diagnosis even after MDD. Therefore, some minor changes suggesting connective tissue disease or hypersensitivity may be better left out or underemphasized.

Acute Exacerbation of Usual Interstitial Pneumonia

Recognition of acute exacerbation in UIP cases is important because most such cases rapidly progress to be lethal, and immediate and intense treatment should be considered.[23,41,42] The prototype of the pathologic pattern of acute exacerbation is a mixture of diffuse alveolar damage (DAD) and UIP[23,24]; however, some variations, such as association of OP or an increase of fibroblast foci, are also reported[43,44] (**Figs. 8A, B**). Although pathologic suggestion to the clinician is meaningful and important, the diagnosis of acute exacerbation of IPF should be a diagnosis after MDD,[45,46] because pathology alone cannot be diagnostic.

Differential Diagnosis of Usual Interstitial Pneumonia

The most common differential diagnoses of UIP are either fibrotic NSIP[40,47,48] or UIP from other

Table 2
Histopathology patterns and features of usual interstitial pneumonia quoted from an official American Thoracic Society/European Respiratory Society/Japanese Respiratory Society/Latin American Thoracic Association clinical practice guideline: diagnosis of idiopathic pulmonary fibrosis

UIP	Probable UIP	Indeterminate for UIP	Alternative Diagnosis
• Dense fibrosis with architectural distortion (ie, destructive scarring and/or honeycombing) • Predominant subpleural and/or paraseptal distribution of fibrosis • Patchy involvement of lung parenchyma by fibrosis • Fibroblast foci • Absence of features to suggest an alternative diagnosis	• Some histologic features from column 1 are present but to an extent that precludes a definite diagnosis of UIP/IPF And • Absence of features to suggest an alternative diagnosis Or • Honeycombing only	• Fibrosis with or without architectural distortion, with features favoring either a pattern other than UIP or features favoring UIP secondary to another cause • Some histologic features from column 1, but with other features suggesting an alternative diagnosis • Some histologic features from column 1, but with other features suggesting an alternative diagnosis	• Features of other histologic patterns of IIPs (eg, absence of fibroblast foci or loose fibrosis) in all biopsies • Histologic findings indicating other diseases (eg, hypersensitivity pneumonitis, Langerhans cell histiocytosis, sarcoidosis, lymphangioleiomyomatosis (LAM))

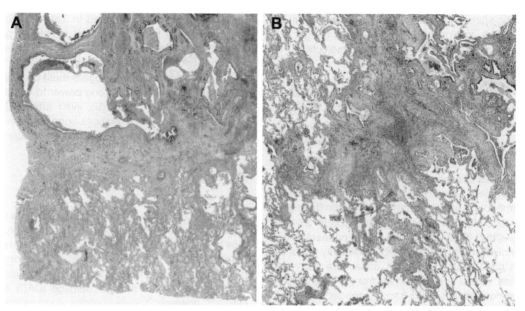

Fig. 8. (*A*) Acute exacerbation of UIP typically shows a mixture of dense fibrosis with honeycomb changes (*left upper region*) and DAD (*lower*). (*B*) Acute exacerbation may present an exaggerated appearance of fibroblastic foci.

causes, such as connective tissue disease,[49–51] asbestosis,[52–55] CHP,[56–58] or idiosyncratic reaction to a drug.[59] Important points in differential diagnosis of UIP are shown in **Table 3**. When looking at the histologic pattern, distinction from fibrotic NSIP is important because of differences in treatment choice and predictive prognosis. The easiest and most important way to distinguish UIP from NSIP is to identify the patchy and peripherally accentuated distribution by scanning magnification. There is 1 exception, which is when tissues are only taken from end-stage honeycomb lung. Microscopic honeycombing is a common and characteristic feature of UIP but is not specific to UIP/IPF. Fibrotic NSIP can show honeycomb changes when it progresses. Abrupt change from disarrayed scar to normal lung is probably the most useful distinguishing point. The application of the IPF guideline[18] is problematic for fibrotic NSIP cases, because most cases are in the categories of either probable UIP or indeterminate for UIP. Consideration of NSIP diagnosis should be mentioned at the time of MDD.

Aside from idiopathic causes, connective tissue disease (especially rheumatoid arthritis[60]) and CHP,[56–58] are responsible for the presence of UIP pattern. Features suggestive of rheumatoid arthritis are the presence of lymphoid follicles with germinal centers, and plasma cell infiltration. There are several other histologic features suggested by different experts, such as presence of pleuritis, bronchiolitis, and the perivascular

fibrosis; however, many of them are based on empiric impressions, not on evidence. One report suggests the use of Web-based calculation using a formula extracted by their cohort of ILD cases.[61] ATS/ERS has proposed putting cases with autoimmune characteristics into the category of interstitial pneumonia with autoimmune features (IPAF).[62] However, evidence is still limited, and this category is still tentative.

Cases with asbestos exposure should be evaluated carefully to look for asbestos bodies. Iron staining to highlight asbestos bodies is recommended for suspected cases. Presence of more than 2 asbestos bodies in 1 biopsy specimen may qualify for the diagnosis of asbestosis; however, the distinction from cases of IPF arising in patients with asbestos exposure is difficult with such subtle pathology. Additional clues for asbestosis are airway-centered accentuation of fibrosis, and fibrous pleural plaques identified by radiology or histology.[63,64]

Distinction of UIP from CHP is currently a large problem in the respiratory community. Interobserver agreement is low not only by pathology but also by radiology and even by MDD. Pathologically, the judgment of airway-centered accentuation is the most unreliable factor to skew the diagnosis.[65] The presence of nonnecrotizing granuloma is one of the strongest features supporting a CHP diagnosis[58]; however, incidental granulomas can be seen in various other situations, including IPF. There is no ground truth to clearly separate

Table 3
Tips to separate common differential diagnosis of usual interstitial pneumonia

Differential Diagnosis	Suggestive Findings	Opposed Findings (More Suggestive for UIP)
Fibrotic NSIP	Diffuse distribution, loose fibrosis, cellular infiltration	Abrupt change, fibroblast foci, patchy distribution, peripheral accentuation
Smoking-related IP	ACA, marked pigmented macrophages, hyalinized acellular fibrosis, marked emphysema, large cysts simulating bullae	Abrupt change, fibroblast foci, marked dense fibrosis, patchy distribution, perilobular accumulation of elastic fibers
Connective tissue disease: RA, SSc	LYGC, plasmacytosis, cellular/follicular bronchiolitis, cellular/fibrinous pleuritis, vascular thickening in normal lung area	Fibroblast foci, subpleural fat metaplasia
Asbestosis	Asbestos body, ACA, loose fibrosis, hemosiderosis, frequent foci of OP	Marked architectural destruction, fibroblastic foci
Chronic hypersensitivity pneumonitis	ACC, poorly formed granuloma, interstitial giant cell with cholesterol cleft, cellular interstitial pneumonia in nonfibrotic area, marked bronchiolitis	None
Drug-induced ILD	Foamy atypical type II pneumocyte, wide area of bronchial/squamous metaplasia, vascular intimal injury, diffuse distribution, frequent OP	Adjacent completely normal lung area, fibroblastic foci

Abbreviations: ACA, airway-centered accentuation; LYGC, lymphoid follicle with germinal center; RA, rheumatoid arthritis; SSc, systemic scleroderma.

IPF and UIP of CHP. Claims including challenge test and immune test for immunoglobulin (Ig) Gs are still not solely reliable. The recommendation for diagnostic pathologists is to describe the factors suggestive of CHP, and include the possibility of IPF for therapeutic choice if the changes are not diagnostic for definitive CHP.

The Hypothetical Idea of the Usual Interstitial Pneumonia Bucket

There is a hypothesis that UIP pattern fibrosis from different causes may all be the same disease, but the causes of its initiation and progression are different (**Fig. 9**).[66] Based on the analogy of the UIP bucket, once UIP starts in the patient's lung, it progresses differently based on the patient's underlying and superimposed conditions. In this analogy, the lungs are represented as a bucket of water. As additional insults are produced (eg,

smoking, antigen inhalation, connective tissue disease), figurative stones are added to the bucket, causing it to overflow and have decreased capacity. In patients with UIP, the eventual end stage is honeycomb lung. Removing causes of deterioration may slow down the progression of UIP, but eventually it will proceed to lethal honeycomb fibrosis. Given this hypothesis, patients with UIP secondary to known causes may benefit from antifibrotic agents that are currently used for IPF.

NONSPECIFIC INTERSTITIAL PNEUMONIA (NSIP)

History and Clinical Features of Nonspecific Interstitial Pneumonia

The idea of NSIP was first proposed by Katzenstein and colleagues[67] in 1994 for cases that did not fit into any specific diagnostic category. In the 2002 classification of IIPs,[8] NSIP was included

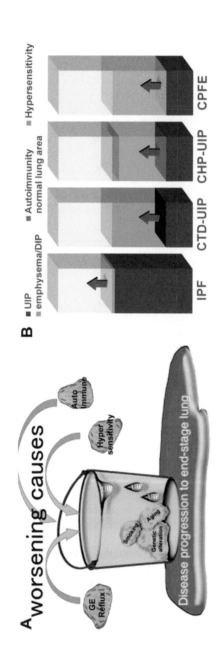

Fig. 9. The UIP bucket analogy. (*A*) Once UIP development is initiated with a mixed cause of genetic abnormalities, tobacco smoking, senescence, and so on, multiple factors such as gastroesophageal reflux accelerate the process. Each additional factor causes the water level of UIP to rise and eventually overflow, resulting in end-stage honeycomb fibrosis. (*B*) UIP progression in the lungs of patients with UIP with various causes. The bars indicate abnormality inside the total lung. Patients with connective tissue disease (CTD)-UIP and CHP-UIP have both UIP and CTD–related ILD and hypersensitivity pneumonitis-related ILD. Prolonged inflammation caused by autoimmunity or hypersensitivity reaction leads to an increased proportion of UIP lesions and eventually kills the patients. CPFE, combined pulmonary fibrosis and emphysema; GE, gastroesophageal.

as a provisional disease. In 2008, the ATS stated that idiopathic NSIP is an independent disease that shows different clinical behavior from other diseases.[68] Compared with IPF, idiopathic NSIP is seen in younger patients (around 50 years old), women more than men, and those with less smoking history.[68,69] HRCT features are also different from IPF and show bilateral ground-glass attenuation as a predominant feature accentuated around the bronchovascular bundle.[70,71] Subpleural sparing is also frequent on CT scan.[68,72]

Histopathologic features of Nonspecific Interstitial Pneumonia

Pathologic features of NSIP are diffuse and uniform distribution of abnormalities throughout the biopsy. The basic architecture of the lung is mostly preserved, and alveolar septa are thickened by either cellular infiltration or fibrosis[67] (**Figs. 10A, B**).

Cellular NSIP shows inflammatory cell infiltration, mainly lymphocytes and plasma cells, as the predominant pathology. Focal areas of OP may be seen but should not occupy more than 20% of the region of disease. Fibrotic NSIP often shows a mixture of lymphoplasmacytic infiltration and interstitial fibrosis. There may be some peripheral accentuation (**Fig. 10C**), but, importantly, completely normal lung is usually absent. Microscopic honeycombing or UIP pattern can be present as a minor component (**Fig. 10D**). When it exceeds 20% of areas, the prognosis may worsen to one similar to UIP.[68] Whether radiology shows UIP features or not with HRCT may be helpful for the diagnosis. As mentioned, histologic distinction from UIP is difficult in some cases. Some other helpful findings to differentiate NSIP from UIP are absence or paucity of both smooth muscle hyperplasia and fibroblast foci.[48]

There are cases of NSIP associated with extensive overlapping areas of OP. Those cases may show clinical features of myositis, and serum tests may be positive for anti-aminoacyl tRNA synthetase (ARS) or anti-melanoma differentiation associated gene 5 (MDA5) antibodies[62,73] (**Figs. 10E, F**). These cases often progress rapidly to respiratory failure; therefore, careful observation and use of high-dose steroids along with other immunosuppressants are often required. Because of a wide range of clinical behavior, these cases may better be separated from the category of NSIP.

Differential Diagnosis of Nonspecific Interstitial Pneumonia

The differential diagnosis of NSIP is broad; among cases with pathologic NSIP, idiopathic disease may be a minor component. There are broad causes that present with an NSIP pattern including connective tissue disease[74] as a leading consideration, followed by hypersensitivity pneumonitis,[57] radiation pneumonitis, eosinophilic pneumonia, and lymphoproliferative disorder. Important points in the differential diagnosis of NSIP are shown in **Table 4**. NSIP in patients with connective tissue disease shows more lymphoid follicles, plasma cell infiltration, and airspace fibrin, and less fibroblast foci, fatty metaplasia, and dense fibrosis.[75] Separation from hypersensitivity pneumonitis may be difficult. Presence of granulomas or airway-centered accentuation are major elements in hypersensitivity pneumonitis, but are not always identified. A final diagnosis of idiopathic NSIP should be given after MDD by pulmonary experts.

ORGANIZING PNEUMONIA (OP), AND ORGANIZING PNEUMONIA VARIANTS (FIBROSING ORGANIZING PNEUMONIA, CICATRICIAL VARIANT OF ORGANIZING PNEUMONIA)

The key pathologic feature of OP is airspace filling by plugs of young fibroplasia mixed with myofibroblasts and stromal edema. Eosinophilic collagenous fibrosis is usually missing or limited. Inflammatory cells can be seen but are usually scant. OP can be seen in various situations, such as infection[76] and drug injury,[77] as well as surrounding areas of other disease such as cancer.[78] The focus here is on the idiopathic form, cryptogenic OP (COP). COP usually has a patchy distribution and involves several secondary lobules to create a consolidated lesion. The border of the lesion is often clear, usually adjacent to normal lung. There is no architectural destruction; therefore, basic structure is clear when observed by elastic fiber staining (EVG). OP does not create any elastic fibers and is easily identified by elastic staining (**Figs. 11A, B**). It is often associated with a mild to moderate level of lymphoplasmacytic infiltration in the adjacent thickened alveolar septa, but not so much in the area of OP plugs. The prototypical shape of the OP plug is a polypoid protrusion into the airspace with a thin stalk (**Fig. 11C**). There are several variations in shape. Some show multibranching and extend from one alveolus to the next through interalveolar fenestrae. Others show incorporation into alveolar septa and show a crescentic shape, which can be difficult to distinguish from fibroblast foci seen in UIP (**Fig. 11D**). The natural history of OP is dissolution to complete disappearance. On the way, it may show small eosinophilic particles surrounded by pneumocytes, referred to as collagen globules.[79]

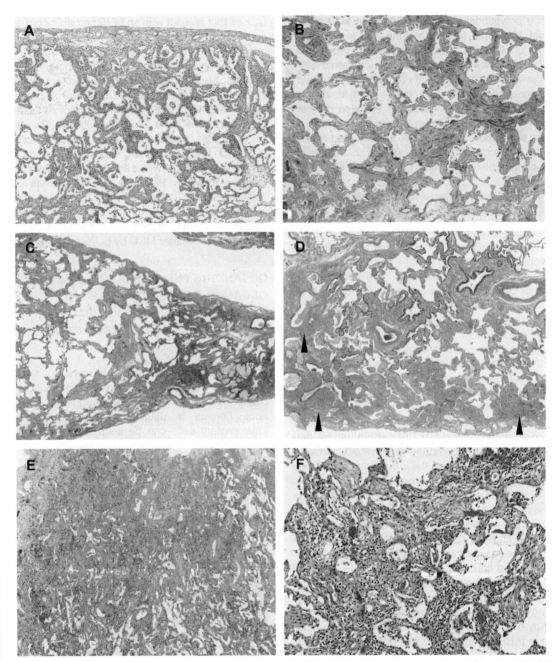

Fig. 10. Pathology images of NSIP. (*A*) Low-power view of cellular NSIP. (*B*) Low-power view of fibrotic NSIP. (*C*) Slight peripheral accentuation can be seen in fibrotic NSIP. (*D*) Some structural destruction similar to UIP (*arrow-heads*) can be seen as a part of NSIP. When it dominates, the diagnosis of UIP is preferable. (*E*, *F*) NSIP admixed with foci of OP. This patient did not have a well-characterized connective tissue disease, but his blood serum test was positive for anti-aminoacyl tRNA synthetase (ARS) antibody.

The last area to resolve is located around interlobular septa, around lymphatic vessels. This situation can provide the radiological reversed halo sign in HRCT (**Fig. 11E**).

According to case reports, there are some OP cases with worse prognosis.[80–82] On histology, some cases show marked fibrin along with OP[83] and are called acute fibrinous OP. This variant was classified as a rare histologic pattern in the ATS and ERS classification in 2013.[9] Other cases, called fibrosing variant of OP, show a mixed pattern of fibrotic NSIP and OP, and are mentioned in the ATS and ERS classification.[9] These cases are often found to have underlying polymyositis

Table 4
Tips to separate common differential diagnosis of nonspecific interstitial pneumonia

Differential Diagnosis	Suggestive Findings	Opposed Findings (More Suggestive for NSIP)
UIP (see Table 3)		
OP	Masson body, patchy distribution, foamy macrophages	Diffuse distribution, septal thickening by fibrosis
DAD	Hyaline membrane, marked fibrin, widening of alveolar septa, pleural thickening, edema, foamy macrophage	Interstitial fibrosis
Connective tissue disease	LYGC, plasmacytosis, diffuse vascular wall thickening, wide area of OP	None
CHP	Airway-centered distribution, granuloma, giant cell with cholesterol cleft	None
Eosinophilic pneumonia	Tissue eosinophilia, pink macrophages, airspace fibrin, type II pneumocyte atypia, OP	None
Drug-induced ILD	Foamy atypical type II pneumocyte, foamy macrophages, vascular injury	None
Radiation pneumonitis	Fibroelastosis, hyalinized vascular injury, bizarre pneumocytes	None

or antisynthetase syndrome[84] and show a worse prognosis than COP. Rarely, OP ends up with scar-like fibrosis; this is referred to as cicatricial variant of OP and can be difficult to distinguish from UIP[85,86](Fig. 11F). It is unclear whether this variant shows disease progression or not at this time.

The differential diagnosis of OP can be broad, and includes cellular NSIP, DAD, infection,[76] connective tissue disease manifesting in the lung,[87] eosinophilic pneumonia,[88] drug injury,[89] radiation pneumonitis, and vasculitis. Important points in differential diagnosis of OP are shown in **Table 5**. The histologic picture of OP is dynamic and it may show completely different patterns depending on the time of biopsy. The later phase of COP may show prototypic cellular and fibrotic NSIP. Recognition of the dynamic quality of OP is important, and can be correlated with the radiological finding of waxing and waning opacities. Difficulties may be encountered in separating OP from organizing DAD. The different prognoses of COP and DAD make distinction important. The useful key to distinguishing COP from organizing DAD is its distribution. Organizing DAD often shows complete replacement by disease within

the entire tissue and does not show an associated normal lung component. Distortion of alveolar septa is more severe in organizing DAD as well. There are some cases showing a mixture of OP, DAD, and NSIP, and these can represent myositis-related lung disease as described earlier,[73,84] and serum testing for anti-ARS and anti-MDA5 antibodies should be recommended.

DIFFUSE ALVEOLAR DAMAGE (DAD)

The histologic picture of DAD varies largely by time course, which is divided into 3 phases: exudative, organizing, and fibrotic.[90,91] In the exudative phase, major findings are stromal and airspace edema, epithelial hypertrophy and denudation, hyaline membrane formation, and collapse of alveolar sacs resulting in simplification of the lung or widening of the alveolar duct[91] (Fig. 12A). In the organizing phase, collapse of alveolar spaces is more obvious and fibroblasts start to appear in the thickened stroma. Type II cell hyperplasia is common and may show atypia simulating neoplasia.[92] Squamous metaplasia is also a common finding at this phase. Hyaline membranes are

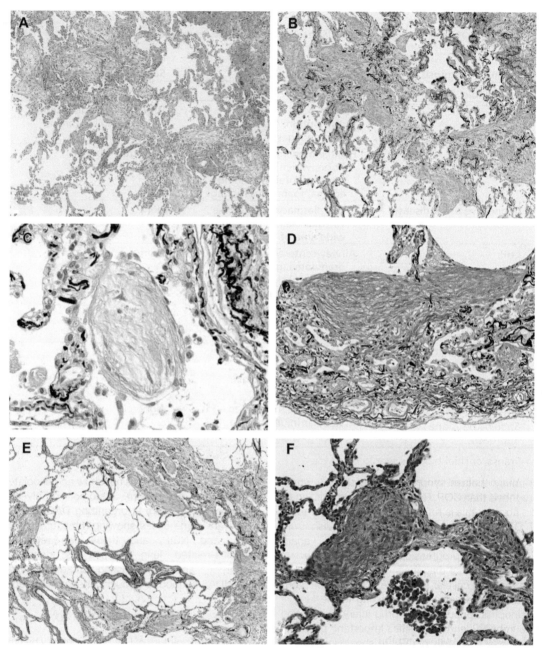

Fig. 11. OP and its variants. (*A, B*) Typical appearance of OP in hematoxylin-eosin and EVG staining. (*C*) Classic appearance of polypoid organization. It usually shows fibroplasia without elastic fibers. (*D*) Incorporated type of OP, which attached to alveolar septa in a wider area than polypoid type. (*E*) OP foci can be arranged in perilobular areas around the lymphatic routes, which manifest as reversed halo sign in CT imaging. (*F*) Scarred (cicatricial) form of OP.

usually not found or are uncommon (**Fig. 12**B). Biopsies for DAD often are performed in this phase, in which case distinction from OP is the major issue. In the fibrotic phase, the changes described earlier are absent and the pathology resembles that of fibrotic NSIP or even honeycomb lung of UIP. Knowledge of the clinical course and radiological findings are critical to give a diagnosis of the fibrotic phase of DAD.

Important points in differential diagnosis of DAD are shown in **Table 6**. One of the most important differential diagnoses of DAD is acute exacerbation in a previously unrecognized chronic fibrotic disease such as UIP.[46] Presence or absence of

Table 5
Tips to separate common differential diagnosis of organizing pneumonia

Differential Diagnosis	Suggestive Findings	Opposed Findings (More Suggestive for OP)
Cellular NSIP (see **Table 4**)		
DAD	Hyaline membrane, marked fibrin, DID, dilatation of alveolar ducts, fibrin thrombus, epithelial denudation, SQM, widened alveolar septa	Masson body, adjacent complete normal lung
Connective tissue disease	LYGC, plasmacytosis, DID, focal chronic fibrosis, bronchiolitis	Patchy distribution
Chronic eosinophilic pneumonia	Tissue eosinophilia, pink macrophage, type II cell atypia	—
Hypersensitivity pneumonitis	Airway-centered interstitial fibrosis, granuloma, giant cell with cholesterol cleft, PBM	Complete alveolar filling by organization
Radiation pneumonitis	Fibroelastosis, marked vascular injury	None
Drug-induced ILD	Foamy atypical type II pneumocyte, diffuse distribution, hemorrhage	None

Abbreviations: DID, diffuse distribution; SQM, squamous metaplasia; PBM, peribronchial metaplasia.

UIP in the whole biopsied sample should be carefully examined. There are many causes known to produce secondary DAD, including infection, connective tissue disease (especially myositis and systemic lupus erythematosus), disseminated intravascular coagulation, septic shock, drug injury, high concentration of inspired oxygen, and burn injury. DAD is more destructive compared with OP and NSIP, so epithelial changes and disarray of elastic fibers stand out.

DESQUAMATIVE INTERSTITIAL PNEUMONIA (DIP)

The main pathologic feature of DIP is diffuse airspace filling by pigmented macrophages (**Figs. 13A, B**). These macrophages are often positive to periodic acid–Schiff and iron staining. Background lung shows various levels of fibrosis along with emphysematous changes.[13] The fibrosis is usually hyalinized, uniform, and does not show architectural destruction other than emphysematous changes. Inflammatory cell infiltration is generally faint but rarely present. Ironically, lymphoid follicles with germinal centers are common. Diffuse hyperplasia of type II cell is almost always present, which is the cause of the erroneous

nomenclature, desquamative[8,93] (**Fig. 13B**). If fibrosis shows even a slight hint of UIP, reconsideration of diagnosis from DIP to UIP may be needed. Careful comparison with HRCT is a strong recommendation.

The differential diagnosis of DIP includes DIP reaction in fibrotic NSIP or UIP, eosinophilic pneumonia, asbestosis, diffuse alveolar hemorrhage, giant cell interstitial pneumonia/hard metal pneumoconiosis, and Langerhans cell histiocytosis (LCH).

RESPIRATORY BRONCHIOLITIS–ASSOCIATED INTERSTITIAL LUNG DISEASE (RB-ILD)

Most of the pathologic features of respiratory bronchiolitis (RB) ILD overlap with those of DIP. The difference is that RB-ILD is accentuated in peribronchiolar alveoli, adjacent to airways[94,95] (**Fig. 13D**). Therefore, radiological images of RB-ILD, unlike those of DIP, show upper lung–predominant centrilobular nodules.[96–98] The pathologic diagnosis should be RB,[8,9] and the term RB-ILD should be used only after MDD. There may be some inflammatory cell infiltration and fibrosis accentuated in the respiratory bronchioles, often associated with centriacinar emphysema.

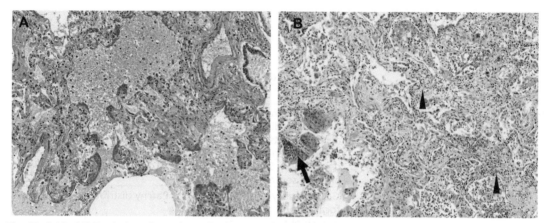

Fig. 12. DAD. (*A*) Exudative phase shows hyaline membrane along the widened alveolar duct. (*B*) Organizing DAD shows diffuse organization not only inside the airspace but also inside the alveolar septa thickened by young fibroplasia (*arrowheads*). Squamous metaplasia (*arrow*) is a common finding in organizing DAD.

Differential diagnosis of RB-ILD includes DIP, asbestosis, LCH, and other small airway diseases.

LYMPHOCYTIC INTERSTITIAL PNEUMONIA (LIP)

The histopathology of LIP is characterized by severe infiltration of the interstitium and alveolar spaces of the lung by lymphocytes along with plasma cells[8,9] (**Figs. 14**A, B). Airspace exudate with eosinophilic proteinaceous liquid, positive for anti-IgG immunostaining, is common. Some cases may be associated with lymphoid follicles with germinal centers. Giant cells with cytoplasmic cholesterol clefts and/or nonnecrotizing poorly

formed granuloma are often present. Lymphocyte infiltration penetrating the pleura or interlobular septa is rare, but, if present along with lack of germinal centers in lymphoid aggregates, lymphoma should be considered as a likely possibility (**Fig. 14**C). The idiopathic form of LIP is extremely rare, and most cases are cellular NSIP, hypersensitivity pneumonitis, lymphoproliferative disorder, connective tissue disease such as Sjögren syndrome, or immune deficiency–related conditions.

Important points in the differential diagnosis of LIP are shown in **Table 7**. Diffuse lymphoid hyperplasia and nodular lymphoid hyperplasia are in this spectrum and usually show more lymphoid follicles and prominent plasmacytosis along lymphatic

Table 6
Tips to separate common differential diagnosis of diffuse alveolar damage

Differential Diagnosis	Suggestive Findings	Opposed Findings (More Suggestive for DAD)
OP	Masson body	Hyaline membrane, alveolar edema
NSIP	Interstitial fibrosis,	Hyaline membrane, alveolar edema
IPF/UIP acute exacerbation	Dense fibrosis, architectural destruction	None
Connective tissue disease	LYGC, plasmacytosis, cellular/ fibrinous pleuritis, focal fibrosis	None
Eosinophilic pneumonia	Tissue eosinophilia, pink macrophage, type II cell atypia, marked fibrin	Hyaline membrane
Secondary DAD: infection, high oxygen concentration, burn	Extensive hyaline membrane, neutrophil, extensive epithelial denudation, bronchial erosion	None

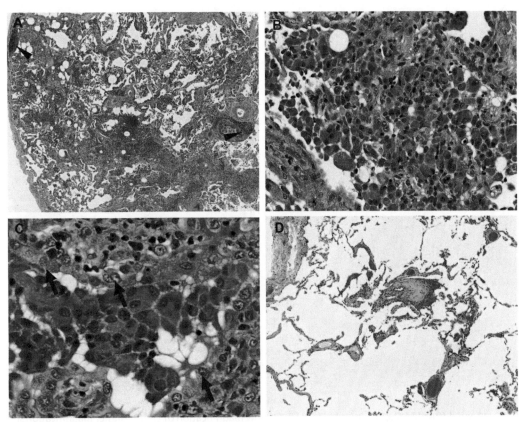

Fig. 13. DIP and respiratory bronchiolitis (RB). (*A*) Low magnification of DIP, which shows diffuse airspace filling by alveolar macrophages along with scattered lymphoid follicles (*arrowheads*). (*B*) Higher magnification of alveolar macrophages with characteristic light-brown pigment. (*C*) DIP is often associated with hyperplastic type II pneumocytes (*arrows*). (*D*) RB shows limited areas of airspace filling of macrophages around alveolar ducts. It may show inflammatory changes, such as airspace organization.

routes (**Fig. 14**D). A critical distinction is for malignant lymphoma, especially marginal zone B cell lymphoma.[99,100] Lymphoma commonly shows extension along lymphatic routes and shows monotonous features. Staining for immunoglobulin kappa/lambda light chains, may not be conclusive, and, in such cases, genetic analysis of heavy-chain restriction may be required for diagnosis.[101] The prognosis of marginal zone B cell lymphoma is often favorable and may not progress for decades. Use of chemotherapy is often not the primary recommendation, but follow-up to monitor the transformation into a diffuse large B cell lymphoma is suggested.

PLEUROPULMONARY FIBROELASTOSIS (PPFE)

PPFE was first proposed by Frankel and colleagues[102] as a form of ILD. With several subsequent pivotal reports, idiopathic PPFE was listed as one of the rare IIPs in the revised classification.[9] PPFE presents as an upper lobe–dominant progressive pulmonary fibrosis that often results in

shrinkage of upper lung and flattening of the chest. The reported prognosis of PPFE is poor, with a median survival of around 2 to 5 years.[103–105] Most PPFE cases are idiopathic; however, there are cases of PPFE secondary to bone marrow transplant as a manifestation of graft-versus-host disease (GVHD)[106] and CHP.[107,108]

The pathologic features of PPFE include linear or wedge-shaped dense elastofibrosis without visible residual alveolar sacs, complete filling of alveolar spaces by collagenous and elastic fibers, and often traction bronchiolectasis inside the fibrotic area (**Figs. 15**A, B). There is usually no architectural destruction and no breakdown of elastic fibers, a feature that can be highlighted by elastic staining. There is no obvious inflammatory infiltration and no honeycomb formation. The overlying pleura can be thickened by hyalinized fibrosis (**Fig. 15**C). PPFE is occasionally associated with interstitial emphysema, a cystic lesion surrounded by collagen and lacking epithelial covering. This occurrence of interstitial emphysema, alternatively called interstitial air cysts, can result in pneumothorax or

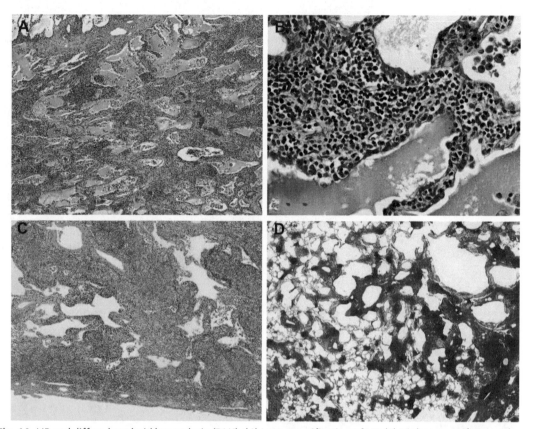

Fig. 14. LIP and diffuse lymphoid hyperplasia (DLH). (*A*) Low magnification of LIP. (*B*) Higher magnification shows compact lymphocytic infiltration along with plasma cells. Pink airspace exudate, often containing immune globulin, is a frequent finding. (*C*) Lymphoma often shows uniform-looking lymphocytic infiltration and involves the pleura. (*D*) Typical appearance of DLH. Note frequent lymphoid follicles with germinal center along the lymphatic route.

pneumomediastinum, and may be lethal. Donor lymphocyte attack of host pneumocytes has been reported as an event of GVHD resulting in wide denudation of epithelium and alveolar collapse[109] (**Fig. 15**D). Similar epithelial denudation may relate to idiopathic PPFE as a hypothetical pathogenesis.

Apical cap is a well-known and nonspecific finding in the lobar apices, mostly related to aging.[110] The histologic features of PPFE completely overlap with apical cap and their separation solely based on pathology is difficult or impossible. Another challenge is that PPFE can be associated with UIP or NSIP fibrosis in the lower lung.[111] There is little consensus on how those cases should be classified at this point.

RARE HISTOLOGIC PATTERNS, ACUTE FIBRINOUS AND ORGANIZING PNEUMONIA (AFOP), AND BRONCHIOLOCENTRIC PATTERN OF INTERSTITIAL PNEUMONIA

Two new categories are currently considered as provisional because there is insufficient clinical and radiological data available to establish them as new disease entities.

Acute Fibrinous and Organizing Pneumonia (AFOP)

AFOP is a histologic condition proposed by Beasley and colleagues[83] that shows acute lung injury pattern that does not fit neatly into DAD, OP, or eosinophilic pneumonia. As the name indicates, marked accumulation of intra-alveolar fibrin is observed, along with OP. The prototypical feature is appearance of a fibrin ball inside the airspace (**Fig. 16**A). The distribution of fibrin should be significant, occupying more than 50% of airspaces within the lesion. One important differential diagnosis is DAD, which is recognized by even a faint level of hyaline membrane formation. When a pattern of AFOP is found, prior consideration should be given to infection, such as *Pneumocystis*, and vasculitis including granulomatous polyangiitis, before considering idiopathic AFOP.

Bronchiolocentric Pattern of interstitial Pneumonia, Alternatively Airway-centered interstitial Fibrosis

Bronchiolocentric pattern of interstitial pneumonia (**Fig. 16**B) was recently proposed by 4 different groups under various names, such as

Table 7
Tips to separate common differential diagnosis of lymphoid interstitial pneumonia

Differential Diagnosis	Suggestive Findings	Opposed Findings (More Suggestive for DAD)
Cellular NSIP	OP	Pink airspace fluid, cystic change without fibrosis
Lymphoma	Pleural invasion, lymphatic accentuation, nodular change, necrosis, granuloma	Germinal center, fibrosis
LPD: MCD, and so forth	Frequent Russel bodies, LYGC	None
Connective tissue disease: SjS, RA	LYGC, dense fibrosis without cellular infiltration, honeycombing	None
CHP	Interstitial giant cell with cholesterol cleft, granuloma, PBM	Cystic change without fibrosis
HIV infection	Granuloma, foamy macrophage, edema	None
IgG4-related lung disease	Frequent Russel bodies, thickening/fibrosis of interlobular septa, nodular fibrosis	None

Abbreviations: HIV, human immunodeficiency virus; LPD, lymphoproliferative disease; MCD, multicentric Castleman disease; SjS, Sjögren syndrome.

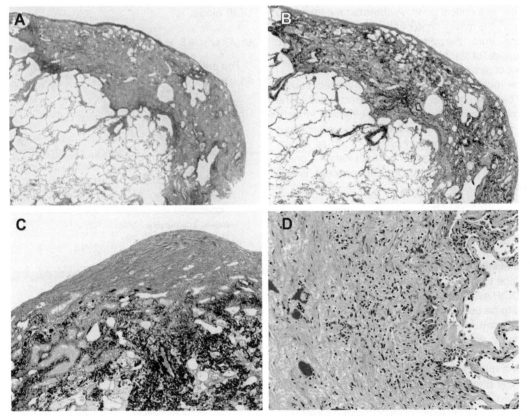

Fig. 15. PPFE. (*A*) Typical appearance of PPFE. (*B*) EVG staining highlights accumulation of elastic fibers. (*C*) Hyalinized thickening of pleura is a frequent event in PPFE. (*D*) PPFE caused by GVHD. The lymphocytes are infiltrating into epithelial cells, resulting in denudation of the pneumocytes.

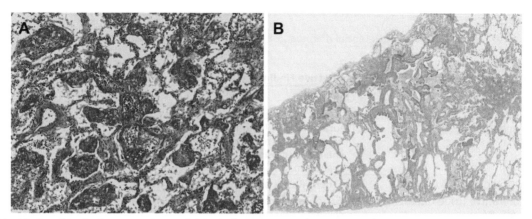

Fig. 16. Rare histologic patterns in IIPs. (*A*) Typical appearance of AFOP. Note the airspace filled with large fibrin balls. There is no associated architectural destruction. (*B*) Airway-centered interstitial fibrosis. Fibrotic areas are located away from pleura and involve respiratory bronchioles. Clear recognition of airway by bronchiolar metaplasia is a critical part of the identification of airway-centered accentuation.

bronchiolocentric interstitial pneumonia,[112] airway-centered interstitial fibrosis,[113] and peribronchiolar metaplasia (PBM) ILD.[114] There are significant overlaps among these reports; however, PBM-ILD may be different with regard to the lack of interstitial fibrosis. There are debates about whether those diseases are different from UIP. There are not enough data to give an answer, but accurate recognition of what designates the airway center is a critical point. A common mistake is to specify the airway center according to a gap or distance from the pleura or interlobular septa. Because of its complexity, interobserver agreement of airway-centered location is low.[115] Perivenular regions along the lymphatic vessels should not be misjudged as airway-centered lesions. The primary consideration of airway-centered interstitial pneumonia is not an idiopathic condition but injury associated with inhalation, such as hypersensitivity pneumonia or aspiration pneumonia.[116] Similar to AFOP, the concept is still provisional.

UNCLASSIFIABLE IDIOPATHIC INTERSTITIAL PNEUMONIAS (UCIP)

Pathologists sometimes confront cases that are difficult to categorize and that are in the category of UCIP even after MDD. UCIP is not recommended to be used as a pathologic diagnosis; however, it may be used in cases whose pathologic patterns do not fit into any specific type, those with a pattern indicating a new entity, or those with a mixture of more than 1 pattern. Examples are the previously discussed fibrosing OP[83] as a new entity, and mixture of UIP and PPFE.[111]

More common types of UCIP include cases that have features of either autoimmunity or hypersensitivity pneumonitis. Cases that are not fully diagnostic of connective tissue disease but show features of autoimmunity are currently clinically categorized as IPAF[62]; however, there is no such group for cases with features of hypersensitivity pneumonitis. At this point, a tentative diagnosis closest to the condition is preferable (ie, probable IPF, IPAF, or probable hypersensitivity pneumonitis), rather than giving a diagnosis of UCIP alone.

DISCLOSURE

The authors have no conflicts of interest for this article.

REFERENCES

1. Fernandez Perez ER, Daniels CE, Schroeder DR, et al. Incidence, prevalence, and clinical course of idiopathic pulmonary fibrosis: a population-based study. Chest 2010;137:129–37.
2. Bjoraker JA, Ryu JH, Edwin MK, et al. Prognostic significance of histopathologic subsets in idiopathic pulmonary fibrosis. Am J Respir Crit Care Med 1998;157:199–203.
3. King TE Jr, Tooze JA, Schwarz MI, et al. Predicting survival in idiopathic pulmonary fibrosis: scoring system and survival model. Am J Respir Crit Care Med 2001;164:1171–81.
4. Mapel DW, Hunt WC, Utton R, et al. Idiopathic pulmonary fibrosis: survival in population based and hospital based cohorts. Thorax 1998;53:469–76.
5. Schwartz DA, Helmers RA, Galvin JR, et al. Determinants of survival in idiopathic pulmonary fibrosis. Am J Respir Crit Care Med 1994;149:450–4.
6. Taniguchi H, Ebina M, Kondoh Y, et al, Pirfenidone Clinical Study Group in J. Pirfenidone in idiopathic pulmonary fibrosis. Eur Respir J 2010;35:821–9.

7. Richeldi L, du Bois RM, Raghu G, et al. Efficacy and safety of nintedanib in idiopathic pulmonary fibrosis. N Engl J Med 2014;370:2071–82.

8. American Thoracic S, European Respiratory S. American Thoracic Society/European Respiratory Society International Multidisciplinary Consensus Classification of the Idiopathic Interstitial Pneumonias. This joint statement of the American Thoracic Society (ATS), and the European Respiratory Society (ERS) was adopted by the ATS board of directors, June 2001 and by the ERS Executive Committee, June 2001. Am J Respir Crit Care Med 2002;165:277–304.

9. Travis WD, Costabel U, Hansell DM, et al. An official American Thoracic Society/European Respiratory Society statement: update of the international multidisciplinary classification of the idiopathic interstitial pneumonias. Am J Respir Crit Care Med 2013;188:733–48.

10. Yoshikawa A, Sato S, Tanaka T, et al. Breakdown of lung framework and an increase in pores of Kohn as initial events of emphysema and a cause of reduction in diffusing capacity. Int J Chron Obstruct Pulmon Dis 2016;11:2287–94.

11. Miller MS. The Lung. 2nd edition. Springfield (IL): Charles C. Thomas; 1947.

12. Basset F, Ferrans VJ, Soler P, et al. Intraluminal fibrosis in interstitial lung disorders. Am J Pathol 1986;122:443–61.

13. Katzenstein AL, Myers JL. Idiopathic pulmonary fibrosis: clinical relevance of pathologic classification. Am J Respir Crit Care Med 1998;157:1301–15.

14. Heppleston AG. The pathology of honeycomb lung. Thorax 1956;11:77–93.

15. Westcott JL, Cole SR. Traction bronchiectasis in end-stage pulmonary fibrosis. Radiology 1986;161:665–9.

16. Barcia SM, Kukreja J, Jones KD. Pulmonary interstitial emphysema in adults: a clinicopathologic study of 53 lung explants. Am J Surg Pathol 2014;38:339–45.

17. Tachibana Y, Taniguchi H, Kondoh Y, et al. Pulmonary interstitial emphysema is a risk factor for poor prognosis and a cause of air leaks. Respir Investig 2019;57(5):444–50.

18. Raghu G, Remy-Jardin M, Myers JL, et al, American Thoracic Society ERSJRS, Latin American Thoracic S. Diagnosis of idiopathic pulmonary fibrosis. An Official ATS/ERS/JRS/ALAT clinical practice guideline. Am J Respir Crit Care Med 2018;198:e44–68.

19. Walsh SLF, Wells AU, Desai SR, et al. Multicentre evaluation of multidisciplinary team meeting agreement on diagnosis in diffuse parenchymal lung disease: a case-cohort study. Lancet Respir Med 2016;4:557–65.

20. Song JW, Do KH, Kim MY, et al. Pathologic and radiologic differences between idiopathic and collagen vascular disease-related usual interstitial pneumonia. Chest 2009;136:23–30.

21. Ohtani Y, Saiki S, Kitaichi M, et al. Chronic bird fancier's lung: histopathological and clinical correlation. An application of the 2002 ATS/ERS consensus classification of the idiopathic interstitial pneumonias. Thorax 2005;60:665–71.

22. Churg A, Muller NL, Flint J, et al. Chronic hypersensitivity pneumonitis. Am J Surg Pathol 2006;30:201–8.

23. Kondoh Y, Taniguchi H, Kawabata Y, et al. Acute exacerbation in idiopathic pulmonary fibrosis. Analysis of clinical and pathologic findings in three cases. Chest 1993;103:1808–12.

24. Parambil JG, Myers JL, Ryu JH. Histopathologic features and outcome of patients with acute exacerbation of idiopathic pulmonary fibrosis undergoing surgical lung biopsy. Chest 2005;128:3310–5.

25. Babiak A, Hetzel J, Krishna G, et al. Transbronchial cryobiopsy: a new tool for lung biopsies. Respiration 2009;78:203–8.

26. Pajares V, Puzo C, Castillo D, et al. Diagnostic yield of transbronchial cryobiopsy in interstitial lung disease: a randomized trial. Respirology 2014;19:900–6.

27. Ravaglia C, Bonifazi M, Wells AU, et al. Safety and diagnostic yield of transbronchial lung cryobiopsy in diffuse parenchymal lung diseases: a comparative study versus video-assisted thoracoscopic lung biopsy and a systematic review of the literature. Respiration 2016;91:215–27.

28. Johannson KA, Marcoux VS, Ronksley PE, et al. Diagnostic yield and complications of transbronchial lung cryobiopsy for interstitial lung disease. a systematic review and metaanalysis. Ann Am Thorac Soc 2016;13:1828–38.

29. Carrington CB, Gaensler EA, Coutu RE, et al. Natural history and treated course of usual and desquamative interstitial pneumonia. N Engl J Med 1978;298:801–9.

30. Raghu G, Weycker D, Edelsberg J, et al. Incidence and prevalence of idiopathic pulmonary fibrosis. Am J Respir Crit Care Med 2006;174:810–6.

31. Behr J, Kreuter M, Hoeper MM, et al. Management of patients with idiopathic pulmonary fibrosis in clinical practice: the INSIGHTS-IPF registry. Eur Respir J 2015;46:186–96.

32. Raghu G, Collard HR, Egan JJ, et al, Fibrosis AE-JACoIP. An official ATS/ERS/JRS/ALAT statement: idiopathic pulmonary fibrosis: evidence-based guidelines for diagnosis and management. Am J Respir Crit Care Med 2011;183:788–824.

33. American Thoracic Society. Idiopathic pulmonary fibrosis: diagnosis and treatment. International consensus statement. American Thoracic Society

(ATS), and the European Respiratory Society (ERS). Am J Respir Crit Care Med 2000;161: 646–64.

34. Raghu G, Amatto VC, Behr J, et al. Comorbidities in idiopathic pulmonary fibrosis patients: a systematic literature review. Eur Respir J 2015;46: 1113–30.

35. Ozawa Y, Suda T, Naito T, et al. Cumulative incidence of and predictive factors for lung cancer in IPF. Respirology 2009;14:723–8.

36. Douglas WW, Ryu JH, Schroeder DR. Idiopathic pulmonary fibrosis: impact of oxygen and colchicine, prednisone, or no therapy on survival. Am J Respir Crit Care Med 2000;161:1172–8.

37. Nagao T, Nagai S, Hiramoto Y, et al. Serial evaluation of high-resolution computed tomography findings in patients with idiopathic pulmonary fibrosis in usual interstitial pneumonia. Respiration 2002; 69:413–9.

38. Katzenstein AL, Zisman DA, Litzky LA, et al. Usual interstitial pneumonia: histologic study of biopsy and explant specimens. Am J Surg Pathol 2002; 26:1567–77.

39. Flaherty KR, Colby TV, Travis WD, et al. Fibroblastic foci in usual interstitial pneumonia: idiopathic versus collagen vascular disease. Am J Respir Crit Care Med 2003;167:1410–5.

40. Travis WD, Matsui K, Moss J, et al. Idiopathic nonspecific interstitial pneumonia: prognostic significance of cellular and fibrosing patterns: survival comparison with usual interstitial pneumonia and desquamative interstitial pneumonia. The Am J Surg Pathol 2000;24:19–33.

41. Collard HR, Moore BB, Flaherty KR, et al, Idiopathic Pulmonary Fibrosis Clinical Research Network I. Acute exacerbations of idiopathic pulmonary fibrosis. Am J Respir Crit Care Med 2007;176: 636–43.

42. Collard HR, Ryerson CJ, Corte TJ, et al. Acute exacerbation of idiopathic pulmonary fibrosis. An international working group report. Am J Respir Crit Care Med 2016;194:265–75.

43. Ambrosini V, Cancellieri A, Chilosi M, et al. Acute exacerbation of idiopathic pulmonary fibrosis: report of a series. Eur Respir J 2003;22:821–6.

44. Silva CI, Muller NL, Fujimoto K, et al. Acute exacerbation of chronic interstitial pneumonia: high-resolution computed tomography and pathologic findings. J Thorac Imaging 2007;22:221–9.

45. Sakamoto K, Taniguchi H, Kondoh Y, et al. Acute exacerbation of idiopathic pulmonary fibrosis as the initial presentation of the disease. Eur Respir Rev 2009;18:129–32.

46. Kondoh Y, Taniguchi H, Kataoka K, et al, Tokai Diffuse Lung Disease Study Group. Prognostic factors in rapidly progressive interstitial pneumonia. Respirology 2010;15:257–64.

47. Rudd RM, Haslam PL, Turner-Warwick M. Cryptogenic fibrosing alveolitis. Relationships of pulmonary physiology and bronchoalveolar lavage to response to treatment and prognosis. Am Rev Respir Dis 1981;124:1–8.

48. Fukuda Y, Mochimaru H, Terasaki Y, et al. Mechanism of structural remodeling in pulmonary fibrosis. Chest 2001;120:41S–3S.

49. Urisman A, Jones KD. Pulmonary pathology in connective tissue disease. Semin Respir Crit Care Med 2014;35:201–12.

50. Omote N, Taniguchi H, Kondoh Y, et al. Lung-dominant connective tissue disease: clinical, radiologic, and histologic features. Chest 2015;148:1438–46.

51. Churg A, Wright JL, Ryerson CJ. Pathologic separation of chronic hypersensitivity pneumonitis from fibrotic connective tissue disease-associated interstitial lung disease. Am J Surg Pathol 2017;41: 1403–9.

52. Attanoos RL, Alchami FS, Pooley FD, et al. Usual interstitial pneumonia in asbestos-exposed cohorts - concurrent idiopathic pulmonary fibrosis or atypical asbestosis? Histopathology 2016;69:492–8.

53. Wick MR, Kendall TJ, Ritter JH. Asbestosis: demonstration of distinctive interstitial fibroelastosis: a pilot study. Ann Diagn Pathol 2009;13: 297–302.

54. Kawabata Y, Shimizu Y, Hoshi E, et al. Asbestos exposure increases the incidence of histologically confirmed usual interstitial pneumonia. Histopathology 2016;68:339–46.

55. Roggli VL, Gibbs AR, Attanoos R, et al. Pathology of asbestosis- an update of the diagnostic criteria: Report of the asbestosis committee of the college of american pathologists and pulmonary pathology society. Arch Pathol Lab Med 2010;134:462–80.

56. Chiba S, Tsuchiya K, Akashi T, et al. Chronic hypersensitivity pneumonitis with a usual interstitial pneumonia-like pattern: correlation between histopathologic and clinical findings. Chest 2016;149: 1473–81.

57. Ochi J, Ohtani Y, Takemura T, et al. Histological variability and consequences in chronic bird-related hypersensitivity pneumonitis. Respirology 2017;22:1350–6.

58. Selman M, Pardo A, King TE Jr. Hypersensitivity pneumonitis: insights in diagnosis and pathobiology. Am J Respir Crit Care Med 2012;186: 314–24.

59. Trahan S, Hanak V, Ryu JH, et al. Role of surgical lung biopsy in separating chronic hypersensitivity pneumonia from usual interstitial pneumonia/idiopathic pulmonary fibrosis: analysis of 31 biopsies from 15 patients. Chest 2008;134:126–32.

60. Yousem SA, Colby TV, Carrington CB. Lung biopsy in rheumatoid arthritis. Am Rev Respir Dis 1985; 131:770–7.

61. Ozasa M, Ichikawa H, Sato S, et al. Proposed method of histological separation between connective tissue disease-associated interstitial pneumonia and idiopathic interstitial pneumonias. PLoS One 2018;13:e0206186.

62. Fischer A, Antoniou KM, Brown KK, et al, CTD-ILD EATFoUFo. An official European Respiratory Society/American Thoracic Society research statement: interstitial pneumonia with autoimmune features. Eur Respir J 2015;46:976–87.

63. Akira M. High-resolution CT in the evaluation of occupational and environmental disease. Radiol Clin North Am 2002;40:43–59.

64. Staples CA. Computed tomography in the evaluation of benign asbestos-related disorders. Radiol Clin North Am 1992;30:1191–207.

65. Morisset J, Johannson KA, Jones KD, et al. Identification of diagnostic criteria for chronic hypersensitivity pneumonitis: an international modified delphi survey. Am J Respir Crit Care Med 2018; 197:1036–44.

66. Tabata K, Fukuoka J. Histopathologic features of usual interstitial pneumonia and related patterns: what is important for radiologists? Semin Ultrasound CT MR 2014;35:2–11.

67. Katzenstein AL, Fiorelli RF. Nonspecific interstitial pneumonia/fibrosis. Histologic features and clinical significance. Am J Surg Pathol 1994;18:136–47.

68. Travis WD, Hunninghake G, King TE Jr, et al. Idiopathic nonspecific interstitial pneumonia: report of an American Thoracic Society project. Am J Respir Crit Care Med 2008;177:1338–47.

69. Park IN, Jegal Y, Kim DS, et al. Clinical course and lung function change of idiopathic nonspecific interstitial pneumonia. Eur Respir J 2009; 33:68–76.

70. Hartman TE, Swensen SJ, Hansell DM, et al. Nonspecific interstitial pneumonia: variable appearance at high-resolution chest CT. Radiology 2000;217:701–5.

71. Johkoh T, Muller NL, Colby TV, et al. Nonspecific interstitial pneumonia: correlation between thin-section CT findings and pathologic subgroups in 55 patients. Radiology 2002;225:199–204.

72. Silva CI, Muller NL, Hansell DM, et al. Nonspecific interstitial pneumonia and idiopathic pulmonary fibrosis: changes in pattern and distribution of disease over time. Radiology 2008;247:251–9.

73. Suzuki A, Kondoh Y, Taniguchi H, et al. Lung histopathological pattern in a survivor with rapidly progressive interstitial lung disease and anti-melanoma differentiation-associated gene 5 antibody-positive clinically amyopathic dermatomyositis. Respir Med Case Rep 2016;19:5–8.

74. Tzelepis GE, Toya SP, Moutsopoulos HM. Occult connective tissue diseases mimicking idiopathic interstitial pneumonias. Eur Respir J 2008;31:11–20.

75. Honda T, Imaizumi K, Yokoi T, et al. Differential Th1/Th2 chemokine expression in interstitial pneumonia. Am J Med Sci 2010;339:41–8.

76. Drakopanagiotakis F, Polychronopoulos V, Judson MA. Organizing pneumonia. Am J Med Sci 2008;335:34–9.

77. Prasad R, Gupta P, Singh A, et al. Drug induced pulmonary parenchymal disease. Drug Discov Ther 2014;8:232–7.

78. Romero S, Barroso E, Rodriguez-Paniagua M, et al. Organizing pneumonia adjacent to lung cancer: frequency and clinico-pathologic features. Lung Cancer 2002;35:195–201.

79. Fukuda Y, Ishizaki M, Kudoh S, et al. Localization of matrix metalloproteinases-1, -2, and -9 and tissue inhibitor of metalloproteinase-2 in interstitial lung diseases. Lab Invest 1998;78:687–98.

80. Cohen AJ, King TE Jr, Downey GP. Rapidly progressive bronchiolitis obliterans with organizing pneumonia. Am J Respir Crit Care Med 1994;149:1670–5.

81. Epler GR. Bronchiolitis obliterans organizing pneumonia. Arch Intern Med 2001;161:158–64.

82. Nizami IY, Kissner DG, Visscher DW, et al. Idiopathic bronchiolitis obliterans with organizing pneumonia. An acute and life-threatening syndrome. Chest 1995;108:271–7.

83. Beasley MB, Franks TJ, Galvin JR, et al. Acute fibrinous and organizing pneumonia: a histological pattern of lung injury and possible variant of diffuse alveolar damage. Arch Pathol Lab Med 2002;126:1064–70.

84. Fischer A, Swigris JJ, du Bois RM, et al. Anti-synthetase syndrome in ANA and anti-Jo-1 negative patients presenting with idiopathic interstitial pneumonia. Respir Med 2009;103:1719–24.

85. Churg A, Wright JL, Bilawich A. Cicatricial organising pneumonia mimicking a fibrosing interstitial pneumonia. Histopathology 2018;72:846–54.

86. Yousem SA. Cicatricial variant of cryptogenic organizing pneumonia. Hum Pathol 2017;64:76–82.

87. Yoo JW, Song JW, Jang SJ, et al. Comparison between cryptogenic organizing pneumonia and connective tissue disease-related organizing pneumonia. Rheumatology 2011;50:932–8.

88. Olopade CO, Crotty TB, Douglas WW, et al. Chronic eosinophilic pneumonia and idiopathic bronchiolitis obliterans organizing pneumonia: comparison of eosinophil number and degranulation by immunofluorescence staining for eosinophil-derived major basic protein. Mayo Clinic Proc 1995;70:137–42.

89. Lohr RH, Boland BJ, Douglas WW, et al. Organizing pneumonia. Features and prognosis of cryptogenic, secondary, and focal variants. Arch Intern Med 1997;157:1323–9.

90. Beasley MB. The pathologist's approach to acute lung injury. Arch Pathol Lab Med 2010;134:719–27.

91. Tomashefski JF Jr. Pulmonary pathology of acute respiratory distress syndrome. Clin Chest Med 2000;21:435–66.

92. Ware LB. Pathophysiology of acute lung injury and the acute respiratory distress syndrome. Semin Respir Crit Care Med 2006;27:337–49.

93. Liebow AA, Steer A, Billingsley JG. Desquamative interstitial pneumonia. Am J Med 1965;39:369–404.

94. Myers JL, Veal CF Jr, Shin MS, et al. Respiratory bronchiolitis causing interstitial lung disease. A clinicopathologic study of six cases. Am Rev Respir Dis 1987;135:880–4.

95. Yousem SA, Colby TV, Gaensler EA. Respiratory bronchiolitis-associated interstitial lung disease and its relationship to desquamative interstitial pneumonia. Mayo Clinic Proc 1989;64:1373–80.

96. Hidalgo A, Franquet T, Gimenez A, et al. Smoking-related interstitial lung diseases: radiologic-pathologic correlation. Eur Radiol 2006;16: 2463–70.

97. Moon J, du Bois RM, Colby TV, et al. Clinical significance of respiratory bronchiolitis on open lung biopsy and its relationship to smoking related interstitial lung disease. Thorax 1999;54:1009–14.

98. Park JS, Brown KK, Tuder RM, et al. Respiratory bronchiolitis-associated interstitial lung disease: radiologic features with clinical and pathologic correlation. J Comput Assist Tomogr 2002;26:13–20.

99. Addis BJ, Hyjek E, Isaacson PG. Primary pulmonary lymphoma: a re-appraisal of its histogenesis and its relationship to pseudolymphoma and lymphoid interstitial pneumonia. Histopathology 1988;13:1–17.

100. Herbert A, Walters MT, Cawley MI, et al. Lymphocytic interstitial pneumonia identified as lymphoma of mucosa associated lymphoid tissue. J Pathol 1985;146:129–38.

101. Cazzola M. Introduction to a review series: the 2016 revision of the WHO classification of tumors of hematopoietic and lymphoid tissues. Blood 2016;127:2361–4.

102. Frankel SK, Cool CD, Lynch DA, et al. Idiopathic pleuroparenchymal fibroelastosis: description of a novel clinicopathologic entity. Chest 2004;126: 2007–13.

103. Ishii H, Watanabe K, Kushima H, et al. Pleuroparenchymal fibroelastosis diagnosed by multidisciplinary discussions in Japan. Respir Med 2018; 141:190–7.

104. Kato M, Sasaki S, Kurokawa K, et al. Usual interstitial pneumonia pattern in the lower lung lobes as a prognostic factor in idiopathic pleuroparenchymal fibroelastosis. Respiration 2019;97:319–28.

105. Watanabe K. Pleuroparenchymal fibroelastosis: its clinical characteristics. Curr Respir Med Rev 2013;9, 299-237.

106. Mariani F, Gatti B, Rocca A, et al. Pleuroparenchymal fibroelastosis: the prevalence of secondary forms in hematopoietic stem cell and lung transplantation recipients. Diagn Interv Radiol 2016;22: 400–6.

107. Khiroya R, Macaluso C, Montero MA, et al. Pleuroparenchymal fibroelastosis: a review of histopathologic features and the relationship between histologic parameters and survival. Am J Surg Pathol 2017;41:1683–9.

108. Reddy TL, Tominaga M, Hansell DM, et al. Pleuroparenchymal fibroelastosis: a spectrum of histopathological and imaging phenotypes. Eur Respir J 2012;40:377–85.

109. Oo ZP, Bychkov A, Zaizen Y, et al. Combination of pleuroparenchymal fibroelastosis with non-specific interstitial pneumonia and bronchiolitis obliterans as a complication of hematopoietic stem cell transplantation - Clues to a potential mechanism. Respir Med Case Rep 2019;26:244–7.

110. Yousem SA. Pulmonary apical cap: a distinctive but poorly recognized lesion in pulmonary surgical pathology. Am J Surg Pathol 2001;25:679–83.

111. Enomoto N, Kusagaya H, Oyama Y, et al. Quantitative analysis of lung elastic fibers in idiopathic pleuroparenchymal fibroelastosis (IPPFE): comparison of clinical, radiological, and pathological findings with those of idiopathic pulmonary fibrosis (IPF). BMC Pulm Med 2014;14:91.

112. Yousem SA, Dacic S. Idiopathic bronchiolocentric interstitial pneumonia. Mod Pathol 2002;15: 1148–53.

113. Churg A, Myers J, Suarez T, et al. Airway-centered interstitial fibrosis: a distinct form of aggressive diffuse lung disease. Am J Surg Pathol 2004;28:62–8.

114. Fukuoka J, Franks TJ, Colby TV, et al. Peribronchiolar metaplasia: a common histologic lesion in diffuse lung disease and a rare cause of interstitial lung disease: clinicopathologic features of 15 cases. Am J Surg Pathol 2005;29:948–54.

115. Hashisako M, Tanaka T, Terasaki Y, et al. Interobserver agreement of usual interstitial pneumonia diagnosis correlated with patient outcome. Arch Pathol Lab Med 2016;140:1375–82.

116. Kuranishi LT, Leslie KO, Ferreira RG, et al. Airway-centered interstitial fibrosis: etiology, clinical findings and prognosis. Respir Res 2015;16:55.

Lung Transplant Pathology
An Overview on Current Entities and Procedures

Christopher Werlein[a],*, Allison Seidel[a,b],
Gregor Warnecke, MD[b,c], Jens Gottlieb, MD[b,d],
Florian Laenger, MD[a,b,1], Danny Jonigk, FRCPath[a,b,1]

KEYWORDS

- Acute cellular rejection • Acute antibody-mediated rejection • Chronic lung allograft dysfunction
- Lung transplant • Alveolar fibroelastosis

Key points

- Acute cellular and antibody-mediated rejection lead to acute graft dysfunction and predisposition to chronic lung allograft dysfunction.

- Histopathologic analysis of biopsy material remains the gold standard for the diagnosis of acute cellular rejection because no other reliable and specific clinical tests are available so far.

- Acute antibody-mediated rejection is a widely recognized entity requiring comprehensive analysis of clinical, serologic, microbial, and histopathologic results for its correct diagnosis.

- Important differential diagnoses for acute rejection are infections and posttransplant lymphoproliferative disorder, whose identification can be challenging by conventional histopathology.

- Specialized histologic tools such as immunohistochemistry and molecular pathology can significantly improve the diagnostic reliability regarding differentiation between alloimmune reactions and infections or other causes, and their integration into the diagnostic work-up is strongly recommended.

ABSTRACT

Alloimmune reactions are, besides various infections, the major cause for impaired lung allograft function following transplant. Acute cellular rejection is not only a major trigger of acute allograft failure but also contributes to development of chronic lung allograft dysfunction. Analogous to other solid organ transplants, acute antibody-mediated rejection has become a recognized entity in lung transplant pathology. Adequate sensitivity and specificity in the diagnosis of alloimmune reactions in the lung can only be achieved by synoptic analysis of histopathologic, clinical, and radiological findings together with serologic and microbiologic findings.

Contributors: C. Werlein prepared the images. A. Seidel and J. Gottlieb prepared the tables. C. Werlein, A. Seidel, J. Gottlieb, G. Warnecke, F. Laenger, and D. Jonigk wrote the article. Grant numbers and sources of support: Sonderforschungsbereich, SFB' 738 (Projekt B9) of the German Research Foundation to D. Jonigk and F. Laenger. The grants of the European Research Council (ERC); European Consolidator Grant, XHale to D. Jonigk (ref. no.771883).
[a] Institute for Pathology, OE 5110, Hannover Medical School, Carl-Neuberg-Str. 1, Hannover 30625, Germany; [b] Biomedical Research in Endstage and Obstructive Lung Disease Hannover (BREATH); [c] Department of Cardiac, Thoracic, Transplantation and Vascular Surgery, OE6210, Hannover Medical School, Carl-Neuberg-Str. 1, Hannover 30625, Germany; [d] Department of Pneumology, OE6210, Hannover Medical School, Carl-Neuberg-Str. 1, Hannover 30625, Germany
[1] These authors contributed equally and share last authorship.
* Corresponding author.
E-mail address: Werlein.Christopher@mh-hannover.de

Surgical Pathology 13 (2020) 119–140
https://doi.org/10.1016/j.path.2019.11.003

Abbreviations

ACR	Acute cellular rejection
AFE	Alveolar fibroelastosis
AMR	Antibody-mediated rejection
ARAD	Azithromycin-responsive allograft dysfunction
BAL	Broncho alveolar lavages
BO	Bronchiolitis obliterans
BOS	Bronchiolitis obliterans syndrome
C4d	Complement Compound 4d
CD3	Cluster of Differentiation 3
CD8	Cluster of Differentiation 8
CLAD	Chronic lung allograft dysfunction
CMV	Cytomegalovirus
Col-V	Collagen V
COPD	Chronic obstructive pulmonary disease
C-X-C motif	C-X-C motif chemokine
CXCL-1	C-X-C motif chemokine ligand 1
CXCR2	C-X-C motif chemokine receptor 2
DSA	Donor-specific antigens
EBV	Epstein-Barr virus
FEV1	Forced expiratory volume in 1 second
FVC	Forced vital capacity
GERD	Gastroesophageal reflux disease
HLA	Human leukocyte antigens
HRCT	High-resolution computed tomography
HSV	Herpes simplex virus
IL-17	Interleukin 17
IL-8	Interleukin-8
ISHLT	International Society of Heart and Lung Transplantation
Kα1T	K-alpha 1 tubulin
LuTx	Lung transplant
NRAD	Neutrophilic reversible allograft dysfunction
oCLAD	Obstructive chronic lung allograft dysfunction
OP	Organizing pneumonia
P2X7	P2X purinoceptor 7
PAS	Periodic acidic shift
PGD	Primary graft dysfunction
PPFE	Pleuroparenchymal fibroelastosis
PTLD	Posttransplant lymphoproliferative disorder
pVOD	Pulmonary veno-occlusive disease
RAS	Restrictive allograft syndrome
ROS	Reactive oxygen species
SAG	Self-antigen
TGF-β	Transforming growth factor β
WHO	World Health Organization

OVERVIEW

Since the first human lung transplant (LuTX) in 1963,[1] LuTX has been established as the only definite treatment modality for end-stage lung disease. Overall survival of LuTx recipients increased from 4.2 years in the 1990s to 6.1 years in the 2000s.[2] Standardized and improved surgical techniques, immunosuppressive regimens, as well as clinical follow-up reduced the mortality and morbidity within the first year post-transplant, contributing to survival rates of 80% to 90%.[3] However, the incidence and detrimental role of chronic lung allograft dysfunction (CLAD) remains the major limiting factor for survival of LuTX patients and is the major reason why the survival rates are still significantly lower compared with other solid organ transplant recipients. Main causes of death within 30 days after LuTx are graft failure (24.7%), infections (19.6%), cardiovascular complications (10.9%), technical complications (11%), acute rejection (3.4%), malignancies (0.2%), and other causes (29.8%). In contrast, 1 year after LuTx, CLAD is by far the most common cause of death, followed by infections, allograft failure of other causes besides CLAD, and malignancy (**Table 1**).[4] So far no clinical testing alone allows the determination of the possible causes of lung function impairment of LuTx patients, thus histopathologic assessment of posttransplant lung biopsies is a main element of the interdisciplinary diagnostic work-up and correct treatment of both acute graft rejection and chronical failure. In this article, the major histopathologic changes and criteria for infection, acute rejection, and CLAD are discussed.

EARLY COMPLICATIONS FOLLOWING TRANSPLANT

Primary graft dysfunction (PGD) is the most important early postoperative complication,[5] followed by pneumonia, rare hyperacute rejection, and scarce surgery-associated complications, especially dehiscence or necrosis of the bronchial anastomosis (see **Table 1**).[6,7] Ischemic reperfusion injury with subsequent cellular oxidative stress, induction of apoptosis, as well as increased leukocyte adhesion with activation of the complement system levels is the trigger for PGD. On the histomorphologic level, this results in an acute lung injury pattern with endothelial and epithelial necrosis, interstitial edema, and intra-alveolar fibrin deposition, summarized as diffuse alveolar damage.[8,9] These findings are not pathognomonic for PGD but may be seen as the sequelae of infection (see **Fig. 9**) and of high-grade acute cellular rejection (ACR) as well (discussed later). Hyperacute graft rejection as another potential cause for PGD would be caused by acute antibody-mediated rejection (AMR; discussed later), which is seen extremely rarely these days because of improved compatibility pretransplant testing.[9] However, in these situations, biopsy material is only sampled in rare cases because the correct diagnosis can usually be obtained by the clinical and radiological findings and because the biopsy procedure–associated morbidity in these critically ill patients is unacceptably high.

ALLOIMMUNE RESPONSE

Alloimmune responses can lead to acute rejection (eg, ACR and AMR; discussed later) and

---

Table 1
Causes of deaths for adult lung transplant recipients

Cause of Death	0–30 d (%)	>1–3 y (%)	> 3–5 y (%)	>5–10 y (%)	>10 y (%)
Bronchiolitis	0.3	25.9	29.0	25.4	20.9
Acute rejection	3.4	1.5	0.7	0.6	0.2
Malignancy	0.2	9.4	12.4	15.0	16.0
Infection	19.6	38	19.5	18.2	17.2
Graft failure	24.7	16.7	18.0	17.8	17.4
Cardiovascular	10.9	4.8	4.9	5.1	6.5
Technical	11.0	3.4	0.6	0.8	0.9
Other	29.8	25.6	15.1	17.0	20.9

Data from Yusen RD, Christie JD, Edwards LB, et al. The registry of the international society for heart and lung transplantation: Thirtieth adult lung and heart-lung transplant report - 2013; Focus theme: Age. *J Hear Lung Transplant.* 2013;32(10):965-978.

contribute to chronic lung dysfunction (eg, CLAD; discussed later). The correct histologic identification of respective histologic injury patterns as well as the differentiation from other disorders in lung biopsy samples is of the utmost importance.

An analysis of more than 500 patients transplanted at Hannover School of Medicine between 2009 and 2013 showed that approximately 30% of LuTx recipients are affected by an acute graft rejection within the first year posttransplant.[10] According to the International Society of Heart and Lung Transplantation (ISHLT), acute graft rejection accounts for 3.8% and 1.8% of deaths within the first month posttransplant and between 1 month and 1 year after transplant, respectively.[11,12] Acute graft rejection can be either cell mediated (ACR) or antibody related (AMR). ACR is mainly mediated via T lymphocytes recognizing primarily human leukocyte antigens (HLAs) and other donor-mediated antigens,[11] whereas, in AMR, preformed or de novo–synthetized antibodies directed against recipient antigens as well as HLAs are thought to be the driving cause of rejection.[11] Clinically, a decrease in forced expiratory volume in 1 second (FEV1) is the major symptom and can be accompanied by dyspnea, fever, and leukocytosis. This symptom is very sensitive but lacks specificity; thus, the clinical differentiation between acute graft rejection and other complications or diseases (eg, pulmonary infections) is very challenging. Therefore, the histopathologic examination of biopsy samples in concert with clinical, radiological, microbiological, and serologic findings is the gold standard for the correct subdiagnosis of acute graft rejection.

Transbronchial biopsies should consist of at least 5 aerated tissue samples and should be fixated in 5% buffered formaldehyde immediately after acquisition before paraffin embedding. Gentle agitation of the sample vial may contribute to better unfolding of the alveoli. At least 3 cuts of each paraffin block should be stained, besides standard hematoxylin-eosin, with periodic acid–Schiff (PAS) reaction, as well as a staining for connective tissues (eg, elastica van Gieson). Additional staining for specific pathogens (eg, Ziehl-Neesen, Grocott), immunohistochemical staining for viral pathogens (eg, cytomegalovirus [CMV], herpes simplex virus [HSV], adenovirus), and detection of T-lymphocyte presence (CD3) or complement activation (C4d) are optional and should be considered according to clinical and histomorphologic findings.

In 2007, the ISHLT published an update of the Working Formulation for the Standardization of Nomenclature in the Diagnosis of Lung Rejection, a structured guideline for the assessment of inflammatory and structural changes taking into account characteristics, extent, and anatomic localization of changes in posttransplant lung biopsy samples: (1) acute rejection, (2) small airway inflammation, (3) chronic airway rejection (eg, obliterative bronchiolitis), (4) chronic vascular rejection (accelerated graft vascular sclerosis), and (5) large bronchial inflammation.[13,14] Although there is a significant interobserver and intraobserver variability in grading, which has been shown to potentially affect treatment and outcome,[11,15–18] the ISHLT grading system is still the recommended tool to evaluate posttransplant lung transbronchial biopsies in a standardized manner.

GRADE A: ACUTE CELLULAR REJECTION

Correct grading of ACR (A0–A4) is of utmost importance because treatment regimens differ drastically between mild and severe ACR. ACR grading is primarily based on the degree of perivascular inflammation in the alveolar parenchyma and secondly on the presence or absence of adjacent injury patterns in the lung (Fig. 1, Table 2).

Grade A0 (no ACR) is defined as normal parenchyma without evidence of mononuclear cell infiltration, hemorrhage, or necrosis. In grade A1 (minimal ACR), focal circular mononuclear cell infiltrates of up to 3 layers wide are seen around small blood vessels, usually without evidence for endothelialitis (discussed later) or concomitant eosinophils. Grade A2 (mild ACR) manifests as a mononuclear cell infiltrate around blood vessels visible at scanning magnification, potentially accompanied by infiltration of the perivascular stroma. Furthermore, endothelialitis, characterized by subendothelial lymphocytes, signs of endothelial activation, and eosinophils, can be present. Concurrent lymphocytic bronchiolitis is more often present in grade A2 rejection, compared with grade A1. The extent of mononuclear cell infiltrates increases in grade A3 (moderate ACR), showing an expansion into the adjacent peribronchial alveolar septa and spaces, as well as infiltrates of neutrophils and eosinophils. Endothelialitis is a common finding. Moreover, aggregates of intra-alveolar macrophages in the areas of septal infiltration and type 2 cell hyperplasia may be present. Diffuse perivascular, interstitial, and air-space infiltrates by mononuclear cells with prominent alveolar epithelial damage and endothelialitis are correlates of grade A4 (severe ACR). In addition, intra-alveolar necrotic epithelial cells, macrophages, hyaline membranes, hemorrhage, and neutrophils, as well as parenchymal necrosis, infarction, or necrotizing

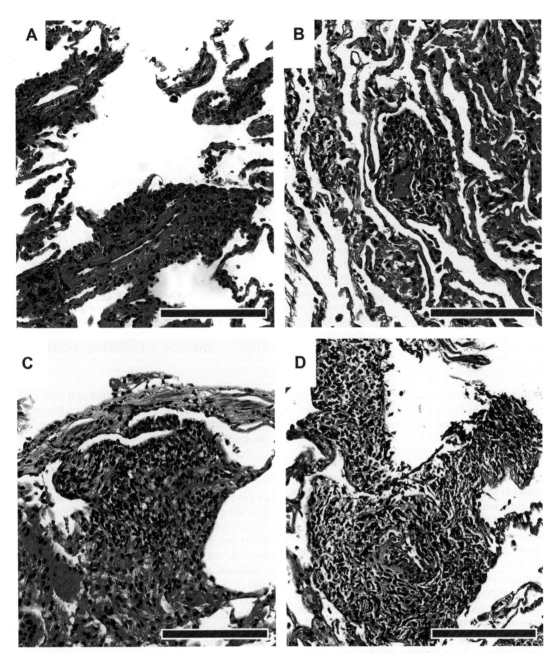

Fig. 1. Grading of ACR (ISHLT grade A). (*A*) Minimal acute cellular rejection (ACR) (A1): focal circular mononuclear cell infiltrates of up to 3 layers around small blood vessels without evidence for endothelialitis. (*B*) Mild ACR (A2): mononuclear cell infiltrate around blood vessels visible at scanning magnification and accompanied by infiltration of the perivascular stroma and endothelialitis, with subendothelial lymphocytes. (*C*) Mild ACR (A2): more severe case of a grade A2 rejection. Note that the mononuclear cell infiltrate does not spill over into the adjacent alveolar spaces, so the case was not classified as grade A3. (*D*) Moderate ACR (A3): mononuclear cell infiltrates increase in grade A3, showing an expansion into the adjacent peribronchial alveolar septa and spaces, accompanied by neutrophils and eosinophils as well as by endothelialitis (hematoxylin-eosin, original magnification ×100; scale bar, 300 μm).

vasculitis, may be found. The histomorphology of grade A4 rejection in part resembles acute posttransplant lung injury, and these entities must be strictly distinguished, because therapeutic consequences greatly diverge. Grade AX is assigned if there is no, or only scarce, alveolar parenchyma present in the biopsy material.[11,13] However, the described pattern of lymphocytic

Table 2
Histopathologic criteria for graduation of acute cellular rejection (International Society of Heart and Lung Transplantation A)

A0 (no ACR)	Normal parenchyma without evidence of mononuclear cell infiltration, hemorrhage or necrosis
AX (no evaluation possible)	No or only scarce lung parenchyma in the received biopsy material
A1 (minimal ACR)	Focal circular mononuclear cell infiltrates of up to 3 layers around small blood vessels are present without evidence for endothelialitis or eosinophils
A2 (mild ACR)	Mononuclear cell infiltrate around blood vessels visible on scanning magnification and potential infiltration of the perivascular stroma without alveolar infiltrates. Endothelialitis and eosinophils can be present
A3 (moderate ACR)	The degree of mononuclear cell infiltrates increases in grade A3, showing an expansion into adjacent peribronchial alveolar septae and spaces as well as infiltrates of neutrophils and eosinophils. Endothelialitis is a common finding. Moreover, aggregates of intra-alveolar macrophages in the zones of septal infiltration and type 2 alveolar cell hyperplasia may be present
A4 (severe ACR)	Diffuse perivascular, interstitial, and intra-alveolar aggregates of mononuclear cells with prominent pneumocyte damage and endothelialitis. In addition, intra-alveolar necrotic epithelial cells, macrophages, hyaline membranes, hemorrhage, and neutrophils as well as parenchymal necrosis, infarction, or necrotizing vasculitis can be found

infiltration is by itself not pathognomonic for the diagnosis of ACR because especially viral infection can closely mimic these patterns.

GRADES B AND E: AIRWAY INFLAMMATION

Inflammation of the small, noncartilaginous bronchioles is scored as B grade, inflammation of large cartilaginous bronchi is addressed in grade E (discussed later). Because pulmonary infections associated with airway inflammation are a common complication in transplanted patients, acute infection must be excluded before ascribing the histomorphologic findings to an alloimmune reaction. Following the ACR definitions, grade Bx describes biopsies limited by sampling problems, infection, tangential cutting, and so forth, and grade B0 is assigned in cases lacking evidence of bronchiolar inflammation. The former separation into 4 different levels of severity (B1–B4) was abandoned for only 2 grades (B1R and B2R) for the sake of improved reproducibility. Grade B1R (low-grade small airway inflammation) is defined by mononuclear infiltrates of the bronchiolar submucosa (either partial or circumferential), submucosal eosinophils, and only rare intraepithelial lymphocytes, whereas epithelial damage is absent. In contrast, in grade B2R (high-grade small airway inflammation), mononuclear infiltrates show signs of activation with an increase of eosinophils and plasmacytoid cells. In addition, intraepithelial lymphocytes and epithelial damage in the form of metaplasia and necrosis are found and can, in severe cases, lead to epithelial ulceration, fibrinopurulent exudate, intraluminal cellular detritus, and neutrophilic granulocytes (**Fig. 2, Table 3**). Disproportionally high numbers of neutrophilic granulocytes, compared with the submucosal mononuclear cell infiltrate, are highly suggestive of infection rather than an alloimmune response.[19] In these cases, an interdisciplinary synopsis of histomorphologic findings, bronchoalveolar lavage (BAL) results, clinical assessment, and serologic findings are useful to make the correct diagnosis.

Of note, inflammatory infiltrates of the bronchioles (B1R or B2R) can expand to alveolar vessels in the direct vicinity, mimicking ACR. Henceforth, ACR should only be addressed in these cases if there is at least 1 layer of inflammation-free alveoli between the inflammatory infiltrates of the bronchioles and the arteriole. Otherwise, it should be classified as B1R/B2R and A0.

GRADE C: OBLITERATIVE BRONCHIOLITIS

In biopsy specimens, bronchiolitis obliterans (BO) is characterized by an eccentric/concentric submucosal deposition of extracellular matrix with bronchial stenosis and infiltration by mononuclear cells as well as smooth muscle layer/elastic fiber destruction, accompanied by hypertrophy and hyperplasia of the remaining smooth muscle cells (**Fig. 3**). Furthermore, bronchiolar ectasia with or without mucostasis and squamous cell metaplasia can be found. However,

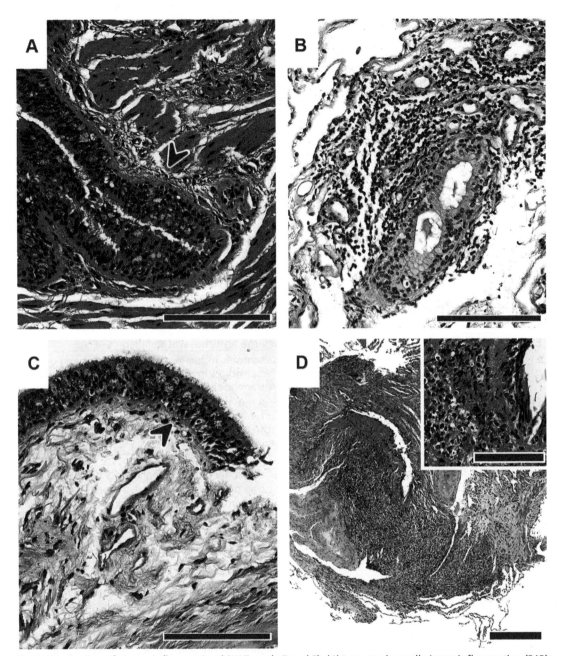

Fig. 2. Graduation of airway inflammation (ISHLT grade B and E). (*A*) Low-grade small airway inflammation (B1R): mononuclear infiltrates of the bronchiolar submucosa, either infrequent or circumferential; submucosal eosinophils; and only singular intraepithelial lymphocytes without signs of epithelial damage. Arrowhead points to submucosal mononuclear cells (hematoxylin-eosin, original magnification ×100; scale bar 300 μm). (*B*) High-grade small airway inflammation (B2R): mononuclear infiltrates show signs of activation with an increase of eosinophils, plasmacytoid cells, and intraepithelial lymphocytes (hematoxylin-eosin, original magnification ×100; scale bar 300 μm). (*C*) Low-grade large-airway inflammation (E1): mild chronic inflammation with a sparse band of lymphocytes in the subepithelium and occasional intraepithelial lymphocytes. Arrowhead points to submucosal mononuclear cells (hematoxylin-eosin, original magnification ×100; scale bar 300 μm). (*D*) High-grade large-airway inflammation (E2): moderate to severe chronic inflammation with a prominent subepithelial band of lymphocytes, scattered intraepithelial lymphocytes, and focal epithelial cell necrosis (hematoxylin-eosin, original magnification ×50; scale bar, 300 μm). (*Inset*) Higher magnification of (*D*) with distinct intraepithelial lymphocytes (hematoxylin-eosin, original magnification ×200; scale bar, 50 μm).

Table 3
Histopathologic criteria for the graduation of acute airway inflammation (lymphocytic bronchiolitis and bronchitis) (International Society of Heart and Lung Transplantation B/E)

Graduation of small-airway lymphocytic bronchitis	
Grade B0 (no bronchiolar inflammation)	No bronchiolar inflammation
BX (sampling error)	Biopsies limited by sampling errors, infection, tangential cutting and so forth
B1R (low-grade small airway inflammation)	Infrequent mononuclear infiltrates of the submucosa in small bronchioli, submucosal eosinophils, and only rarely intraepithelial lymphocytes. No completely missing epithelial damage
B2R (high-grade small airway inflammation)	Mononuclear infiltrates show signs of activation with an increase in eosinophils and plasmacytoid cells. In addition, intraepithelial lymphocytes and epithelial damage in the form of metaplasia and necrosis are found and can, in severe cases, lead to epithelial ulceration, fibrinopurulent exudate and intraluminal cellular debris, and neutrophil granulocytes
Graduation of large-airway lymphocytic bronchitis	
E0	No inflammation
EX	No large bronchus was sampled
E1	Mild chronic inflammation with a thin band of lymphocytes in the subepithelium and occasional intraepithelial lymphocytes
E2	Moderate to severe chronic inflammation with a prominent subepithelial band of lymphocytes, scattered intraepithelial lymphocytes, and epithelial cell necrosis

this process manifests heterogeneously, as Verleden and colleagues[22] have shown: only sparse bronchioles with a diameter more than 2 mm, approximately 50% of bronchioli with a diameter of 1 to 2 mm, and most small bronchioles with a diameter less than 1 mm are affected. Thus, sensitivity for BO in transbronchial biopsies of patients with CLAD is less than 5%,[20–22] and definite histopathologic proof of the diagnosis of BO, a substantial hallmark of obstructive CLAD (oCLAD) (discussed later) can only be attained by a systematic work-up of the (explanted) allograft.[23] However, BO is not exclusively found as a sign of CLAD and can also manifest in the nontransplant setting after viral infection (caused by adenoviruses, measles, influenza, respiratory syncytial virus, mycoplasma[24]) or following chemical exposition to organic ketones[25,26] or mustard gas.[27,28] Furthermore, BO must be histomorphologically separated from the organizing pneumonia (OP) lung injury pattern (formerly BO OP), a common and unspecific epiphenomenon found in various clinical settings.[29,30] On histology OP is characterized by loosely organized granulation tissue and polypoid aggregates of activated myofibroblasts, embedded in extracellular matrix extending into bronchiolar and alveolar airspaces.

Thus, the correct diagnosis of oCLAD is a diagnosis of exclusion and relies mostly on the incorporation of clinical and radiological findings, with transbronchial biopsies being of only minor importance.

GRADE D: CHRONIC VASCULAR REJECTION

Analogous to CLAD, chronic progressive vascular rejection is a multifactorial process, visible on histopathologic examination by fibrotic remodeling of both arteries and veins. Affected veins show a fiber-rich concentric or eccentric intima and media hyperplasia and potential hyaline sclerosis. In accordance with the classification of chronic airway rejection, D0 has no evidence for vascular remodeling, whereas D1 has[13] (**Fig. 4**). Notably, histologic changes of chronic vascular rejection can usually only be properly assessed in lung explants or open lung biopsy specimens.

GRADE E: LARGE-AIRWAY LYMPHOCYTIC BRONCHITIS

Inflammation in large cartilaginous bronchi is represented in grade E and was introduced

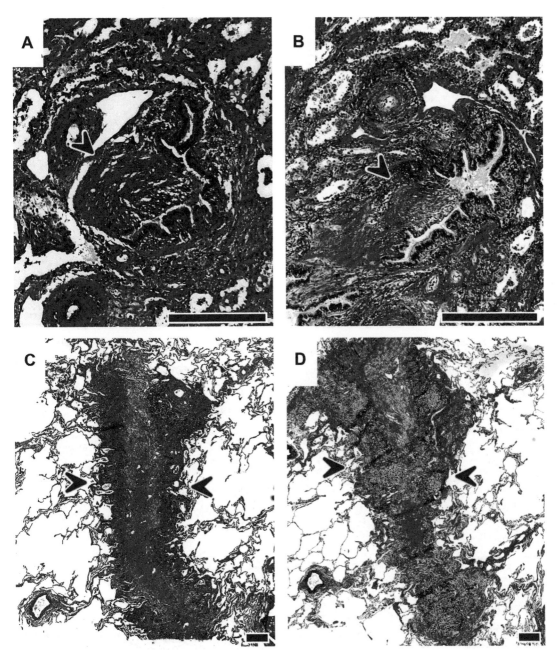

Fig. 3. BO (ISHLT C1). (*A, B*) Incipient BO: eccentric submucosal deposition of extracellular matrix with bronchial stenosis and smooth muscle layer/elastic fiber destruction accompanied by hypertrophy and hyperplasia of the remaining smooth muscle cells. Arrowhead points to submucosal extracellular matrix ([*A*] hematoxylin-eosin, original magnification ×40, scale bar 300 μm; [*B*] elastica van Gieson, original magnification ×40; scale bar, 300 μm. (*C, D*) Advanced BO: complete obliteration of a larger airway with extracellular matrix and smooth muscle cells. Arrowheads trace the airway. ([*C*] hematoxylin-eosin, original magnification ×40, scale bar, 300 μm; [*D*] elastica van Gieson, original magnification ×40; scale bar, 300 μm).

analogous to the ISHLT revised B grading by Greenland and colleagues[14] in 2012. Grade E0 denotes no inflammation; grade E1 is defined by mild chronic inflammation with a sparse band of lymphocytes in the subepithelial space and occasional intraepithelial lymphocytes; in grade E2, moderate to severe chronic inflammation with a prominent subepithelial band of lymphocytes, scattered intraepithelial lymphocytes, and epithelial cell necrosis are found. Grade EX is used if no classifiable bronchus tissue was sampled (see **Fig. 2, Table 3**).

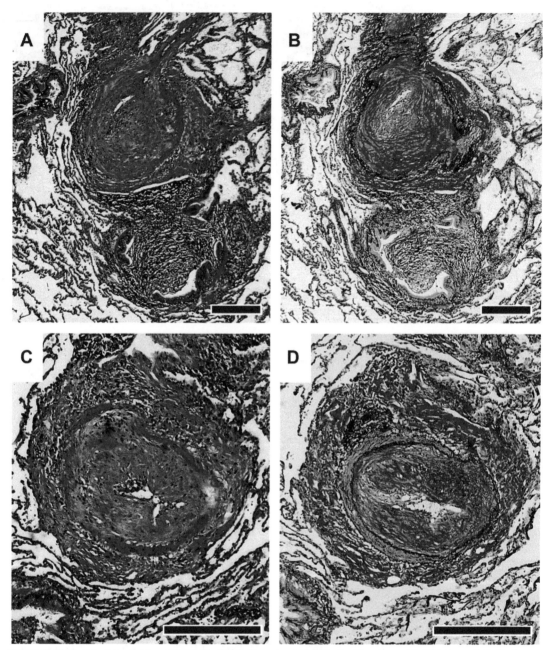

Fig. 4. Chronic vascular rejection (ISHLT D). (*A, B*) Chronic vascular rejection. Eccentric intima and media hyperplasia of a lung artery next to a bronchiole ([*A*] hematoxylin-eosin, original magnification ×20, scale bar, 300 μm; [*B*] elastica van Gieson, original magnification ×20; scale bar, 300 μm). (*C, D*) Chronic vascular rejection. Concentric stenosing intima and media hyperplasia of a pulmonary artery ([*C*] hematoxylin-eosin, original magnification ×20, scale bar 300 μm; [*D*] elastica van Gieson, original magnification ×20; scale bar 300 μm).

ACUTE ANTIBODY-MEDIATED REJECTION

Over the years AMR leading to acute and chronic graft rejection[31] in transplanted lungs grew from a highly controversial concept to an accepted entity. At present, preformed (because of pregnancy, blood transfusions, or previous organ transplant) or de novo–synthesized antibodies of the graft recipient (donor-specific antigens [DSAs]), mainly directed against HLAs on the endothelium of small blood vessels, are thought to play the key role in AMR.[32] One year posttransplant DSAs are detectable in between 10% and 61% of organ recipients,[33,34] although not all DSA-positive recipients develop AMR and there are certain cases of AMR without detectable DSAs against HLA. In these patients, antibodies directed against epithelial cells, referred to as non-HLA DSA or tissue self-antigens (SAGs), such as K-alpha 1 tubulin (Kα1T) and collagen V (Col-V), are being discussed as possible triggers for AMR and subsequent development of CLAD.[35–37] Furthermore, DSAs are also thought to play a role not only in AMR but also in hyperacute rejection.[38–45] Graft injury by pathologic activation of the recipient's immune system via DSA can either occur through activation of the complement system (classic pathway) or through complement-independent attraction and activation of inflammatory cells, such as macrophages, natural killer cells, and neutrophils via the FC-receptor subunit of immunoglobulins.

In contrast with ACR, there are no definite histomorphologic injury patterns associated with AMR. At present, the correct diagnostic of AMR relies on a combination of clinical features, serology, histopathology, and immunologic findings.[11,32] Indicative histologic patterns are the presence of neutrophilic capillaritis with marginalization of neutrophils, arteritis, and necrosis of capillaries and alveolar septae (see **Fig. 6**). Recently, Calabrese and colleagues[46] reported an alveolar septal widening as another potential marker for AMR. C4d as an immunohistochemical marker for complement system activity in pulmonary capillaries is an additional criterion for the presence of AMR (**Fig. 5**). However, C4d staining is rarely positive in transplant transbronchial biopsies. However, lately the role of C4d for the diagnostic identification of AMR has been questioned. There is a high interobserver variability in C4d examination,[47] and positive C4d staining in otherwise diagnosed AMR without evidence for DSA is exceptionally rare.[11,48] Furthermore, there seems to be no definite correlation between positive staining for C4d and the presence of DSA.[48,49] In addition, analogous to ACR, C4d is not specific for AMR but can be found in any process involving complement activation, such as reperfusion injury and infections. Nonetheless C4d staining is recommended as a diagnostic adjunct if specific morphologic findings are present (**Box 1**). Clinical symptoms in AMR are often nonspecific and include an asymptomatic decrease in lung function, cough, dyspnea, fever, and lethargy, which can rapidly progress to respiratory failure.

In 2016, the ISHLT published a consensus for staging of clinical antibody-mediated rejection[32] in which definite AMR consists of the clinical presence of allograft dysfunction (alterations in pulmonary physiology, gas exchange properties, radiologic features, or deteriorating functional performance), DSA, and histopathologic findings, including C4d staining, and is classified as definite AMR if 3 out of 3 criteria are positive, probable AMR with 2 out of 3 positive criteria, and possible AMR if 1 out of 3 criteria is positive[11,50] (**Table 4**).

In summary, AMR remains a diagnosis of exclusion, requiring comprehensive analysis of clinical, serologic, microbial, and histopathologic findings.[51]

CHRONIC GRAFT DYSFUNCTION

Chronic graft dysfunction can either affect small airways (CLAD) or pulmonary vasculature (transplant-associated vasculopathy), resulting either in fibrotic remodeling of the airways or fibrotic vasculopathy.

CHRONIC LUNG ALLOGRAFT DYSFUNCTION

CLAD is an umbrella term for all airway-associated manifestations of chronic graft injury and can be subdivided into different phenotypes.[52] The disease is defined by a persistent decline of pulmonary function (FEV1) to 80% of baseline or less. Predisposing factors for the development of CLAD include immunologic injuries, such as recurrent episodes of acute graft rejection, both ACR and AMR, as well as nonimmunologic factors such as reperfusion injury; prolonged ischemia before transplant; gastroesophageal reflux disease (GERD); and various viral, bacterial, and mycotic infections.[53]

To define CLAD, other factors explaining persistent decline of FEV1, such as neutrophilic reversible allograft dysfunction (NRAD) or azithromycin-responsive allograft dysfunction (ARAD), should be excluded. ARAD needs to be addressed, because it dramatically changes the further therapeutic approach compared with classic CLAD. ARAD is defined by neutrophilia in BAL without evidence for infection and clinical response to azithromycin[54–57] and is thought to represent a potential precursor lesion to oCLAD, because lymphocytic bronchiolitis, a risk factor for developing oCLAD, is associated with increased neutrophil levels in BAL.[55,58]

An obstructive phenotype (BO syndrome [BOS]) is defined by obstructive ventilatory dysfunction and the lack of opacities on imaging. Restrictive allograft syndrome (RAS) is defined by loss of lung volumes (low total lung capacity) and opacities on imaging with the absence of obstructive physiology on pulmonary function. Most recently, mixed and undefined phenotypes, including RAS, have been acknowledged as well.

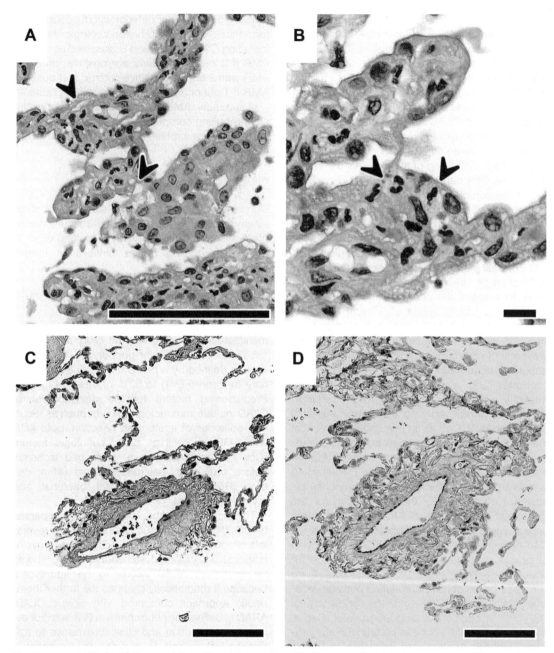

Fig. 5. Acute AMR. (*A, B*) Neutrophil capillaritis in small capillaries. Arrowheads point to neutrophil granulocytes inside the capillary endothelium ([*A*] hematoxylin-eosin, original magnification ×200, scale bar, 100 μm; [*B*] hematoxylin-eosin, original magnification ×400, scale bar 10 μm). (*C*) C4d-positive capillaries. (*D*) C4d-positive endothelial cells ([*C*] hematoxylin-eosin, original magnification ×200, scale bar, 100 μm; [*D*] immunohistochemistry, original magnification ×200, scale bar, 100 μm).

BRONCHIOLITIS OBLITERANS SYNDROME

BOS is clinically defined as persistent obstructive ventilation impairment (≥20% FEV1 decrease compared with the best posttransplant value), a low FEV1/forced vital capacity (FVC) ratio less than 0.7 for at least 3 weeks, and supported by air trapping and atelectasis in computed tomography.[35] Within 5 years after LuTx, approximately 50% of the transplant recipients had oCLAD, and survival after diagnosis of oCLAD ranges from 3 to 5 years.[23] The histomorphologic hallmark for BOS is BO, which predominantly affects only small airways with a diameter less than 1 mm. As

<table>
<tr><td>

Box 1
Indications for C4d immunohistochemistry

Neutrophilic marginalization

Neutrophilic capillaritis

Severe ACR (≥ A3)

Persistent, recurrent rejection (independent from grade)

Diffuse alveolar damage

Severe lymphocytic bronchiolitis (B2R)

BO (grade C1)

Arteritis without evidence of underlying rejection or infection

Graft dysfunction without morphologic tangible cause

Evidence of DSA

C4d staining should be considered as an additional marker for the diagnosis of acute AMR, if 1 or more of the histologic criteria mentioned here are present.

</td></tr>
</table>

a diagnosis of exclusion relying on the clinical presentation of the patient and supporting radiological and histologic findings.

Treatment of BOS is attempted by photopheresis, total lymphoid irradiation, or redo transplant,[35–37] high-dose corticosteroids have proved to be ineffective.[21]

RESTRICTIVE ALLOGRAFT SYNDROME

RAS is clinically defined by a decline in the total lung capacity and, in contrast with BOS, normal ratio of FEV1 to FVC (FEV1/FVC).[59] In high-resolution computed tomography (HRCT) examination, most afflicted patients show patchy pleuroparenchymal consolidation and ground-glass opacities, especially in the upper pulmonary compartments.[35] RAS accounts for up to one-third of all CLAD. Importantly, patients after diagnosis of RAS are limited to a median survival of only 6 to 18 months, only one-third of the median survival of patients with manifest BOS, a prognosis comparable with metastasized malignant neoplasms.[8,60] On the histologic level, RAS predominantly manifests in the form of subpleural, periseptal, and parabronchial alveolar fibroelastosis (AFE) (discussed later).

mentioned earlier, a heterogeneous distribution and preferential location in the peripheral airway segments hamper the diagnosis of BO in biopsy specimens. Thus, the correct diagnosis of BOS is

Table 4
Probability of antibody-mediated rejection

Allograft dysfunction	Exclusion of other causes	Histology	C4d positivity in Biopsy	DSA	Certainty
+	+	+	+	+	definite
+	+	+	?	+	probable
+	+	+	+	?	probable
+	+	?	+	+	probable
+	?	+	+	+	probable
+	+	+	?	?	possible
+	+	?	?	+	possible
+	+	?	+	?	possible
+	?	+	+	?	possible
+	?	+	?	+	possible
+	?	?	+	+	possible

Triple test suggested by the ISHLT consensus for staging of clinical AMR. Herein, the results of a triple test consisting of the clinical presence of allograft dysfunction DSA and histopathologic findings (including C4d staining) are classified as definite (3 out of 3 criteria are positive), probable (2 out of 3 criteria positive) or possible (1 out of 3 criteria).

ALVEOLAR FIBROELASTOSIS

The histologic pattern found in AFE was first described in patients with a variant of idiopathic fibrosis and was initially termed pleuroparenchymal fibroelastosis (PPFE).[61] Later, analogous patterns were identified in patients with pulmonary graft-versus-host disease after hematopoietic stem cell transplant,[62] and, more recently, also in LuTX patients.[55] The characteristic architectural changes were not only found in direct vicinity of the visceral pleura but also next to pleural septa and adjacent to bronchi and bronchioli. The histologic hallmark of fully developed AFE is the fibrotic obliteration of the alveolar parenchyma with concomitant preservation of the elastic fibers in the former alveolar walls (**Figs. 6** and **7**). An additional histologic feature of AFE is an abrupt transition between fibrotic areas and adjacent, nonremodelled alveolar parenchyma.

MISCELLANEOUS POSTTRANSPLANT CONDITIONS

Besides the different manifestations of alloimmunity and recurrences of the underlying disease, there are several other disease entities frequently occurring in the transplanted lung. Because of the required immunosuppressive treatment and reduced mucociliary clearance and coughing reflex, LuTx patients are especially prone to pulmonary infections. In the first 30 days posttransplant, infections are mainly caused by bacteria, whereas between 1 and 6 months after transplant, viruses (**Fig. 8**) (eg, CMV, influenza A/B, parainfluenza, adenoviruses, and rhinoviruses) and fungi (**Fig. 9**) (eg, *Aspergillus* species, *Candida* species, *Cryptococcus neoformans*, and *Pneumocystis jirovecii*) play an important role. As the lung is continuously exposed to the outside, LuTx patients face a lifelong elevated infection rate. Particularly, CMV-associated infections of the lung are a risk factor for the development of both ACR and CLAD.[63–65]

Another rare but important adverse event linked to immunosuppressive treatment is posttransplant lymphoproliferative disorder (PTLD). PTLD occurs in approximately 6% of transplanted patients and is responsible for 2% to 3% of patient deaths in LuTx patients.[66,67] PTLD consists of a spectrum of lymphoproliferative entities, mostly induced by Epstein-Barr virus (EBV) infection. PTLD is most commonly located in the transplanted lung, but can occur in any anatomic compartment, including lymph nodes or mucosa-associated lymphatic tissue in the intestine.[68] Besides positive serology for EBV, histologic examination plays an important role in the correct diagnosis of PTLD. According to the World Health Organization (WHO), PTLD is divided into 4 categories (early, polymorphic, monomorphic, and Hodgkin-like) (see **Fig. 8**). Of note, PTLD can manifest in an angiocentric manner, mimicking ACR or bronchiolar airway inflammation.[9]

RECURRENCE OF PRIMARY DISEASE

Recurrence of the primary disease is overall a rare event, and even more rarely diagnosed via transbronchial biopsy because of sampling limitations. Notable in this context is sarcoidosis, which has a high recurrence rate in the graft of up to 10%, and granulomatous inflammation can regularly be diagnosed by transbronchial lymph node or mucosal biopsies. Cases of recurring lepidic adenocarcinoma, in the context of chronic obstructive pulmonary disease (COPD) or advanced interstitial fibrosis, have been reported, even though these neoplasms were (most likely incorrectly) classified as in situ lesions in the recipient's lung at the time. At present, malignancy excludes potential transplant recipients from LuTx. Other recurring disease entities include lymphangioleiomyomatosis, pulmonary Langerhans-cell histiocytosis, pulmonary veno-occlusive disease (pVOD), and desquamative interstitial pneumonia.[9]

MOLECULAR MECHANISMS OF POSTTRANSPLANT CHANGES IN THE LUNG

In the last decade, fundamental research on the underlying molecular mechanisms has progressed and revealed a multitude of interesting findings.

ROLE OF AUTOCHTHONOUS CELLS: ENDOTHELIUM, BRONCHIAL EPITHELIUM, AND FIBROBLASTS

Experiments in mice showed that the bronchial epithelium, if exposed to various stressors (including HLA, K-alpha1 tubulin, and collagen V), induces fibroblastic growth via interferon γ and interleukin 17+/CD8+.[69] Furthermore, the bronchial epithelium can undergo an epithelial-mesenchymal transition toward a fibroblastlike phenotype if stimulated by transforming growth factor β (TGF-β).[70,71] Another source for the increased number of myofibroblasts in CLAD are bone marrow–derived progenitor cells, which have been shown to be increased in patients with oCLAD.[72] If primary human lung fibroblasts are cultured with medium from damaged bronchial epithelial cells, the fibroblasts express

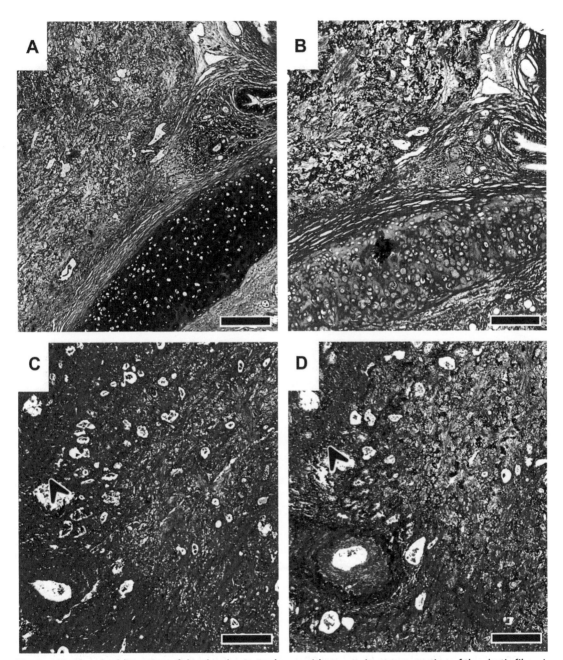

Fig. 6. AFE. Fibrotic obliteration of the alveolar parenchyma with concomitant preservation of the elastic fibers in the former alveolar walls. (*A, B*) Parabronchial AFE. (*C, D*) Paravasal and paraseptal alveolar fibroelastosis. Arrowhead points to the pulmonary septum [*A, C*] hematoxylin-eosin, original magnification ×20, scale bar, 30 μm; [*B, D*] elastica van Gieson, original magnification ×20, scale bar, 30 μm.

proinflammatory cytokines such as interleukin 6, interleukin 8, monocyte chemoattractant protein-1, and granulocyte macrophage colony-stimulating factor,[20] emphasizing the importance of the bronchial epithelium not only as a first line of defense against exogenous stimuli but also as a stimulant for chronic and progressive lung remodeling. In particular, high levels of antibodies against HLA, collagen V, and K-alpha1 tubulin, and high levels of DSA seem to be associated with a higher risk of developing CLAD.[35–37,42–45] Besides the bronchial epithelium, persistent injury to lung allograft induces the upregulation of several chemokines interacting with CXCR2-expressing endothelial cells, leading to aberrant vascular remodeling and

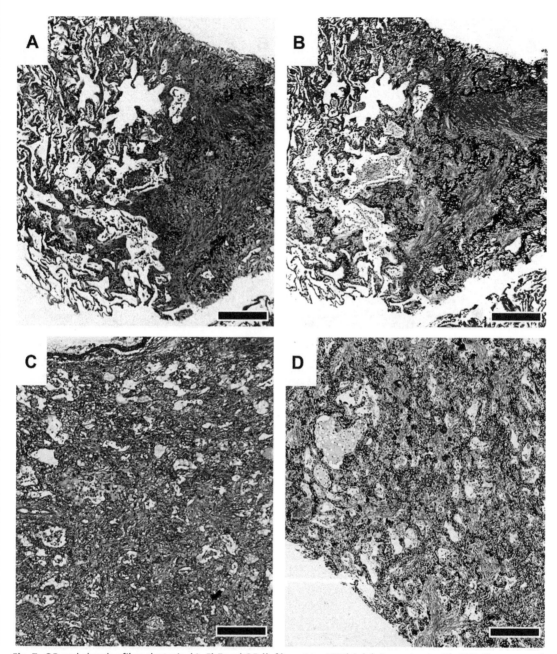

Fig. 7. OP and alveolar fibroelastosis. (*A, B*) Focal OP (*left*) next to AFE (*right*). In contrast with AFE, there are only scarce and thin collagen bundles inside the alveolar spaces in OP and clusters of macrophages are regularly seen. (*C, D*) Broad area of OP that might be mistaken for genuine AFE. Note the incomplete lining of the alveolar spaces with collagen; aggregates of macrophages; and normal, nonhypertrophic, elastotic fibers [*A, C*] hematoxylin-eosin, original magnification ×20, scale bar, 300 μm; [*B, D*] elastica van Gieson, original magnification ×20, scale bar, 300 μm.

formation of granulation tissue around smaller airways.[73] In addition, an enhanced peribronchial microcirculation in damaged lung allografts has been described[74] and microvascular damage (eg, via C3 proteins of the complement system) seems to be another factor in the development of CLAD.[75,76]

ROLE OF NONAUTOCHTHONOUS CELLS: MACROPHAGES AND NEUTROPHILS

Besides endothelial cells and the bronchial epithelium, nonautochthonous cells, especially neutrophils and macrophages, have been reported to play a substantial role in CLAD and ACR.

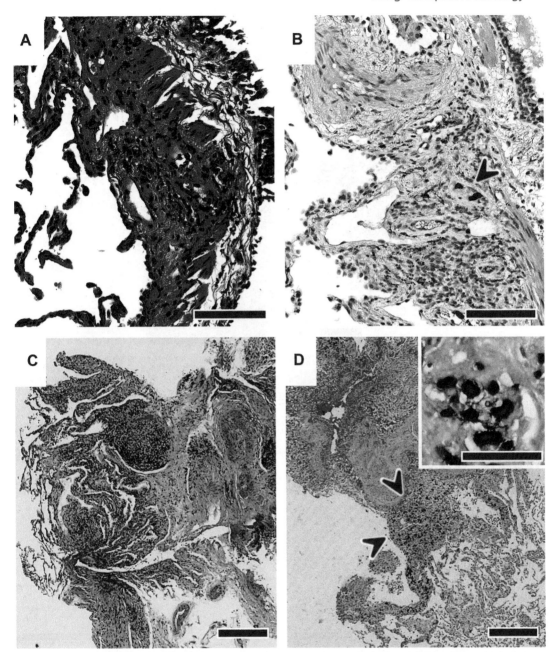

Fig. 8. Viral infections and lymphoproliferative disorders in lung allografts. (*A, B*) CMV infection of the lung showing a subepithelial mononuclear cell–rich infiltrate (*A*) and immunohistochemical positivity (*arrowhead*) for CMV (*B*) mimicking alloimmunogenic airway inflammation (ISHLT B). (*C, D*) Posttransplant lymphoproliferative disorder (PTLD). Atypical infiltrate of lymphocytes affecting the entire bronchus of the graft (*C*). Immunohistochemical positivity for Epstein-Barr virus nucleic acids inside these lymphocytes (*arrowheads*). (*Inset*) Higher magnification of immunohistochemical positivity for Epstein-Barr virus nucleic acids (*D*). [*A*] hematoxylin-eosin, original magnification ×200, scale bar, 100 mm; [*B*] Immunhistochemical staining against cytomegalovirus, original magnification × 200, scale bar, 100 mm; [*C*] hematoxylin-eosin, original magnification 20, scale bar, 300 mm; [*D*] immunohistochemical staining against Epstein-Barr virus nucleic acids, original magnification ×20, scale bar, 300 mm; [*inset*] original magnification ×200, scale bar, 50 µm).

In PGD, recipients' circulating neutrophils adhere to the graft endothelium and release tissue-destructive proteases, reactive oxygen species (ROS), and cytokines, leading to tissue damage.[77] As mentioned earlier, neutrophils play an important role in a particular subset of oCLAD referred to as ARAD. It has been shown that T lymphocytes, macrophages, and epithelial cells on

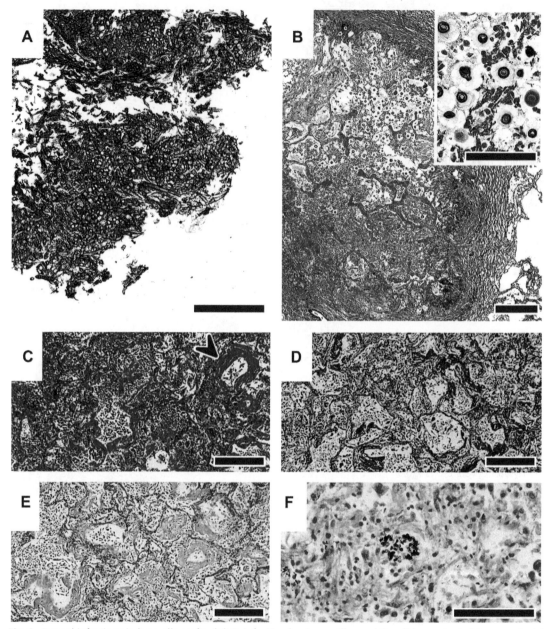

Fig. 9. Fungal infections in lung allografts. (*A*) Coinfection by *Aspergillus* and *Candida* species in biopsy material without detectable lung parenchyma. (*B*) Cryptococcosis. Round encapsulated fungal forms accompanied by a loose fibrinous exudate. (*Inset*) The fungal forms. (*C–F*) *Pneumocystis jirovecii* pneumonia in lung transplant patient. Diffuse alveolar damage with hyaline membranes (*arrowhead*) and accumulation of macrophages (*C*). No PAS-positive fungi (*D*). No signs of fibrotic remodeling in the elastica von Gieson staining (*E*). On silver staining (Grocott), round, approximately 8-μm to 10-μm fungal organisms can easily be identified (*F*) ([*A*] PAS, original magnification ×200, scale bar, 100 μm, [*B*] hematoxylin-eosin, original magnification ×40, scale bar, 300 μm; [*inset*] hematoxylin-eosin, original magnification ×200 scale bar, 100 μm); [*C*] original magnification ×20, scale bar, 300 μm; [*D*] original magnification ×20, scale bar, 300 μm; [*E*] original magnification ×20, scale bar, 300 μm; [*F*] original magnification ×100, scale bar, 100 μm).

chronic lung injury release chemokine (C-X-C motif) ligand 1 (CXCL-1) and interleukin 8 (IL-8), thereby recruiting neutrophils to the site of injury.[78,79] In addition, neutrophils and macrophages delicately sense stress-released ATP, which is commonly found in sites of tissue damage, via P2X7 purinergic receptors, leading to increased levels of interleukin 17 (IL-17). IL-17 stimulates smooth muscle cells and epithelial cells to produce IL-8, leading to further increase of neutrophils and at the same time decreased numbers of regulatory T lymphocytes, leading to disinhibition of neutrophils, and henceforth promoting further tissue damage.[80]

Macrophages can be grossly divided into 2 phenotypes: classically activated, proinflammatory, M1 macrophages, responsible for wound healing after alveolar epithelial injury; and alternatively activated, antiinflammatory, M2 macrophages, responsible for the termination of inflammatory responses in the lung.[81] In LuTx patients, M1 macrophages are mainly thought to be involved in acute rejection, clearing of bacterial infections, and epithelial-mesenchymal transition of the bronchial epithelium.[82] The role of M2 macrophages in CLAD is mainly unknown and is controversial. There is a subset of patients with late-onset CLAD who show a shift toward M2 macrophages in the graft. However, it is unclear whether M2 macrophages in this scenario eventually stimulate or prohibit fibrotic remodeling and extracellular matrix deposition.[60]

ROLE OF THE MICROBIOME

The microbiome also seems to play a role in CLAD, especially in association with macrophages. The composition of the microbiome in the graft changes after transplant, leading to a shift toward M2 macrophages in BAL, possibly contributing to fibrotic remodeling.[83] Further, certain microorganisms (eg, *Pseudomonas aeruginosa* and *Aspergillus* species) are frequently found in patients with manifest CLAD, whereas asymptomatic patients show a different microbiome composition.[84–86] In addition, the reestablishment of the recipients' microbiota in the graft airways can potentially lead to an increased graft survival.[87]

MOLECULAR BIOMARKERS AS A DIAGNOSTIC TOOL FOR CHRONIC LUNG ALLOGRAFT DYSFUNCTION

As mentioned earlier, lung biopsy samples alone are not sensitive enough for a reliable detection of BO, the histopathologic hallmark of CLAD. Retrospective messenger RNA expression level analysis in LuTx patients identified 5 genes from the transforming growth factor-β axis (BMP4, IL6, MMP1, SMAD1, and THBS1) with distinguishable expression patterns between LuTx patients with and without CLAD.[60] Based on relative messenger RNA expression levels of the 5 genes mentioned earlier, a scoring system for an early diagnosis of CLAD was developed and showed promising

results in separating patients developing CLAD from stable patients. Furthermore, patients classified as stable 220 days after LuTx did not develop CLAD in the follow-up period.[60] However, despite the advances regarding the underlying molecular mechanism on ACR and CLAD, until now, no thoroughly reliable predictive, prospectively evaluated test in BAL, blood samples, or biopsy material has been established.[51,60,88–91]

ACKNOWLEDGMENTS

The authors thank Regina Engelhardt, Annette Mueller Brechlin, Christina Petzold, and Valentina Osmani for their excellent technical support, and Jill Barry for editing the article.

DISCLOSURE

The authors have nothing to disclose.

REFERENCES

1. Hardy JD, Webb WR, Dalton ML, et al. Lung homotransplantation in man. Transplantation 1963; 186(12):1065–74.
2. Thabut G, Mal H. Outcomes after lung transplantation. J Thorac Dis 2017;9(8):2684–91.
3. Wohlschlaeger J, Laenger F, Gottlieb J, et al. Lungentransplantation. Pathologe 2019. https://doi.org/10.1007/s00292-019-0598-z.
4. Yusen RD, Christie JD, Edwards LB, et al. The registry of the international society for heart and lung transplantation: thirtieth adult lung and heart-lung transplant report - 2013; focus theme: age. J Heart Lung Transplant 2013;32(10):965–78.
5. Lee JC, Christie JD. Primary graft dysfunction. Clin Chest Med 2011;32(2):279–93.
6. Porhownik NR. Airway complications post lung transplantation. Curr Opin Pulm Med 2013;19(2): 174–80.
7. Santacruz JF, Mehta AC. Airway complications and management after lung transplantation: ischemia, dehiscence, and stenosis. Proc Am Thorac Soc 2009;6(1):79–93.
8. Wohlschläger J, Sommerwerck U, Jonigk D, et al. Lungentransplantation und AbstoßungLung transplantation and rejection. Pathologe 2011;32(2):104–12.
9. Farver C, Wallace WD. The pathology of lung transplantation. In: Ruiz P, editor. Transplantation pathology. 2nd edition. Cambridge (England): Cambridge University Press; 2018. p. 156–82.
10. Ius F, Sommer W, Tudorache I, et al. Early donor-specific antibodies in lung transplantation: risk factors and impact on survival. J Heart Lung Transplant 2014;33(12):1255–63.
11. Roden AC, Kern RM, Aubry MC, et al. Transbronchial cryobiopsies in the evaluation of lung

allografts: do the benefits outweigh the risks? Arch Pathol Lab Med 2016;140(4):303–11.

12. Yusen RD, Edwards LB, Kucheryavaya AY, et al. The Registry of the International Society for Heart and Lung Transplantation: thirty-second official adult heart transplantation report - 2015; focus theme: early graft failure. J Heart Lung Transplant 2015; 34(10):1244–54.

13. Stewart S, Fishbein MC, Snell GI, et al. Revision of the 1996 working formulation for the standardization of nomenclature in the diagnosis of lung rejection. J Heart Lung Transplant 2007;26(12):1229–42.

14. Greenland JR, Jones KD, Hays SR, et al. Association of large-airway lymphocytic bronchitis with bronchiolitis obliterans syndrome. Am J Respir Crit Care Med 2012;187(4):417–23.

15. Chakinala MM, Ritter J, Gage BF, et al. Reliability for grading acute rejection and airway inflammation after lung transplantation. J Heart Lung Transplant 2005;24(6):652–7.

16. Stephenson A, Flint J, English J, et al. Interpretation of transbronchial lung biopsies from lung transplant recipients: inter- and intraobserver agreement. Can Respir J 2005;12(2):75–7.

17. Colombat M, Groussard O, Lautrette A, et al. Analysis of the different histologic lesions observed in transbronchial biopsy for the diagnosis of acute rejection. Clinicopathologic correlations during the first 6 months after lung transplantation. Hum Pathol 2005;36(4):387–94.

18. Bhorade SM, Husain AN, Liao C, et al. Interobserver variability in grading transbronchial lung biopsy specimens after lung transplantation. Chest 2013; 143(6):1717–24.

19. Husain AN, Garrity ER. Lung transplantation: the state of the airways. Arch Pathol Lab Med 2016;140(3):241–4.

20. Suwara MI, Vanaudenaerde BM, Verleden SE, et al. Mechanistic differences between phenotypes of chronic lung allograft dysfunction after lung transplantation. Transpl Int 2014;27(8):857–67.

21. Vos R, Verleden SE, Verleden GM. Chronic lung allograft dysfunction: evolving practice. Curr Opin Organ Transplant 2015;20(5):483–91.

22. Verleden SE, Vasilescu DM, McDonough JE, et al. Linking clinical phenotypes of chronic lung allograft dysfunction to changes in lung structure. Eur Respir J 2015;46(5):1430–9.

23. Kuehnel M, Maegel L, Robertus JL, et al. Airway remodelling in the transplanted lung. Cell Tissue Res 2017;367(3):663–75.

24. Yu J. Postinfectious bronchiolitis obliterans in children: lessons from bronchiolitis obliterans after lung transplantation and hematopoietic stem cell transplantation. Korean J Pediatr 2015;58(12):459–65.

25. Kreiss K, Gomaa A, Kullman G, et al. Clinical bronchiolitis obliterans in workers at a microwave-popcorn plant. N Engl J Med 2002;347(5):330–8.

26. Kanwal R. Bronchiolitis obliterans in workers exposed to flavoring chemicals. Curr Opin Pulm Med 2008;14(2):141–6.

27. Thomason JWW, Rice TW, Milstone AP. Bronchiolitis obliterans in a survivor of a chemical weapons attack. J Am Med Assoc 2003;290(5):598–9.

28. Ghanei M, Mokhtari M, Mohammad MM, et al. Bronchiolitis obliterans following exposure to sulfur mustard: chest high resolution computed tomography. Eur J Radiol 2004;52(2):164–9.

29. Epler GR, Colby TV, McLoud TC, et al. Bronchiolitis obliterans organizing pneumonia. N Engl J Med 1985;312(3):152–8. The New England Journal of Medicine Downloaded from nejm.org at MEMORIAL UNIV OF NEWFOUNDLAND on November 10, 2013. For personal use only. No other uses without permission. From the NEJM Archive. Copyright © 2010 Massachusetts Medical Society. All rights.

30. Travis WD, Colby TV, Koss MN, et al. Non-neoplastic disorders of the lower respiratory tract. 1st edition. Washington, DC: American Registry of Pathology; 2002.

31. Roux A, Bendib Le Lan I, Holifanjaniaina S, et al. Antibody-mediated rejection in lung transplantation: clinical outcomes and donor-specific antibody characteristics. Am J Transplant 2016;16(4):1216–28.

32. Levine DJ, Glanville AR, Aboyoun C, et al. Antibody-mediated rejection of the lung: a consensus report of the International Society for Heart and Lung Transplantation. J Heart Lung Transplant 2016; 35(4):397–406.

33. Smith JD, Banner NR, Hamour IM, et al. De novo donor HLA-specific antibodies after heart transplantation are an independent predictor of poor patient survival. Am J Transplant 2011;11(2):312–9.

34. Westall GP, Paraskeva MA, Snell GI. Antibody-mediated rejection. Curr Opin Organ Transplant 2015; 20(5):492–7.

35. Verleden SE, Sacreas A, Vos R, et al. Advances in understanding bronchiolitis obliterans after lung transplantation. Chest 2016;150(1):219–25.

36. Verleden SE, Ruttens D, Vandermeulen E, et al. Predictors of survival in restrictive chronic lung allograft dysfunction after lung transplantation. J Heart Lung Transplant 2016;35(9):1078–84.

37. Verleden SE, Vos R, Vandermeulen E, et al. Parametric response mapping of bronchiolitis obliterans syndrome progression after lung transplantation. Am J Transplant 2016;16(11):3262–9.

38. Colvin RB, Smith RN. Antibody-mediated organ-allograft rejection. Nat Rev Immunol 2005;5(10):807–17.

39. Girnita AL, McCurry KR, Iacono AT, et al. HLA-specific antibodies are associated with high-grade and persistent-recurrent lung allograft acute rejection. J Heart Lung Transplant 2004;23(10):1135–41.

40. Palmer SM, Davis RD, Hadjiliadis D, et al. Development of an antibody specific to major

histocompatibility antigens detectable by flow cytometry after lung transplant is associated with bronchiolitis obliterans syndrome. Transplantation 2002; 74(6):799–804.

41. Hadjiliadis D, Chaparro C, Reinsmoen NL, et al. Pre-transplant panel reactive antibody in lung transplant recipients is associated with significantly worse post-transplant survival in a multicenter study. J Heart Lung Transplant 2005;24(7 Suppl): 249–54.

42. Hagedorn PH, Burton CM, Carlsen J, et al. Chronic rejection of a lung transplant is characterized by a profile of specific autoantibodies. Immunology 2010;130(3):427–35.

43. Kauke T, Kneidinger N, Martin B, et al. Bronchiolitis obliterans syndrome due to donor-specific HLA-antibodies. Tissue Antigens 2015;86(3):178–85.

44. Le Pavec J, Suberbielle C, Lamrani L, et al. De-novo donor-specific anti-HLA antibodies 30 days after lung transplantation are associated with a worse outcome. J Heart Lung Transplant 2016;35(9): 1067–77.

45. Tikkanen JM, Singer LG, Kim JS, et al. De novo DQ-donor-specific antibodies are associated with chronic lung allograft dysfunction after lung transplantation. Am J Respir Crit Care Med 2016; 194(5):596–606.

46. Calabrese F, Hirschi S, Neil D, et al. Alveolar septal widening as an "alert" signal to look into lung antibody-mediated rejection: a multicenter pilot study. Transplantation 2019;103(11):2440–7, 9000;Online Fir. Available at: https://journals.lww.com/transplantjournal/Fulltext/onlinefirst/Alveolar_septal_widening_as_an__alert__signal_to.96181.aspx.

47. Roden AC, Maleszewski JJ, Yi ES, et al. Reproducibility of complement 4d deposition by immunofluorescence and immunohistochemistry in lung allograft biopsies. J Heart Lung Transplant 2014; 33(12):1223–32.

48. Roberts JA, Barrios R, Cagle PT, et al. The presence of anti-HLA donor-specific antibodies in lung allograft recipients does not correlate with C4d immunofluorescence in transbronchial biopsy specimens. Arch Pathol Lab Med 2014;138(8):1053–8.

49. Westall GP, Snell GI, McLean C, et al. C3d and C4d deposition early after lung transplantation. J Heart Lung Transplant 2008;27(7):722–8.

50. Berry G, Burke M, Andersen C, et al. Pathology of pulmonary antibody-mediated rejection: 2012 update from the pathology council of the ISHLT. J Heart Lung Transplant 2013;32(1):14–21.

51. Benzimra M, Calligaro GL, Glanville AR. Acute rejection. J Thorac Dis 2017;9(12):5440–57.

52. Verleden GM, Glanville AR, Lease ED, et al. Chronic lung allograft dysfunction: definition, diagnostic criteria, and approaches to treatment—A consensus report from the pulmonary council of the ISHLT. J Heart Lung Transplant 2019;38(5):493–503.

53. Royer PJ, Olivera-Botello G, Koutsokera A, et al. Chronic lung allograft dysfunction: a systematic review of mechanisms. Transplantation 2016;100(9): 1803–14.

54. Vanaudenaerde BM, Meyts I, Vos R, et al. A dichotomy in bronchiolitis obliterans syndrome after lung transplantation revealed by azithromycin therapy. Eur Respir J 2008;32(4):832–43.

55. Ofek E, Sato M, Saito T, et al. Restrictive allograft syndrome post lung transplantation is characterized by pleuroparenchymal fibroelastosis. Mod Pathol 2013;26(3):350–6.

56. Verleden SE, De Jong PA, Ruttens D, et al. Functional and computed tomographic evolution and survival of restrictive allograft syndrome after lung transplantation. J Heart Lung Transplant 2014; 33(3):270–7.

57. Verleden GM, Raghu G, Meyer KC, et al. A new classification system for chronic lung allograft dysfunction. J Heart Lung Transplant 2014;33(2):127–33.

58. Glanville AR, Aboyoun CL, Havryk A, et al. Severity of lymphocytic bronchiolitis predicts long-term outcome after lung transplantation. Am J Respir Crit Care Med 2008;177(9):1033–40.

59. Glanville AR, Verleden GM, Todd JL, et al. Chronic lung allograft dysfunction: definition and update of restrictive allograft syndrome—A consensus report from the pulmonary council of the ISHLT. J Heart Lung Transplant 2019;38(5):483–92.

60. Jonigk D, Izykowski N, Rische J, et al. Molecular profiling in lung biopsies of human pulmonary allografts to predict chronic lung allograft dysfunction. Am J Pathol 2015;185(12):3178–88.

61. Frankel SK, Cool CD, Lynch DA, et al. Idiopathic pleuroparenchymal fibroelastosis. Chest 2004; 126(6):2007–13.

62. Von Der Thüsen JH, Hansell DM, Tominaga M, et al. Pleuroparenchymal fibroelastosis in patients with pulmonary disease secondary to bone marrow transplantation. Mod Pathol 2011;24(12):1633–9.

63. Paraskeva M, Bailey M, Levvey BJ, et al. Cytomegalovirus replication within the lung allograft is associated with bronchiolitis obliterans syndrome. Am J Transplant 2011;11(10):2190–6.

64. Uhlin M, Mattsson J, Maeurer M. Update on viral infections in lung transplantation. Curr Opin Pulm Med 2012;18(3):264–70.

65. Patel N, Snyder LD, Finlen-Copeland A, et al. Is prevention the best treatment? CMV after lung transplantation. Am J Transplant 2012;12(3):539–44.

66. Reams BD, McAdams HP, Howell DN, et al. Posttransplant lymphoproliferative disorder: incidence, presentation, and response to treatment in lung transplant recipients. Chest 2003;124(4):1242–9.

67. Trulock EP, Edwards LB, Taylor DO, et al. Registry of the International Society for Heart and Lung Transplantation: twenty-third official adult lung and heart-lung transplantation report-2006. J Heart Lung Transplant 2005;25(8):880–92.

68. Evens AM, Roy R, Sterrenberg D, et al. Post-transplantation lymphoproliferative disorders: diagnosis, prognosis, and current approaches to therapy. Curr Oncol Rep 2010;12(6):383–94.

69. Subramanian V, Ramachandran S, Banan B, et al. Immune response to tissue-restricted self-antigens induces airway inflammation and fibrosis following murine lung transplantation. Am J Transplant 2014; 14(10):2359–66.

70. Pain M, Bermudez O, Lacoste P, et al. Tissue remodelling in chronic bronchial diseases: from the epithelial to mesenchymal phenotype. Eur Respir Rev 2014;23(131):118–30.

71. Borthwick LA, Parker SM, Brougham KA, et al. Epithelial to mesenchymal transition (EMT) and airway remodelling after human lung transplantation. Thorax 2009;64(9):770–7.

72. Bröcker V, Länger F, Fellous TG, et al. Fibroblasts of recipient origin contribute to bronchiolitis obliterans in human lung transplants. Am J Respir Crit Care Med 2006;173(11):1276–82.

73. Belperio JA, Ross DJ, Strieter RM, et al. Role of CXCR2/CXCR2 ligands in vascular remodeling during bronchiolitis obliterans syndrome Find the latest version: role of CXCR2/CXCR2 ligands in vascular remodeling during bronchiolitis obliterans syndrome. J Clin Invest 2005;115(5):1150–62.

74. Luckraz H, Goddard M, McNeil K, et al. Microvascular changes in small airways predispose to obliterative bronchiolitis after lung transplantation. J Heart Lung Transplant 2004;23(5):527–31.

75. Khan MA, Nicolls MR. Complement-Mediated Microvascular Injury Leads to Chronic Rejection. Adv Exp Med Biol 2013;735:233–46.

76. Khan MA, Jiang X, Dhillon G, et al. CD4+ T cells and complement independently mediate graft ischemia in the rejection of mouse orthotopic tracheal transplants. Circ Res 2011;109(11):1290–301.

77. Laubach VE, Kron IL. NIH public access. Surgery 2009;146(1):1–4.

78. Saini D, Weber J, Ramachandran S, et al. Alloimmunity-induced autoimmunity as a potential mechanism in the pathogenesis of chronic rejection of human lung allografts. J Heart Lung Transplant 2011;30(6):624–31.

79. Jaramillo A, Smith CR, Maruyama T, et al. Anti-HLA class I antibody binding to airway epithelial cells induces production of fibrogenic growth factors and apoptotic cell death: a possible mechanism for bronchiolitis obliterans syndrome. Hum Immunol 2003;64(5):521–9.

80. Cekic C, Linden J. Purinergic regulation of the immune system. Nat Rev Immunol 2016;16(3): 177–92.

81. Zhang L, Wang Y, Wu G, et al. Macrophages: friend or foe in idiopathic pulmonary fibrosis? Respiratory Research 2018;19:170. https://doi.org/10.1186/s12931-018-0864-2.

82. Borthwick LA, Gardner A, De Soyza A, et al. Transforming growth factor-β1 (TGF-β1) driven epithelial to mesenchymal transition (EMT) is accentuated by tumour necrosis factor α (TNFα) via crosstalk between the SMAD and NF-κB pathways. Cancer Microenviron 2012;5(1):45–57.

83. Bernasconi E, Pattaroni C, Koutsokera A, et al. Airway microbiota determines innate cell inflammatory or tissue remodeling profiles in lung transplantation. Am J Respir Crit Care Med 2016;194(10):1252–63.

84. Weigt SS, Elashoff RM, Huang C, et al. Aspergillus colonization of the lung allograft is a risk factor for bronchiolitis obliterans syndrome. Am J Transplant 2009;9(9):1903–11.

85. Gregson AL, Wang X, Weigt SS, et al. Interaction between pseudomonas and CXC chemokines increases risk of bronchiolitis obliterans syndrome and death in lung transplantation. Am J Respir Crit Care Med 2013;187(5):518–26.

86. Dickson RP, Erb-Downward JR, Freeman CM, et al. Changes in the lung microbiome following lung transplantation include the emergence of two distinct pseudomonas species with distinct clinical associations. PLoS One 2014;9(5). https://doi.org/10.1371/journal.pone.0097214.

87. Willner DL, Hugenholtz P, Yerkovich ST, et al. Reestablishment of recipient-associated microbiota in the lung allograft is linked to reduced risk of bronchiolitis obliterans syndrome. Am J Respir Crit Care Med 2013;187(6):640–7.

88. Vanaudenaerde BM, Dupont LJ, Wuyts WA, et al. The role of interleukin-17 during acute rejection after lung transplantation. Eur Respir J 2006;27(4): 779–87.

89. Bhorade SM, Yu A, Vigneswaran WT, et al. Elevation of interleukin-15 protein expression in bronchoalveolar fluid in acute lung allograft rejection. Chest 2007; 131(2):533–8.

90. Aharinejad S, Taghavi S, Klepetko W, et al. Prediction of lung-transplant rejection by hepatocyte growth factor. Lancet 2004;363:1503–8.

91. Ross DJ, Moudgil A, Bagga A, et al. Lung allograft dysfunction correlates with gamma-interferon gene expression in bronchoalveolar lavage. J Heart Lung Transplant 1999;18:627–36.

Pulmonary Cystic Disease and Its Mimics

Kirk D. Jones, MD

KEYWORDS

- Lymphangioleiomyomatosis • Pulmonary Langerhans cell histiocytosis • Birt-Hogg-Dubé syndrome
- Lymphocytic interstitial pneumonia • Follicular bronchiolitis • Abscess • Cystic fibrosis
- Bronchiectasis

Key points

- Cystic lung diseases are composed of a broad variety of different diseases that can be separated by gross and microscopic features.

- Diagnoses with close resemblance to cystic lung disease include cavitary diseases, cystic bronchiectasis, emphysema, and cystic changes in fibrosing interstitial lung disease.

- Several of the cystic lung diseases, including lymphangioleiomyomatosis, pulmonary Langerhans cell histiocytosis, pleuropulmonary blastoma, and Birt-Hogg-Dubé syndrome, have underlying genetic abnormalities that can aid in diagnosis.

ABSTRACT

Cystic diseases of the lung encompass a fairly broad variety of different diseases with causes including genetic abnormalities, smoking-related problems, developmental disorders, malignant neoplasms, and inflammatory processes. In addition, there are several diagnoses that closely resemble cystic lung disease, including cavitary diseases, cystic bronchiectasis, emphysema, and cystic changes in fibrosing interstitial lung disease. This article provides a review of cystic lung disease and its gross and histologic mimics.

OVERVIEW

Cystic diseases of the lung encompass a fairly broad variety of different diseases with causes including genetic abnormalities, smoking-related problems, developmental disorders, malignant neoplasms, and inflammatory processes. These patients occasionally arrive with stereotypical symptoms, such as pneumothorax or hemoptysis, or more commonly are uncovered by the radiologist after presenting with unrelated symptoms or nonspecific symptoms, such as dyspnea or chest pain. Knowledge of the radiologic features is significant, because many of these lesions are nearly invisible histologically and are only recognized when aware of their possibility.

Various concepts of cysts occur in the medical literature, and these often have slightly different requirements of size, presence of epithelial or other lining membranes, and others. Not every hole in the lung is properly categorized as a cyst. In the clinical literature, the term cyst most commonly refers to a well-defined air-filled space surrounded by a thin wall (fibrous or epithelial).[1] Other causes of parenchymal defects include cavities, dilated airways, emphysema, and air cysts from pulmonary interstitial emphysema. It is probably less important to know how to properly define a cyst than it is to recognize the variety of settings in which pulmonary parenchymal holes can appear. Differential diagnoses in cystic lung disease and its mimics can be developed based on gross and radiologic features of cyst distribution, number, and location within the primary lobule, as well as

---

Department of Pathology, University of California San Francisco, 505 Parnassus Avenue, Room M565, San Francisco, CA 94143, USA

E-mail address: Kirk.jones@ucsf.edu

Surgical Pathology 13 (2020) 141–163

https://doi.org/10.1016/j.path.2019.11.007

Box 1
Terminology for cystic disease and similar disorders

Cyst: Thin-walled, well-defined airspace with adjacent normal-appearing lung tissue.

Cavity: Thick-walled, well-delineated airspace with adjacent normal-appearing lung tissue.

Emphysema: Alveolar airspace enlargement due to alveolar septal destruction.

Bulla: Emphysematous airspace enlargement greater than 1 cm in diameter.

Bleb: An air-filled split of the (often fibrotically thickened) visceral pleura resulting in a dilated space.

Cystic bronchiectasis: Permanently dilated large airways, often with surrounding fibrosis and inflammation.

Honeycomb cyst: Irregular airspaces, lined by bronchial epithelium, surrounded by dense fibrosis, often observed subpleurally in patients with fibrotic lung disease.

Pulmonary interstitial emphysema (also known as air cyst): Dissection of air into the pulmonary interstitium, often with surrounding fibrosis with histiocytic and giant cell reaction.

---

by microscopic features, particularly in relation to the cellular components of the surrounding lung tissue (**Boxes 1** and **2**).

CAVITARY DISEASES

Cavities differ from cysts predominantly in the thickness of their walls, with a usual cutoff of 4 mm.[2] The thicker walls of the cavity are often due to its cause by inflammatory disease or neoplasm, and these lesions often coexist with nodular disease. It can be helpful, when building a differential diagnosis, to know the duration of cavitary disease, because acute diseases have a different etiologic spectrum than chronic diseases.

The most common causes of acute pulmonary cavities are those secondary to infection and may present as necrotizing pneumonias, abscesses, or septic emboli. These infections are most commonly secondary to bacteria, such as *Staphylococcus aureus*, *Streptococcus pneumoniae*, *Klebsiella pneumoniae*, *Haemophilus influenzae*, and *Pseudomonas aeruginosa*.[3] Other less common organisms that should be considered

---

Box 2
Distribution patterns of cystic lung disease

Upper lobe predominant

    Smoking-related emphysema and bullae

    Pulmonary Langerhans cell histiocytosis

Lower lobe predominant

    Birt-Hogg-Dubé

    Honeycombing in idiopathic pulmonary fibrosis

Random/diffuse

    Lymphangioleiomyomatosis

    Lymphocytic interstitial pneumonia/follicular bronchiolitis

    Infection (bacterial, fungal, mycobacterial, parasitic)

Hilar

    Bronchogenic cyst

Peripheral

    Blebs

    Honeycombing in IPF

    Paraseptal emphysema

    Alveolar growth abnormalities (eg, trisomy 21)

Abbreviation: IPF, idiopathic pulmonary fibrosis.

include Nocardia and fungi (particularly in immunocompromised patients or patients with known acute exposures). Chronic cavitary disease may also be secondary to infection and includes tuberculosis, nontuberculous mycobacteria (such as *Mycobacterium avium* in patients with chronic obstructive pulmonary disease), and fungi. Rare infectious causes of pulmonary cavities include parasitic disease, such as paragonimiasis and echinococcosis. Gross examination of infectious pulmonary cavitary disease often shows an irregular thick-walled space with central granular necrotic material (the term "caseous" may be used in these cases with this cheesy gross appearance). On microscopic examination, the lesions will show variable fibroinflammatory changes within the cavity wall with fibrosis, granulation tissue, and mixed acute and chronic inflammation (**Fig. 1**). Necrotizing granulomas will often show small satellite, well-formed tight "sarcoidal" granulomas adjacent to the cavitary mass.[4]

Other causes of chronic pulmonary cavitary disease include both primary lung cancer and metastatic tumors. Squamous cell carcinoma is the most common primary lung cancer to present with cavitary disease.[5] Adenocarcinoma rarely presents with cavitation, but can be cystic in high-grade tumors with necrosis, and occasionally shows a "bubbly" multilocular appearance on computed tomographic (CT) scan in mucinous tumors. Metastatic squamous cell carcinomas from head and neck or skin often show cavitation. Sarcomas can show cavitary or cystic disease. In

cases of neoplasms, histologic examination is often straightforward, with identification of neoplastic cells composing the cyst lining. Sources of error include false-negative results from mistaking neoplastic cells as reactive epithelium or histiocytic granulomatous inflammation,[6] or false-positive results from mistaking squamous metaplasia in cavitary infection (particularly fungus balls) as neoplastic.[7]

Finally, systemic autoimmune diseases or vasculitides may present with cavitary disease. Granulomatosis with polyangiitis (GPA), a systemic autoimmune disease closely associated with anticytoplasmic neutrophilic antibody production, most commonly presents with bilateral multiple nodules.[8] These nodules will often show cavitation, particularly when they exceed 2 cm. They can be difficult to differentiate from infectious lesions on gross examination. Microscopically, these lesions show irregular borders ("geographic necrosis") with granular nuclear debris, lending the necrosis a basophilic quality (**Fig. 2**A, B). The surrounding inflammatory infiltrate is histiocyte rich, but well-formed granulomas are absent to rare. Multinucleate giant cells with crowded hyperchromatic nuclei may be present.[9] Rheumatoid nodules, observed in patients with rheumatoid arthritis, can show similar features to GPA with basophilic necrosis and surrounding palisading histiocytes. These lesions can often be differentiated by clinical evidence of rheumatoid arthritis, including serologic findings and cutaneous rheumatoid nodules.

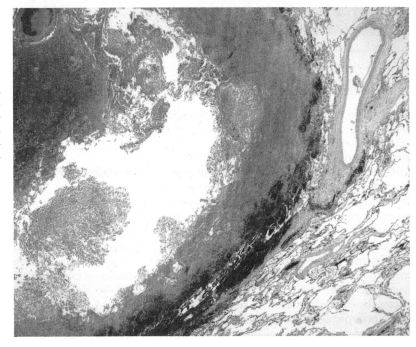

Fig. 1. Abscess. Low magnification reveals a rounded nodule with central necrosis and acute inflammation. The periphery shows granulation tissue and fibrin. This patient had bacterial endocarditis with multiple pulmonary abscesses from septic emboli (hematoxylin-eosin, original magnification ×20).

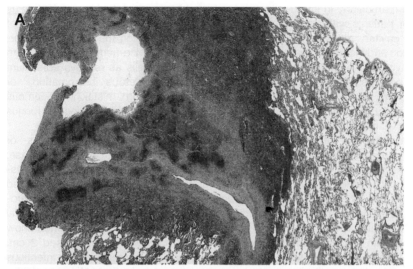

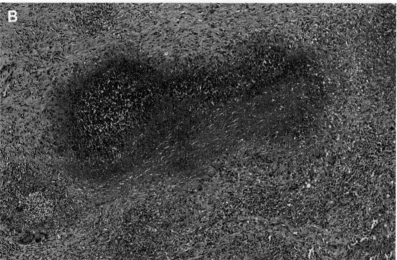

Fig. 2. GPA. (*A*) On low magnification, there is an irregular cavity with marked inflammation and necrosis. The necrotic regions show a variable basophilic appearance (hematoxylin-eosin, original magnification ×20). (*B*) On higher magnification, basophilic geographic necrosis is present with palisading histiocytes, hyper-chromatic multinucleate giant cells, and a surrounding histiocyte-rich mixed inflammatory infiltrate (hematoxylin-eosin, original magnification ×100).

EMPHYSEMA

Emphysema is characterized by enlargement of airspaces secondary to alveolar septal destruction. This common disease is the result of a paradigmatic imbalance of protease over antiprotease and is commonly observed in smokers as centriacinar emphysema and in patients with alpha-1-antitrypsin deficiency as panacinar emphysema. Large spaces of alveolar loss greater than 1 cm are referred to as bullae (singular bulla). Gross examination of the lung in patients with centriacinar emphysema usually shows apically oriented rounded regions of tissue loss, often with pigment deposition (the "dirty holes of emphysema"). Microscopic examination shows alveolar space enlargement with alveolar septal fragmentation resembling free-floating alveolar septa.

Occasionally, one observes an unusual organizational change next to large bullae referred to as placental transmogrification, where the tissue surrounding the bullous change resembles placental villi (**Fig. 3**).[10]

BRONCHIECTASIS

Dilatation of bronchi is termed bronchiectasis, which is a common change observed secondary to postinflammatory remodeling. The differential diagnosis includes disorders of mucociliary clearance from abnormal mucus (as in cystic fibrosis), abnormal cilia (as in ciliary dyskinesia), or cartilage abnormalities (such as Williams-Campbell syndrome).[11] Localized bronchiectasis is commonly observed in postobstructive conditions and may be the result of tumors or foreign bodies.

Fig. 3. Emphysema with placental transmogrification. Typical changes of emphysema include airspace enlargement with alveolar septal fragmentation. There are polypoid plugs of tissue with vascular cores resembling placental villi (*bottom right*). These changes occasionally occur adjacent to large bullae (hematoxylineosin, original magnification ×40).

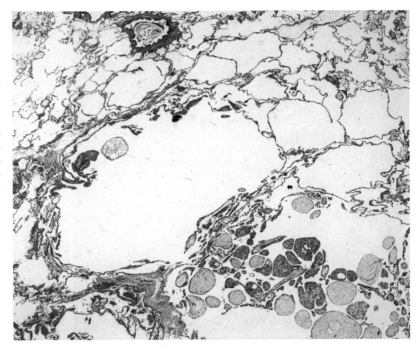

Occasionally, cases of bronchiectasis appeared to be secondary to inflammatory changes from constrictive bronchiolitis. This bronchiectasis/obliterative bronchiolitis complex is commonly observed in chronic rejection followed lung transplant and as the pulmonary manifestation of graft-versus-host disease. Gross examination of lungs with bronchiectasis shows dilated airways, extending from central lung to near the pleural surface, with axial ridges that resemble the interior of an extended accordion (**Fig. 4**A). Microscopy reveals inflamed airways with surrounding changes of chronic pneumonia (**Fig. 4**B).

CYSTIC CHANGES IN FIBROSING INTERSTITIAL PNEUMONIAS

Many cases of pulmonary fibrosis, particularly those with prominent architectural destruction, can present with cystic changes. Two common forms of cystic change in fibrotic lung disease are honeycomb cysts (microscopic honeycombing) and pulmonary interstitial emphysema (air cysts).

In usual interstitial pneumonia, a pattern of fibrosing interstitial lung disease observed in most cases of the clinical entity idiopathic pulmonary fibrosis, there is a peripheral lobular, subpleural, and paraseptal fibrosis with destruction of the typical pulmonary alveolar septal architecture. As the fibrosis progresses, the combination of peripheral fibrosis and central bronchiolar dilatation results in the formation of microscopic honeycombing; characterized histologically as irregular enlarged airspaces, lined by bronchiolar epithelium, often containing mucus and scant inflammatory cells, surrounded by dense fibrosis, often with wisps of smooth muscle (**Fig. 5**). The fibrosis surrounding these cystic spaces extends to the periphery of the lobule (most commonly the pleural surface) and thus differs from severe bronchiolocentric fibrosis, which usually shows residual alveolar spaces between bronchiolectatic spaces and the pleura.[12]

Pulmonary interstitial emphysema, or air cysts, forms when there is dissection of air into the interstitium. Although most commonly described in infants receiving high-pressure ventilation, the finding of interstitial air is relatively common in patients with fibrosing lung diseases, particularly with the pattern of usual interstitial pneumonia.[13,14] Grossly, the lesions vary from rounded to elongated with acute angulated points. Microscopically, the lesions vary according to their chronicity, with acute lesions showing lining by histiocytes, multinucleate giant cells, and eosinophils, and more chronic lesions showing a lamellated fibrosis, nearly devoid of nucleated cells (**Fig. 6**). The histologic changes are similar to those observed in cases of spontaneous pneumothorax and suggest an interstitial fibroinflammatory reaction to components of air.

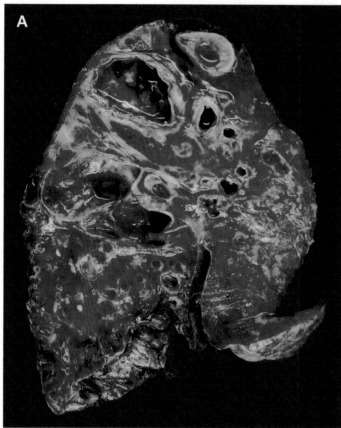

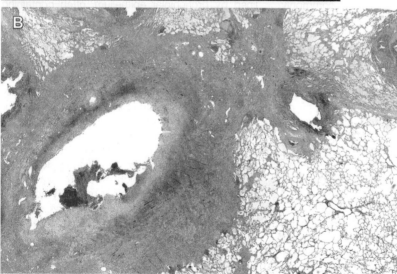

Fig. 4. Bronchiectasis. (*A*) Gross photograph from a 29-year-old with cystic fibrosis showing markedly dilated bronchi extending to near the pleural surface.(*B*) Histology sections show bronchiectasis with associated fibrosis and mixed acute and chronic inflammation (hematoxylin-eosin, original magnification ×20).

DEVELOPMENTAL AND PEDIATRIC CYSTIC LUNG DISEASE

Several cystic diseases arise during fetal lung development and early childhood and include bronchogenic cyst, congenital pulmonary airway malformation (CPAM), and peripheral cystic alveolar growth abnormalities. In addition, pleuropulmonary blastoma, a malignant neoplasm of childhood, should be considered in this differential diagnosis (**Box 3**).

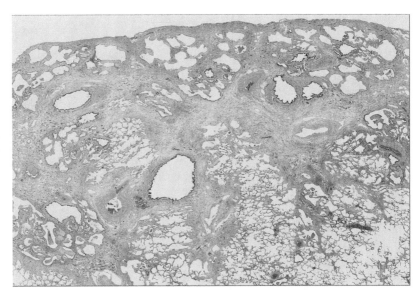

Fig. 5. Microscopic honeycombing. This case of usual interstitial pneumonia in a patient with idiopathic pulmonary fibrosis shows classical microscopic honeycombing with subpleural enlarged irregular airspaces surrounded by dense fibrosis (hematoxylin-eosin, original magnification ×20).

Bronchogenic cysts are congenital cystic lesions that likely arise from abnormal budding of tissue from the primitive foregut. Although they are most commonly identified in the mediastinum, they can occasionally be present along the bronchi. Gross examination shows a solitary ovoid cyst, often filled with mucus. Microscopic evaluation of the cyst wall shows typical layers of the tracheobronchial tree, including cartilage, a single layer of smooth muscle, subepithelial seromucinous glands, and respiratory epithelial lining. The differential diagnosis includes other foregut malformations, such as esophageal duplication cysts.

Congenital pulmonary airway malformations (formerly congenital cystic adenomatoid malformation) refer to a group of variably cystic lesions in the lung characterized by architecturally disordered pulmonary tissue. These lesions are somewhat arbitrarily grouped into types 0 to 4 based on their resemblance to the structures of the tracheobronchial-alveolar airspace continuum. The nomenclature of this lesion was changed due to the fact that only types 1, 2, and 4 are cystic, and only type 3 is adenomatoid. Type 1 lesions show irregular cysts, lined by bronchiolar cuboidal epithelium often with papillary projections, with intervening stromal tissue and a paucity of alveolar structures (**Fig. 7**A). These lesions often show lining of the cyst structures by a bland-appearing mucinous epithelium, which often harbors KRAS mutations, and are morphologically and genetically indistinguishable from mucinous adenocarcinomas (**Fig. 7**B).[15] Type 2 lesions are likely the result of bronchial atresia during early lung development and are characterized by

dilated irregular bronchiole-like structures surrounded by simplified boxlike alveolar structures.[16] Most type 4 lesions likely represent pleuropulmonary blastomas and are discussed as such.

Pleuropulmonary blastoma is a malignant neoplasm of childhood, occurring in the lung. These tumors are classified as types I to III based on the composition of the tumor as cystic or solid. Type I is cystic; type II shows solid nests within the cystic structures, and type III is predominantly solid.[17] Type I pleuropulmonary blastomas are peripherally located and have thin fibrous walls with epithelial lining composed of bronchial, bronchiolar, flattened cuboidal cells, or pneumocytes. The presence of primitive cells in the subepithelial region of the cysts, with hyperchromatic nuclei and increased nuclear to cytoplasmic ratios, aids in the diagnosis. These cells often show rhabdomyomatous differentiation and may show expression of muscle-specific actin and desmin. Occasionally, the cysts show no lesional cells and are referred to as regressed (type IR). In these cases, diagnosis relies heavily on clinical features and genetic testing. There is a strong association of pleuropulmonary blastoma with DICER1 mutations.[18]

Occasionally, cases of numerous peripheral cysts, similar to paraseptal emphysema, but often with mild associated fibrosis, have been described in patients with trisomy 21.[19] These cysts tend to be subpleural, but can be found in both the apex and the base. The origins of cyst formation in these cases are uncertain, but they are usually categorized as a variant of alveolar growth abnormality, such as alveolar hypoplasia.[20]

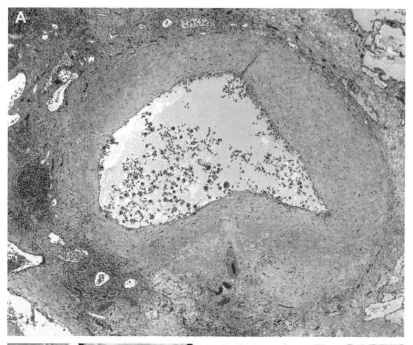

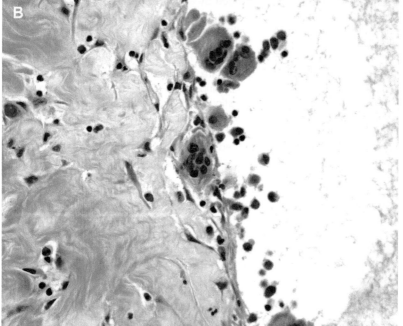

Fig. 6. Pulmonary interstitial emphysema. (*A*) This patient with usual interstitial pneumonia showed several regions of pulmonary interstitial emphysema with interstitial reaction to air ("air cysts"). This rounded cyst shows lamellated dense fibrosis with a lining of multinucleate histiocytes (hematoxylin-eosin, original magnification ×100). (*B*) A higher-power view of the lining shows the histiocytes admixed with eosinophils (hematoxylin-eosin, original magnification ×400).

PULMONARY LANGERHANS CELL HISTIOCYTOSIS

Pulmonary Langerhans cell histiocytosis (PLCH) is a diffuse pulmonary cystic disease that occurs most commonly in smokers. Ninety percent of patients with PLCH are current smokers or have exposure to secondhand smoke.[21] Although some patients present with shortness of breath or cough, many have asymptomatic disease that is discovered incidentally on radiologic imaging.

The imaging and gross features of PLCH are typical of other smoking-related diseases, such as centriacinar emphysema and respiratory bronchiolitis, in that they are accentuated in the apical

Fig. 7. Congenital pulmonary airway malformation. (*A*) On low power, the CPAM, type 1 shows solid regions with undulating ribbons of epithelial cells with admixed cysts (hematoxylin-eosin, original magnification ×20). (*B*) Higher magnification reveals the ciliated lining of the larger cysts, cuboidal lining of the solid components, and scattered nests of mucinous epithelium (hematoxylin-eosin, original magnification ×200).

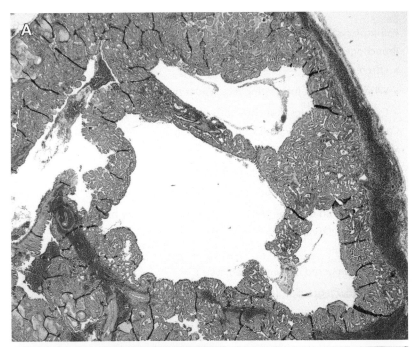

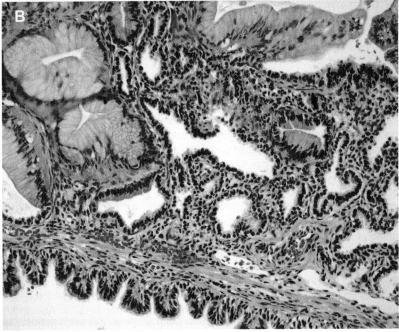

portions of the lungs and in the central portion of the secondary lobule.[22] On CT, one sees irregularly shaped cysts and nodules (often referred to in the radiology literature as "bizarre"). Microscopic evaluation shows that these cysts represent damaged and dilated lumens of former small airways with surrounding cellular infiltration.

This infiltrate is composed of clustered Langerhans cells, a type of histiocyte (tissue-residing cell of monocyte-macrophage lineage) that is involved in immune homeostasis (**Fig. 8**A). These cells are recognized by their ovoid folded nuclei that are reminiscent of dried Medjool dates. They often show punctate nucleoli and have moderate to abundant lightly eosinophilic cytoplasms with somewhat indistinct cell borders (**Fig. 8**B). There are often (but not always) accompanying eosinophils, and this appearance of clustered histiocytes

---

Box 3
Pediatric cystic lung disease

Bronchogenic cyst

- Often central

- When present in mediastinum, consider more generic foregut duplication cyst

- Cyst wall resembles bronchus with single muscular layer, cartilage, and subepithelial glands

Congenital pulmonary airway malformation

- Types 0 to 4

- Type 1 with cysts (usually 0.2–1.0 cm)

- Type 1 can show mucinous epithelium and KRAS mutations

- Type 4 should likely be considered pleuropulmonary blastoma, type I

Pleuropulmonary blastoma

- Types I to III

- Type I composed of thin-walled cysts

- May show regression (type Ir) and lack neoplastic cells

- DICER1 mutations are observed

Alveolar growth abnormalities

- Often asymptomatic

- Present with subpleural cyst formation

- May show associated genetic abnormalities (eg, trisomy 21)

---

and eosinophils was the source of the prior designation of eosinophilic granuloma. The Langerhans cells form rounded airway-centered nodules with peripheral radiating extensions into the adjacent interstitium producing a stellate pattern.[23] Immunohistochemical staining can be helpful in PLCH, because Langerhans cells show robust expression of CD1a and CD207, or Langerin (**Fig. 8**C). It is important to note that smokers will show an increase in resident Langerhans cells, although clustering of these cells is not typical. Because of this overall increase, staining lavage samples for CD1a or CD207 is often discouraged. The lung tissue adjacent to the lesions of PLCH often shows additional smoking-related changes, including respiratory bronchiolitis, centriacinar emphysema, and patchy fibrosis, and in cases of severe respiratory bronchiolitis, careful examination for PLCH should be performed. In many advanced cases, the number of identifiable Langerhans cells decreases and occasionally are not present. These cases show marked airspace enlargement with alveolar septal fibrosis and stellate bronchiolocentric scars (**Fig. 8**D, E). These cases often show pulmonary arterial and venous obliteration, sometimes with mineralization of elastica with associated granulomatous reaction referred to as "endogenous pneumoconiosis" (**Fig. 8**F).[24] These changes reflect the somewhat common finding of clinical hypertension. The author has found that rendering a diagnosis of "burnt-out Langerhans cell histiocytosis" in these cases is somewhat confusing and controversial, currently diagnoses these cases as "airspace enlargement with fibrosis (irregular emphysema)," and discusses the smoking-related cause and the significant risk of pulmonary hypertension.

The nearly ubiquitous association of PLCH with cigarette smoking has led researchers to search for various cytokines that might result in activation of Langerhans cells. These compounds include osteopontin, granulocyte/macrophage colony stimulating factor, and transforming growth factor-beta.[25] An additional concern is whether PLCH is a strictly reactive inflammatory proliferation or whether it represents a neoplastic process. The systemic form of Langerhans cell histiocytosis, more commonly observed in children, is considered a histiocytic malignancy. Approximately half of PLCH cases show mutations in BRAF and MAP2K1.[26,27] These mutations are the same mutations observed in systemic LCH.

Patients with PLCH are treated with smoking cessation and avoidance of secondhand smoke. Occasionally, steroids or chemotherapeutic agents are added, particularly in cases that show

Fig. 8. PLCH. (*A*) A low-power image shows the typical early cellular lesion of PLCH. The nodules tend to be rounded, centered on airways, and often show extension into the interstitium with a stellate pattern (hematoxylin-eosin, original magnification ×20). (*B*) On high magnification, the characteristic nuclear features of the Langerhans cells are noted, including ovoid to reniform shape with occasional clefts and grooves (hematoxylin-eosin, original magnification ×200). (*C*) Immunohistochemical staining for CD1a shows strong membranous expression (diaminobenzidine [DAB] IHC, original magnification × 200.

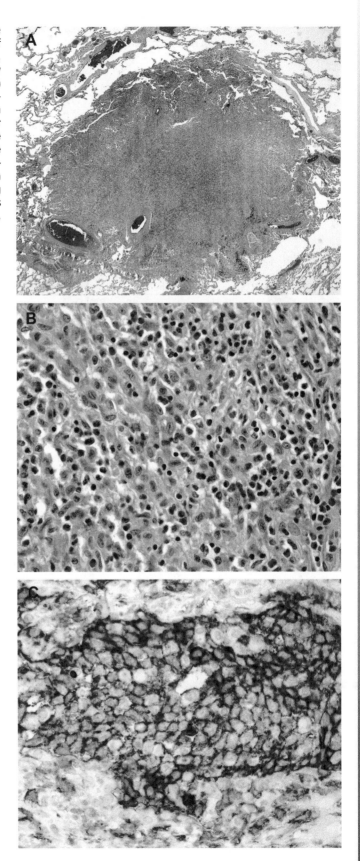

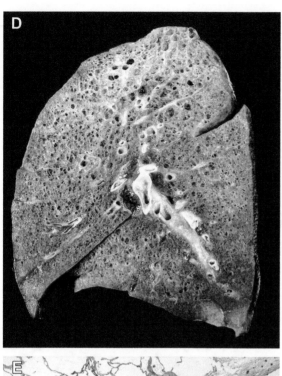

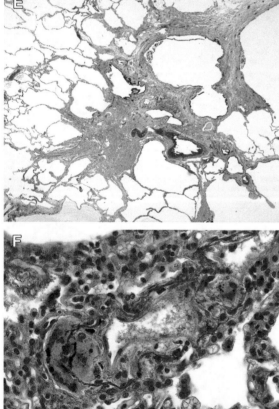

Fig. 8. (*continued*). (*D*) In late stages of the disease, the lung resembles emphysema, but is stiff and fibrous. (*E*) Histologic changes of chronic disease show that the cellular nodules have regressed, leaving fibrotic stellate scars and thickened alveolar septa (hematoxylin-eosin, original magnification ×40). (*F*) Pulmonary vessels may show fibrous obliteration with mineralization of the vascular elastica. This damaged elastica elicits a giant cell reaction (hematoxylin-eosin, original magnification ×200).

extrapulmonary disease or recalcitrance. Patients with advanced disease, including pulmonary hypertension, may require lung transplantation. It is important to note that this disease can recur after transplant, most commonly in patients with extrapulmonary disease or in patients who restart smoking (**Box 4**).

LYMPHANGIOLEIOMYOMATOSIS

Lymphangioleiomyomatosis (LAM) is a rare disease characterized by proliferation of neoplastic smooth muscle-like cells in the lungs and lymphatic spaces. The disease occurs almost exclusively in young women. However, rare cases have been described in men, almost exclusively in the setting of tuberous sclerosis, and occasionally, cases have been described in postmenopausal women, possibly influenced by hormonal therapy.[28-31] LAM shows increased incidence in patients with tuberous sclerosis, in which setting 30% to 40% of adult women develop the disease. Patients with LAM show clinical symptoms of dyspnea, cough, pneumothorax, hemoptysis, and chylothorax.

Gross examination and CT evaluation reveal numerous randomly distributed cysts (**Fig. 9A**). The cysts are rounded with thin walls on CT and range in size from 0.2 to 2 cm in diameter. Microscopic evaluation shows air-filled cysts lined by a variable proliferation of spindled to epithelioid cells characterized by ovoid nuclei with slightly vacuolated chromatin, punctate nucleoli, and moderate amounts of eosinophilic slightly bubbly cytoplasm (**Fig. 9B–D**). Immunohistochemical stains show expression of muscle markers (desmin, actin) and HMB-45, an antibody directed against glycoprotein-100 in the premelanosomal pathway

(**Fig. 9E, F**). Staining for estrogen and progesterone receptors is also frequently positive.

The identification of the origin of the LAM smooth muscle-like cell has been elusive, and localization of an analogous cell in normal lung tissue has been unsuccessful. Recent research using single-cell transcriptomics suggests that the LAM cells are of uterine neural crest origin.[32] This finding supports the hypothesis that LAM possibly represents a form of low-grade metastatic disease and also accounts for the dramatic increased incidence in women.

The prevalence of LAM in patients with tuberous sclerosis is related to the fact that LAM develops secondary to mutations in the 2 TSC genes.[33,34] Mutations of both TSC1 and TSC2 are found in LAM of tuberous sclerosis, and mutations of TSC2 are found in sporadic LAM. Patients with LAM are at increased incidence of angiomyolipoma of the kidney. This hamartomatous tumor is found in most patients with tuberous sclerosis and more than a third of patients with sporadic LAM. A peculiar finding in the lungs of patients with LAM and tuberous sclerosis is the presence of small, rounded proliferations of type 2 pneumocytes, often with mild alveolar septal fibrosis (**Fig. 9G**). This finding has been termed multifocal micronodular pneumocyte hyperplasia and should be differentiated from lesions such as atypical adenomatous hyperplasia.

TSC1 and TSC2 encode the proteins hamartin and tuberin. Abnormalities in these genes result in upregulation of mTOR, which activates several cellular proliferation pathways.[35,36] Notably, one of the effects is increased expression of vascular endothelial growth factors (VEGF) C and D. Serum levels of VEGF-D can be used in diagnosis of patients suspected of having LAM on radiologic findings and can be used in lieu of biopsy in selected

---

Box 4
Pulmonary Langerhans cell histiocytosis

- Upper lobe/zone distribution

- Bronchiolocentric distribution

- Composed of clustered Langerhans cells

- Often shows eosinophils (formerly "eosinophilic granuloma"), but not always

- Related to smoking in nearly all cases

- May show clinical pulmonary hypertension with associated histologic vascular obliteration

- Irregular stellate cellular nodules with cystic change in early active disease

- Stellate bronchiolocentric nodules with "fibrotic emphysema" in later disease

- May show BRAF and/or MAP2K mutations

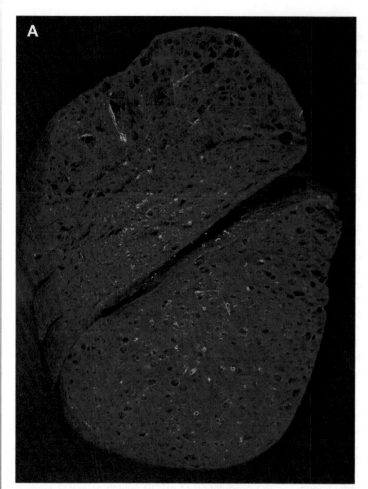

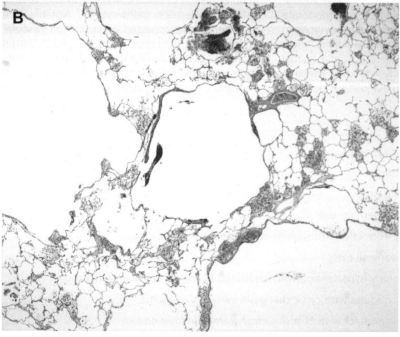

Fig. 9. LAM. (*A*) Gross examination of lungs with LAM shows numerous rounded cysts, extending randomly from apex to base. (*B*) Microscopic evaluation can show numerous cysts with only focal collections of neoplastic cells, as in this case from a 46-year-old woman (hematoxylin-eosin, original magnification ×20).

Fig. 9. (*continued*). (*C*) Alternately, the cysts can show solid larger nests of neoplastic cells (hematoxylin-eosin, original magnification ×20). (*D*) On high magnification, the cytologic features of the neoplastic cells are appreciated with enlarged spindled plump nuclei with occasional small nucleoli, vacuolated chromatin, and moderate amounts of eosinophilic, often coarsely vacuolated, cytoplasm (hematoxylin-eosin, original magnification ×200). (*E*) Immunohistochemical staining reveals expression of HMB-45, often in a patchy distribution (diaminobenzidine [DAB] IHC, original magnification × 100).

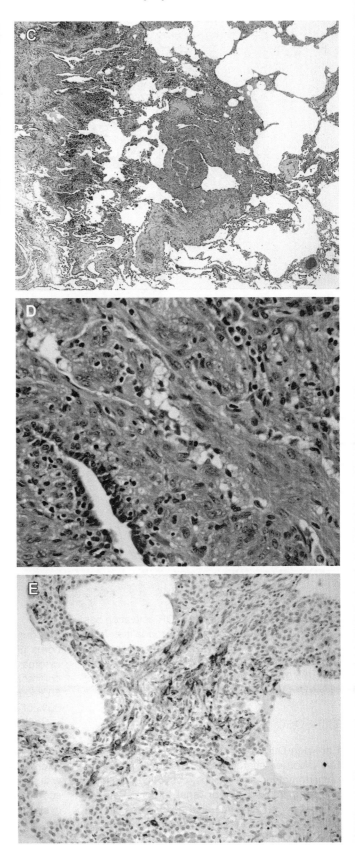

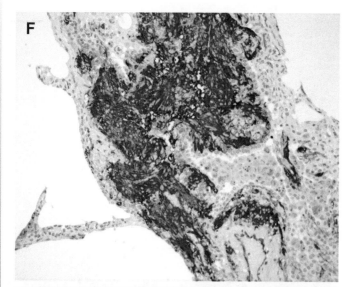

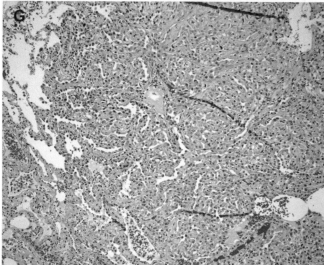

Fig. 9. (*continued*). (*F*) Strong expression of muscle markers is also characteristic of these cells, as seen in this smooth muscle actin stain (diaminobenzidine [DAB] IHC, original magnification × 100). (*G*) Patients with tuberous sclerosis and LAM often show focal proliferation of type 2 pneumocytes termed multifocal micronodular pneumocyte hyperplasia (hematoxylin-eosin, original magnification ×40).

cases.[37] The identification of mTOR activation has led to the migration of treatment modalities from hormonal targeting (which is no longer recommended) to the use of mTOR inhibitors, such as sirolimus.[38,39] This treatment has led to stabilization of disease in many patients (**Box 5**).

BIRT-HOGG-DUBÉ SYNDROME

Birt-Hogg-Dubé syndrome (BHD) is a rare hereditary disorder characterized by development of hamartomatous skin lesions, cystic lung disease, and an increased risk of renal tumors. Patients often show small dome-shaped papules on the face, neck, and upper trunk, which are classified as fibrofolliculomas. Renal tumors develop in approximately a quarter of the patients and consist

predominantly of chromophobe renal cell carcinoma (RCC) or hybrid chromophobe RCC/oncocytoma tumors.[40] Cystic lung disease most commonly develops between the ages of 30 and 50 years, and by the age of 50 years, more than 80% of patients will show cysts.[41]

Radiologic examination shows multiple cysts, predominantly in the basilar subpleural and paraseptal regions. On gross examination, they are often difficult to see. They have no appreciable wall and closely resemble bleb formation. Microscopic evaluation shows similar features.[42,43] The cysts are air filled, often have no associated fibrosis or inflammation, and rarely have a thin wall. The most useful clue to diagnosis is the radiologic information that the lesion is located in the

Fig. 10. LIP/follicular bronchiolitis. (*A*) On low power, sections from a patient with COPA syndrome and cystic disease on imaging show multiple germinal centers surrounding regions of cystic airspace enlargement. There is evidence of remote hemorrhage with hemosiderin-filled macrophages within alveolar spaces (hematoxylin-eosin, original magnification ×20). (*B*) A higher-power view shows the lymphoid aggregates with germinal centers are arranged around bronchovascular bundles, suggesting a diagnosis of follicular bronchiolitis (hematoxylin-eosin, original magnification ×100).

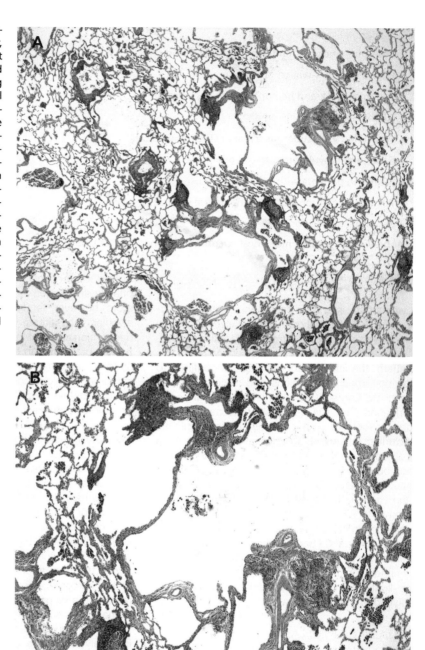

inferior aspect of the lung lobe, rather than the apical bleb formation more commonly observed in typical spontaneous pneumothorax.[44]

BHD is caused by mutations in FLCN, the gene that encodes the protein folliculin.[45] This protein influences mTOR signaling. The pathogenetic cause of cyst formation in BHD is uncertain. Unlike LAM, there does not appear to be a component of cellular proliferation. Rather, there may be cell dropout or weakening of cellular or interstitial integrity, which results in cyst formation.

BHD patients who have experienced pneumothorax are at high risk of additional episodes of pneumothorax, with a recurrence rate of 75%. Most treatments are directed against risk factors of pneumothorax, including avoidance of smoking and scuba diving, and screening for renal tumors (**Box 6**).[41]

> **Box 5**
> **Lymphangioleiomyomatosis**
>
> - Multiple, randomly, and diffusely distributed cysts
> - Round and thin-walled on CT
> - Pneumothorax and hemoptysis not uncommon
> - Almost exclusively in women
> - Associated with tuberous sclerosis (TSC1 and TSC2)
> - Renal angiomyolipomas frequently present
> - MMPH in patients with tuberous sclerosis
> - Possible derivation from uterine neural crest cells
> - Serologic testing for VEGF-D
>
> *Abbreviation*: MMPH, multifocal micronodular pneumocyte hyperplasia.

LYMPHOCYTIC INTERSTITIAL PNEUMONIA

Lymphocytic interstitial pneumonia (LIP) is characterized pathologically by diffuse alveolar septal thickening and robust lymphocytic inflammation. Follicular bronchiolitis is a similar entity, but in this pattern, the inflammatory infiltrate is confined to the peribronchiolar regions and is composed of lymphoid aggregates, often with germinal center formation (**Fig. 10**A,B). These 2 disease patterns are associated with various clinical entities, including autoimmune connective diseases such as Sjogren syndrome and rheumatoid arthritis, immunodeficiency states such as congenital HIV infection and common variable immunodeficiency, and genetic disorders such as COPA syndrome.[46–50] The pathologist is normally less concerned with LIP as a cystic disease, because it is better classified pathologically by the robust inflammation. In these cases, differentiation from lymphoma is useful. In addition, cases of amyloid or light chain deposition disease have been described with cystic change.[51]

METASTATIC NEOPLASMS

Several neoplasms have been reported to cause cystic disease upon metastasis to the lung. In some cases, this is due to necrosis and, given the criteria mentioned previously, is more appropriately designated as cavitary disease. Other tumors, however, tend to show infiltration into the alveolar interstitium, resulting in parenchymal destruction and cyst formation. The most common tumors presenting in this fashion are endometrial stromal sarcoma, epithelioid sarcoma, synovial sarcoma, angiosarcoma, and leiomyosarcoma (benign metastasizing leiomyoma).[52–55] On gross or radiologic examination, there may be a solitary cyst, often subpleural and resembling a bleb. Alternately, there may be numerous nodules with irregular borders. The microscopic appearance varies in accordance with the neoplastic cells. In sarcomas, or low-grade mesenchymal tumors, the lesional cells tend to infiltrate and expand the alveolar or subpleural interstitium (**Fig. 11**A, B). A common presentation is pneumothorax, and the pathologist must be vigilant when confronted with a bleb that shows increased cellularity (**Fig. 11**C–F). In addition, the possibility of metastatic sarcoma should be considered before rendering a diagnosis of the unusual primary pulmonary mesenchymal cystic hamartoma.[56] Typical immunohistochemical stains and molecular analysis can be performed to elucidate the cell of origin and to differentiate these tumors from inflammatory or reactive mesothelial processes.

> **Box 6**
> **Birt-Hogg-Dubé syndrome**
>
> - Lower lobe predominant
> - Histology shows paraseptal tissue loss without significant inflammation or fibrosis
> - Associated with folliculin gene mutations
> - Associated with cutaneous fibrofolliculomas and renal tumors
> - Commonly presents with pneumothorax

Fig. 11. Metastatic sarcoma. (*A*) A low-power view of a metastatic low-grade leiomyosarcoma with multiple nodules. The neoplastic cells infiltrate and expand the alveolar interstitium and result in local architectural destruction with cyst formation (hematoxylin-eosin, original magnification ×20). (*B*) A higher-power view of the leiomyosarcoma shows the expansile interstitial neoplastic growth pattern (hematoxylin-eosin, original magnification ×100). (*C*) A metastatic low-grade endometrial stromal sarcoma shows peripheral subpleural cyst formation (hematoxylin-eosin, original magnification ×40).

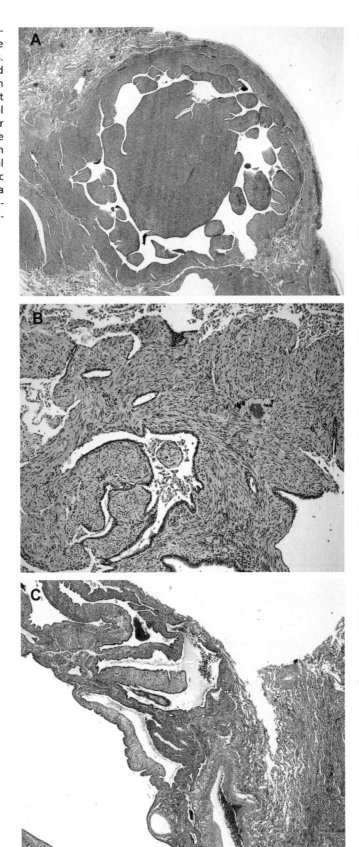

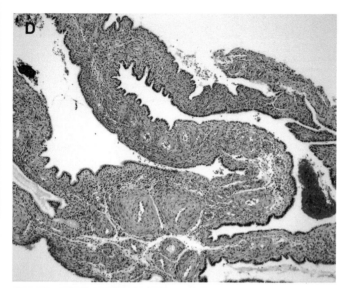

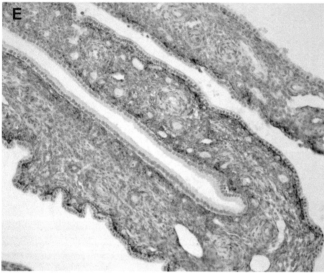

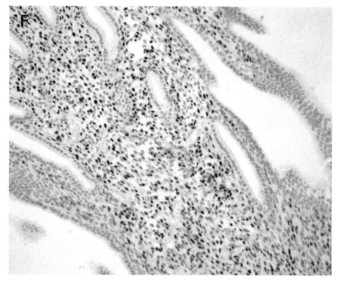

Fig. 11. (*continued*). (*D*) On higher magnification, the cyst lining cells are found to be resident respiratory epithelial cells, whereas the interstitium is expanded by spindled neoplastic tumor cells (hematoxylin-eosin, original magnification ×40). (*E*) Immunohistochemical stains show tumor cell expression of CD10 (diaminobenzidine [DAB] IHC, original magnification × 100), and (*F*) estrogen receptors, supporting the diagnosis of endometrial stromal sarcoma (diaminobenzidine [DAB] IHC, original magnification × 100).

Fig. 12. Respiratory papillomatosis. Histologic evaluation of the cyst walls in respiratory papillomatosis shows papillary projections of keratinizing squamous epithelium with fibrovascular cores (hematoxylin-eosin, original magnification ×20).

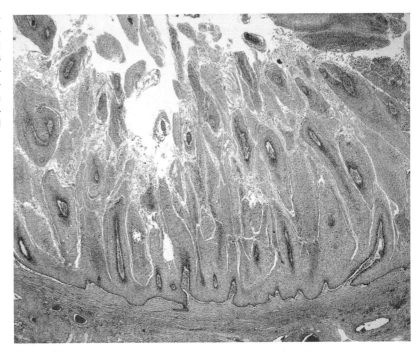

RESPIRATORY PAPILLOMATOSIS

Respiratory papillomatosis, or recurrent respiratory papillomatosis, is a rare disorder characterized by the development of multiple squamous papillomas in the airways, from sinuses to bronchi.[57] The most common sites of these lesions are the larynx and vocal cords (presumably because of their squamous lining), but they can occasionally spread along the tracheobronchial tree and rarely extend to the lungs. In the lungs, the lesions form irregular rounded cysts, likely more accurately cystic dilatation of airways, which are lined by papillary excrescences with fibrovascular cores and lined by squamous epithelium (**Fig. 12**). These lesions are caused by infection with human papillomavirus (HPV), most commonly types HPV6 and HPV11.[58] Treatment of these lesions is difficult and often relies on surgical resection and endobronchial laser ablation.

DISCLOSURE

The author has nothing to disclose.

REFERENCES

1. Raoof S, Bondalapati P, Vydyula R, et al. Cystic lung diseases: algorithmic approach. Chest 2016;150(4): 945–65.
2. Ryu JH, Swensen SJ. Cystic and cavitary lung diseases: focal and diffuse. Mayo Clin Proc 2003;78(6):744–52.
3. Gafoor K, Patel S, Girvin F, et al. Cavitary lung diseases: a clinical-radiologic algorithmic approach. Chest 2018;153(6):1443–65.
4. Ulbright TM, Katzenstein AL. Solitary necrotizing granulomas of the lung: differentiating features and etiology. Am J Surg Pathol 1980;4(1):13–28.
5. Honda O, Tsubamoto M, Inoue A, et al. Pulmonary cavitary nodules on computed tomography: differentiation of malignancy and benignancy. J Comput Assist Tomogr 2007;31(6):943–9.
6. Butnor KJ. Avoiding underdiagnosis, overdiagnosis, and misdiagnosis of lung carcinoma. Arch Pathol Lab Med 2008;132(7):1118–32.
7. Crapanzano JP, Zakowski MF. Diagnostic dilemmas in pulmonary cytology. Cancer 2001;93(6):364–75.
8. Travis WD, Hoffman GS, Leavitt RY, et al. Surgical pathology of the lung in Wegener's granulomatosis. Review of 87 open lung biopsies from 67 patients. Am J Surg Pathol 1991;15(4):315–33.
9. Katzenstein AL, Locke WK. Solitary lung lesions in Wegener's granulomatosis. Pathologic findings and clinical significance in 25 cases. Am J Surg Pathol 1995;19(5):545–52.
10. Fidler ME, Koomen M, Sebek B, et al. Placental transmogrification of the lung, a histologic variant of giant bullous emphysema. Clinicopathological study of three further cases. Am J Surg Pathol 1995;19(5):563–70.
11. Barker AF. Bronchiectasis. N Engl J Med 2002; 346(18):1383–93.
12. Jones KD. Unclassifiable interstitial lung disease: a pathologist's perspective. Eur Respir Rev 2018; 27(147), [pii:170132].

13. Barcia SM, Kukreja J, Jones KD. Pulmonary interstitial emphysema in adults: a clinicopathologic study of 53 lung explants. Am J Surg Pathol 2014;38(3):339–45.

14. Tachibana Y, Taniguchi H, Kondoh Y, et al. Pulmonary interstitial emphysema is a risk factor for poor prognosis and a cause of air leaks. Respir Investig 2019;57(5):444–50.

15. Lantuejoul S, Nicholson AG, Sartori G, et al. Mucinous cells in type 1 pulmonary congenital cystic adenomatoid malformation as mucinous bronchioloalveolar carcinoma precursors. Am J Surg Pathol 2007;31(6):961–9.

16. Fowler DJ, Gould SJ. The pathology of congenital lung lesions. Semin Pediatr Surg 2015;24(4):176–82.

17. Messinger YH, Stewart DR, Priest JR, et al. Pleuropulmonary blastoma: a report on 350 central pathology-confirmed pleuropulmonary blastoma cases by the International Pleuropulmonary Blastoma Registry. Cancer 2015;121(2):276–85.

18. Hill DA, Ivanovich J, Priest JR, et al. DICER1 mutations in familial pleuropulmonary blastoma. Science 2009;325(5943):965.

19. Schloo BL, Vawter GF, Reid LM. Down syndrome: patterns of disturbed lung growth. Hum Pathol 1991;22(9):919–23.

20. Dishop MK. Diagnostic pathology of diffuse lung disease in children. Pediatr Allergy Immunol Pulmonol 2010;23(1):69–85.

21. Vassallo R. Diffuse lung diseases in cigarette smokers. Semin Respir Crit Care Med 2012;33(5):533–42.

22. Hartman TE, Tazelaar HD, Swensen SJ, et al. Cigarette smoking: CT and pathologic findings of associated pulmonary diseases. Radiographics 1997;17(2):377–90.

23. Travis WD, Borok Z, Roum JH, et al. Pulmonary Langerhans cell granulomatosis (histiocytosis X). A clinicopathologic study of 48 cases. Am J Surg Pathol 1993;17(10):971–86.

24. Suri HS, Yi ES, Nowakowski GS, et al. Pulmonary Langerhans cell histiocytosis. Orphanet J Rare Dis 2012;7:16.

25. Gupta N, Vassallo R, Wikenheiser-Brokamp KA, et al. Diffuse cystic lung disease. Part I. Am J Respir Crit Care Med 2015;191(12):1354–66.

26. Alayed K, Medeiros LJ, Patel KP, et al. BRAF and MAP2K1 mutations in Langerhans cell histiocytosis: a study of 50 cases. Hum Pathol 2016;52:61–7.

27. Kamionek M, Ahmadi Moghaddam P, Sakhdari A, et al. Mutually exclusive extracellular signal-regulated kinase pathway mutations are present in different stages of multi-focal pulmonary Langerhans cell histiocytosis supporting clonal nature of the disease. Histopathology 2016;69(3):499–509.

28. Baldi S, Papotti M, Valente ML, et al. Pulmonary lymphangioleiomyomatosis in postmenopausal women: report of two cases and review of the literature. Eur Respir J 1994;7(5):1013–6.

29. Aubry MC, Myers JL, Ryu JH, et al. Pulmonary lymphangioleiomyomatosis in a man. Am J Respir Crit Care Med 2000;162(2 Pt 1):749–52.

30. Schiavina M, Di Scioscio V, Contini P, et al. Pulmonary lymphangioleiomyomatosis in a karyotypically normal man without tuberous sclerosis complex. Am J Respir Crit Care Med 2007;176(1):96–8.

31. Ishii H, Kushima H, Watanabe K, et al. Two cases of pulmonary lymphangioleiomyomatosis in postmenopausal women. Respir Investig 2014;52(4):261–4.

32. Guo M, Yu JJ, Perl AK, et al. Identification of the lymphangioleiomyomatosis cell and its uterine origin. bioRxiv 2019;784199.

33. Smolarek TA, Wessner LL, McCormack FX, et al. Evidence that lymphangiomyomatosis is caused by TSC2 mutations: chromosome 16p13 loss of heterozygosity in angiomyolipomas and lymph nodes from women with lymphangiomyomatosis. Am J Hum Genet 1998;62(4):810–5.

34. Strizheva GD, Carsillo T, Kruger WD, et al. The spectrum of mutations in TSC1 and TSC2 in women with tuberous sclerosis and lymphangiomyomatosis. Am J Respir Crit Care Med 2001;163(1):253–8.

35. Inoki K, Li Y, Zhu T, et al. TSC2 is phosphorylated and inhibited by Akt and suppresses mTOR signaling. Nat Cell Biol 2002;4(9):648–57.

36. Tee AR, Fingar DC, Manning BD, et al. Tuberous sclerosis complex-1 and -2 gene products function together to inhibit mammalian target of rapamycin (mTOR)-mediated downstream signaling. Proc Natl Acad Sci U S A 2002;99(21):13571–6.

37. Young LR, Vandyke R, Gulleman PM, et al. Serum vascular endothelial growth factor-D prospectively distinguishes lymphangioleiomyomatosis from other diseases. Chest 2010;138(3):674–81.

38. McCormack FX, Gupta N, Finlay GR, et al. Official American Thoracic Society/Japanese Respiratory Society clinical practice guidelines: lymphangioleiomyomatosis diagnosis and management. Am J Respir Crit Care Med 2016;194(6):748–61.

39. Gupta N, Finlay GA, Kotloff RM, et al. Lymphangioleiomyomatosis diagnosis and management: high-resolution chest computed tomography, transbronchial lung biopsy, and pleural disease management. An official American Thoracic Society/Japanese Respiratory Society Clinical Practice Guideline. Am J Respir Crit Care Med 2017;196(10):1337–48.

40. Pavlovich CP, Walther MM, Eyler RA, et al. Renal tumors in the Birt-Hogg-Dube syndrome. Am J Surg Pathol 2002;26(12):1542–52.

41. Gupta N, Sunwoo BY, Kotloff RM. Birt-Hogg-Dube syndrome. Clin Chest Med 2016;37(3):475–86.

42. Butnor KJ, Guinee DG Jr. Pleuropulmonary pathology of Birt-Hogg-Dube syndrome. Am J Surg Pathol 2006;30(3):395–9.

43. Koga S, Furuya M, Takahashi Y, et al. Lung cysts in Birt-Hogg-Dube syndrome: histopathological characteristics and aberrant sequence repeats. Pathol Int 2009;59(10):720–8.

44. Fabre A, Borie R, Debray MP, et al. Distinguishing the histological and radiological features of cystic lung disease in Birt-Hogg-Dube syndrome from those of tobacco-related spontaneous pneumothorax. Histopathology 2014;64(5):741–9.

45. Nickerson ML, Warren MB, Toro JR, et al. Mutations in a novel gene lead to kidney tumors, lung wall defects, and benign tumors of the hair follicle in patients with the Birt-Hogg-Dube syndrome. Cancer Cell 2002;2(2):157–64.

46. Howling SJ, Hansell DM, Wells AU, et al. Follicular bronchiolitis: thin-section CT and histologic findings. Radiology 1999;212(3):637–42.

47. Cha SI, Fessler MB, Cool CD, et al. Lymphoid interstitial pneumonia: clinical features, associations and prognosis. Eur Respir J 2006;28(2):364–9.

48. Panchabhai TS, Farver C, Highland KB. Lymphocytic interstitial pneumonia. Clin Chest Med 2016; 37(3):463–74.

49. Tsui JL, Estrada OA, Deng Z, et al. Analysis of pulmonary features and treatment approaches in the COPA syndrome. ERJ Open Res 2018;4(2).

50. Chung A, Wilgus ML, Fishbein G, et al. Pulmonary and bronchiolar involvement in Sjogren's syndrome. Semin Respir Crit Care Med 2019;40(2):235–54.

51. Baqir M, Kluka EM, Aubry MC, et al. Amyloid-associated cystic lung disease in primary Sjogren's syndrome. Respir Med 2013;107(4):616–21.

52. Mehzad M. Leiomyosarcoma of the uterus presenting with pneumothorax. Br J Dis Chest 1977;71(2):132–4.

53. Aubry MC, Myers JL, Colby TV, et al. Endometrial stromal sarcoma metastatic to the lung: a detailed analysis of 16 patients. Am J Surg Pathol 2002; 26(4):440–9.

54. Murakami A, Hayashi T, Terao Y, et al. Cystic, nodular and cavitary metastases to the lungs in a patient with endometrial stromal sarcoma of the uterus. Intern Med 2014;53(9):1001–5.

55. Hoshi M, Oebisu N, Iwai T, et al. An unusual presentation of pneumothorax associated with cystic lung metastasis from epithelioid sarcoma: a case report and review of the literature. Oncol Lett 2018;15(4):4531–4.

56. van der Heijden EH, Kaal SE, Hassing HH, et al. Mesenchymal cystic hamartoma? A revised diagnosis after 23 years. Thorax 2014;69(1):84–5.

57. Ivancic R, Iqbal H, deSilva B, et al. Current and future management of recurrent respiratory papillomatosis. Laryngoscope Investig Otolaryngol 2018;3(1):22–34.

58. Fortes HR, von Ranke FM, Escuissato DL, et al. Recurrent respiratory papillomatosis: a state-of-the-art review. Respir Med 2017;126:116–21.

Connective Tissue Disease Related Interstitial Lung Disease

Jefree J. Schulte, MD[a],*, Aliya N. Husain, MD[b]

KEYWORDS

- Interstitial lung disease • Connective tissue disease • Collagen vascular disease
- Interstitial pneumonia with autoimmune features • Usual interstitial pneumonia
- Nonspecific interstitial pneumonia

Key points

- Connective tissue diseases may present with pulmonary involvement and includes multiple patterns ranging from acute lung injury to diffuse fibrosing processing.

- There is significant histologic overlap between the different connective tissue diseases with pulmonary involvement, but certain patterns and findings can suggest a specific etiology.

- Identification of histologic patterns suggestive of connective tissue disease related interstitial lung disease is important to help distinguish from idiopathic interstitial lung disease, as treatments may differ.

ABSTRACT

Patients with connective tissue diseases may have pulmonary involvement, including interstitial lung disease. Various patterns of interstitial lung disease have been classically described in certain connective tissue diseases. It is now recognized that there is significant overlap between patterns of interstitial lung disease observed in the various connective tissue diseases. Differentiating idiopathic from connective tissue disease-related interstitial lung disease is challenging but of clinical importance. New concepts in the diagnosis of connective tissue disease related interstitial lung disease may prove useful in making the diagnosis.

OVERVIEW

Connective tissue diseases (CTD), also referred to as collagen vascular diseases, are rheumatologic conditions afflicting the proteins that function to create the connective tissue framework of the body. A precise calculation of the incidence and prevalence of interstitial lung disease (ILD) remains elusive, but the disease seems to be more common than once thought.[1] The degree to which this increase in incidence and prevalence may be attributed to CTD is unclear. It is estimated that approximately 15% of patients with ILD have an underlying CTD.[2] Generally, CTD-ILD enters into the differential when the patient is a woman and/or younger than 50 years old, but CTD-ILD can occur in both men and women, and young and old. Although not an exhaustive list of conditions where CTD-ILD may be observed, rheumatoid arthritis (RA), systemic lupus erythematosus (SLE), mixed CTD (MCTD), Sjögren syndrome (SS), polymyositis/dermatomyositis, and systemic sclerosis (scleroderma [SCL]) have classically reported histopathologic features (Table 1). CTD-ILD may show significant clinical, radiographic, and histopathologic overlap with well-defined patterns of ILD and various patterns of ILD have been reported in patients with CTD. Manifestations of CTD-ILD range from changes associated with acute lung injury (ALI) and organizing pneumonia (OP), to diffuse interstitial processes including usual interstitial pneumonia (UIP), nonspecific

---

[a] Department of Pathology, University of Chicago, 5841 South Maryland Avenue, MC6101, Chicago, IL 60637, USA; [b] Department of Pathology, University of Chicago, 5841 South Maryland, Room S627, MC6101, Chicago, IL 60637, USA
* Corresponding author.
E-mail address: Jefree.Schulte@uchospitals.edu

Surgical Pathology 13 (2020) 165–188
https://doi.org/10.1016/j.path.2019.11.005

Table 1
Classically reported patterns in CTD-related ILD

CTD	Classic Histologic ILD Patterns
RA	Rheumatoid nodules UIP
Systemic lupus erythematosus	Acute lupus pneumonitis
Mixed CTD	Cellular NSIP
Sjögren syndrome	NSIP LIP
Polymyositis/ dermatomyositis	NSIP Superimposed acute changes
Scleroderma	Fibrotic NSIP

Overview Key Points

- Significant overlap between idiopathic ILD and CTD-ILD
- Distinguishing between the 2 entities is difficult
- Important to recognize CTD-ILD
  - Different treatments
  - Maybe first manifestation of CTD
  - Prognostic implications

QUICK OVERVIEW OF INTERSTITIAL LUNG DISEASE DIAGNOSIS

BIOPSY AND HISTOPATHOLOGIC DIAGNOSIS

The diagnosis of ILD remains a challenge. Classification of interstitial processes into the various categories of ILD depends on how strict the diagnostician follows published guidelines and those who choose to render a diagnosis by adhering strictly to guidelines (or without sufficient clinical, radiologic, or histopathologic data), may be more apt to render a diagnosis of chronic interstitial pneumonia, unclassifiable.[5] How to classify nonidiopathic ILD complicates the situation further. When contemplating an ILD diagnosis, the pathologist should consider if the biopsy is adequate for assessment, and may choose to provided commentary on the adequacy of the biopsy. Surgical lung biopsy, open, or more commonly video-assisted thorascopic surgery, is the ideal specimen to assess for an interstitial process.[6–8] Ideally, multiple sites from different lobes would be sampled. Although a transbronchial biopsy may be diagnostic in certain conditions (eg, sarcoidosis), in general, it should not be used in the setting of ILD.[6,9]

MULTIDISCIPLINARY APPROACH TO DIAGNOSIS

Clinical and HRCT findings are specific and highly reproducible in certain conditions, including respiratory bronchiolitis ILD and UIP, and emerging data suggest that certain HRCT patterns may be helpful in the diagnosis of CTD-ILD.[10–13] If histopathology differs from the clinical or radiographic impression, the treating physician is obligated to consider other etiologies.[10] In this setting, one may consider CTD-ILD. The facts that no diagnostic modality is perfect and that the diagnostician not uncommonly lacks pertinent clinical information, underline the point made by consensus documents which highlight the importance of a multidisciplinary approach to the diagnosis of ILD.[10,14,15]

interstitial pneumonia (NSIP), and lymphocytic interstitial pneumonia (LIP), among others. Some patients with CTD-ILD present with unclassifiable chronic interstitial pneumonia. Lung biopsy rates are decreasing secondary to improved imaging diagnostics, most notably with advances in high-resolution computed tomography (HRCT) scanning, as well as advances in the pharmacologic management of CTD and ILD. Nonetheless, it remains imperative for the pathologist to recognize features of CTD-ILD. Although most nonacademic pathologists encounter lung specimens in the setting of a lung malignancy, there is often background non-neoplastic lung submitted for histopathologic interpretation. Medical lung disease, including ILD, may be present in these non-neoplastic lung sections. Recognizing early changes of classic ILD can be challenging in and of itself, but a pathologist cognizant of CTD-ILD features may suggest the diagnosis and could help detect an unrecognized CTD; ILD could be the first manifestation of an occult CTD. Although patients with CTD-ILD tend to do better than patients with idiopathic ILD, recognizing CTD-ILD is important because it is reported to be an adverse prognostic indicator in patients with CTD and results in significant morbidity and mortality.[3,4] Last, as treatment paradigms for idiopathic ILD have shifted away from traditional anti-inflammatory therapies toward antifibrotic agents, the distinction between idiopathic ILD and CTD-ILD has increased significance, because CTD-ILD patients are typically not treated with antifibrotic therapy. This review focuses on the diagnosis of CTD-ILD in common CTD, commonalities with idiopathic interstitial fibrosis, as well as an introduction and review of interstitial pneumonia with autoimmune features (IPAF) and new and emerging topics in the field.

RHEUMATOID ARTHRITIS

OVERVIEW

RA is a chronic inflammatory condition that typically manifests with symptoms related to joint damage secondary to overproduction of tumor necrosis factor and activation of other inflammatory cascades.[16,17] The disease afflicts up to 1% of the population of industrialized countries.[16] Involvement of the lung is not uncommon in RA with up to 58% of patients with RA having some indication (usually subclinical) of pulmonary involvement.[18–20] The manifestations of RA in the lung are myriad. Common features of pulmonary involvement by RA include:

- Rheumatoid nodules
- ALI (diffuse alveolar damage [DAD], drug reaction)
- Follicular bronchiolitis
- UIP

RHEUMATOID NODULES

A classic manifestation of RA in the soft tissue is the rheumatoid nodule. Rheumatoid nodules have been reported in the lungs of patients with RA and share a similar histopathology with their soft tissue counterpart (**Fig. 1**).[21–23] Rheumatoid nodules are granulomatous nodules with central fibrinoid necrosis with a peripheral rim of palisaded, epithelioid histiocytes. An outer rim of lymphoplasmacytic inflammation may also be observed. Rheumatoid nodules are typically bilateral, numerous, and present in a subpleural and/or septal distribution. Rheumatoid nodules may present as a diagnostic challenge. Other causes of granulomatous nodules, including infection and vasculitis, should be excluded. Prior or concurrent rheumatoid nodules in the soft tissue, as well as clinical and/or serologic findings supportive of a diagnosis of RA, may prove helpful in making the diagnosis. Numerous rheumatoid-like nodules may be seen in patients with RA who also have coal worker's pneumoconiosis; a condition named rheumatoid pneumoconiosis (or the eponymous Caplan syndrome).[24]

ACUTE LUNG INJURY

ALI is another pattern of pulmonary involvement in RA. The ALI typically presents as DAD (**Fig. 2**).[20,25,26] Without a history of RA, or serologic studies suggestive of RA, the cause of the lung injury may be difficult to ascertain. It was not uncommon for patients with RA to be

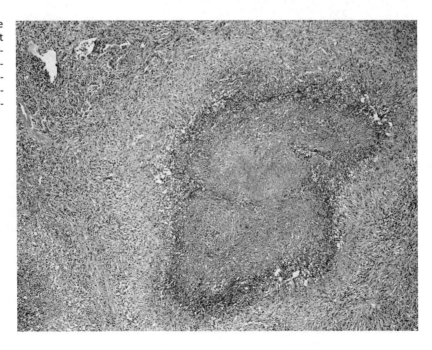

Fig. 1. Rheumatoid nodule in a lung from a patient with RA. There is a necrobiotic center with a peripheral rim of epithelioid histiocytes (stain: hematoxylin and eosin; original magnification ×40).

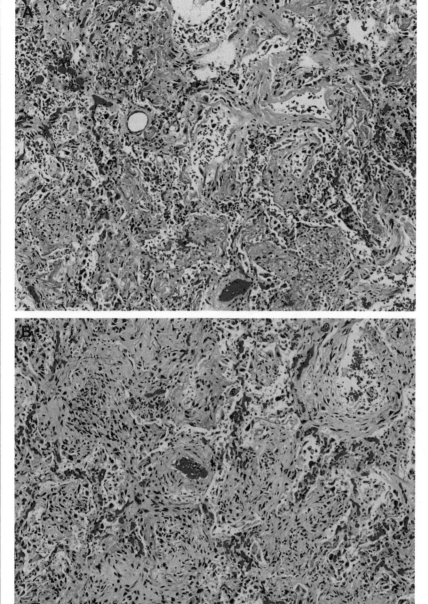

Fig. 2. DAD largely obscuring any background lung pathology (*A*) with hyaline membrane formation and sloughing of epithelium into alveolar spaces observed in acute DAD (stain: hematoxylin and eosin; original magnification ×100). (*B*) Organizing phase of DAD with plugs of granulation tissue filling alveolar spaces (stain: hematoxylin and eosin; original magnification ×100).

treated with methotrexate. Methotrexate and other newer drugs may also induce ALI.[27–30] Although methotrexate ALI may present as DAD, a drug reaction pattern may also be observed. Drug reactions may present as OP or eosinophilic pneumonia (**Fig. 3**).[31] In the setting of a drug reaction, OP may have admixed eosinophils (see **Fig. 3**C). Whether the pathologist diagnoses OP with eosinophils or eosinophilic pneumonia is likely of little consequence because both conditions would be treated with

corticosteroids. Methotrexate does occasionally cause a somewhat more specific pattern of lung injury with interstitial giant cells and/or poorly formed granulomas (**Fig. 4**).[32]

FIBROSING DISEASE IN RHEUMATOID ARTHRITIS INTERSTITIAL LUNG DISEASE

Albeit nonspecific, chronic changes in the lungs of patients with RA include 2 main patterns, follicular bronchiolitis and UIP.[20] Follicular bronchiolitis is

Fig. 3. Patterns of ALI attributed to drug reaction. (*A*) OP characterized by intra-alveolar Masson bodies (*black arrow*; stain: hematoxylin and eosin; original magnification ×100). (*B*) Eosinophilic pneumonia with sheets of eosinophils filling alveolar spaces (stain: hematoxylin and eosin; original magnification ×200). (*C*). Mixed OP with eosinophils (stain: hematoxylin and eosin; original magnification ×200).

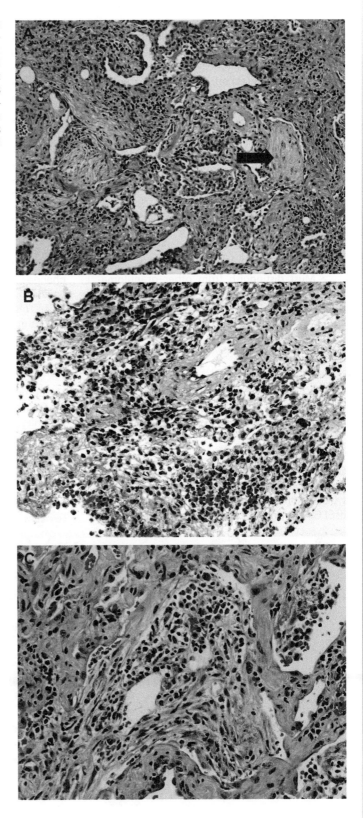

characterized by prominent bronchial-associated lymphoid tissue with or without germinal center formation (**Fig. 5**). The differential diagnosis for follicular bronchiolitis is quite broad and includes other CTD-ILDs, infection, and airway hypersensitivity. UIP pattern fibrosis represents end-stage fibrotic lung in patients with RA and is the most common reported chronic lung disease observed in patients with RA (**Fig. 6**).[33] Certain clues may suggest a diagnosis of RA/CTD-ILD in this setting, including younger age of presentation, combined NSIP pattern, and increased lymphoid follicles when compared with idiopathic UIP (**Fig. 7**).

Rheumatoid Arthritis Interstitial Lung Disease Key Points

- Rheumatoid nodules
  - Must distinguish from other granulomatous lesions
- DAD not uncommon
- Most common chronic changes:
  - Follicular bronchiolitis
  - UIP

SYSTEMIC LUPUS ERYTHEMATOSUS

OVERVIEW

SLE is a chronic inflammatory disease caused by auto-antibodies directed against various tissues, typically with anti-nuclear antibodies. The prevalence of SLE in the United States is approximately 52 cases per 100,000 people.[34] Although clinically apparent, pulmonary disease is less common in SLE than in other CTD-ILDs and most patients will eventually develop some form of pulmonary involvement.[35,36] Pulmonary involvement in SLE classically presents with ALI, termed acute lupus pneumonitis.[37]

ACUTE LUPUS PNEUMONITIS

Acute lupus pneumonitis shows various pathologic changes often with systemic clinical findings, including fever, dyspnea, cough, and hypoxemia. These histopathologic changes are numerous and range from interstitial inflammation to capillaritis with or without diffuse alveolar hemorrhage (**Fig. 8**).[38,39] Hemosiderin-laden macrophages may also be observed in acute lupus pneumonitis (**Fig. 9**). It is not uncommon for the pulmonary changes seen in SLE to be confined to the vascular compartment and not the interstitium; these changes include hypertensive changes, plexiform lesions, and thrombosis (**Fig. 10**).[39–41]

FIBROSING DISEASE IN LUPUS INTERSTITIAL LUNG DISEASE

The chronic changes observed in SLE are usually in the form of cellular NSIP characterized by lymphoplasmacytic interstitial inflammation (**Fig. 11**) with variable fibrosis, or UIP.[38,39,42] The differential diagnosis of pulmonary involvement by SLE is broad.

DIFFERENTIAL DIAGNOSIS

Acute lupus pneumonitis is most challenging because it presents with ALI and should be

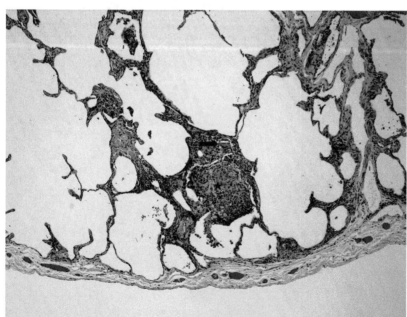

Fig. 4. Interstitial granuloma in a patient treated with methotrexate. There is an associated foreign body giant cell (*black arrow*) which is situated next to a poorly formed granuloma (black star; stain: hematoxylin and eosin; original magnification ×4).

differentiated from infectious processes, vasculitis conditions, and other causes of acute respiratory distress syndrome. The pulmonary changes in chronic SLE may be subtle, especially given the aforementioned fact that SLE is less likely to have clinically apparent disease, but a thorough review of clinical data should help to cinch the diagnosis.

Systemic Lupus Erythematosus Interstitial Lung Disease Key Points

- Acute lupus pneumonitis
  - Presents as a form of ALI
- Most common chronic process is cellular NSIP

MIXED CONNECTIVE TISSUE DISEASE

OVERVIEW

MCTD is characterized by numerous findings typically observed in a number of CTD, but with seropositivity for anti–U1-ribonuclearprotein. Common clinical findings include polyarthritis, Raynaud phenomenon, and sclerodactyly, among others.[43] MCTD affects approximately 2 persons per 100,000 people per year.[44] Pulmonary involvement is observed in the majority (85%) of patients.[43]

Fig. 5. Patterns of follicular bronchiolitis. (*A*) Dense lymphoid aggregates with germinal center formation in a patient with UIP (stain: hematoxylin and eosin; original magnification ×40). (*B*) Lymphoid cells are largely confined to the subepithelial space (stain: hematoxylin and eosin; original magnification ×100).

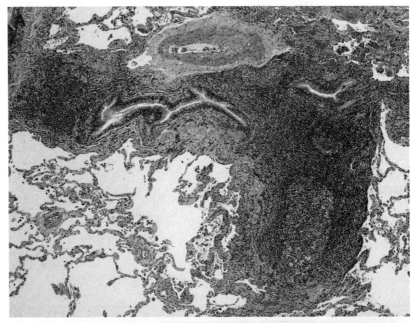

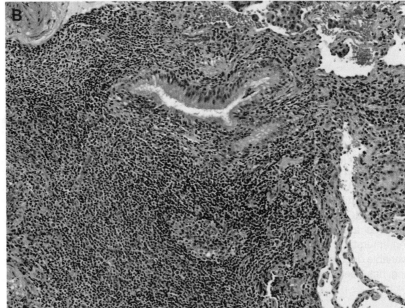

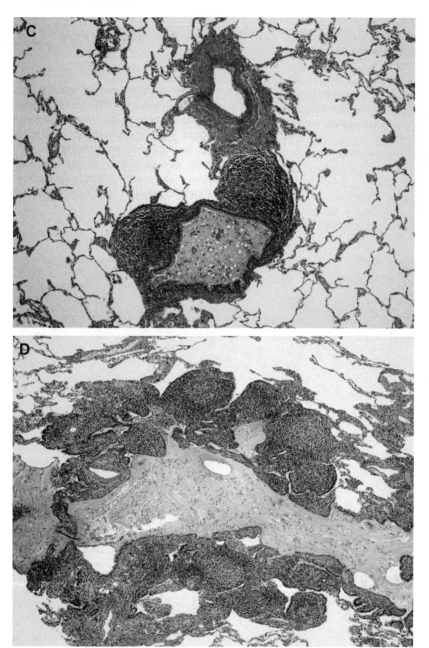

Fig. 5. (*continued*). (*C*) Peribronchiolar lymphoid aggregates in a patient treated with methotrexate (stain: hematoxylin and eosin; original magnification ×40). (*D*) Same patient as seen in *C* with more abundant lymphocytes with germinal center formation (stain: hematoxylin and eosin; original magnification ×40).

PATTERNS OF INTERSTITIAL LUNG DISEASE IN MIXED CONNECTIVE TISSUE DISEASE

ALI, including acute interstitial pneumonia, diffuse alveolar hemorrhage, OP, and DAD, has been reported, but are rare.[45–47] The literature is sparse on the patterns of pulmonary interstitial damage seen in MCTD. Some authors write that ILD may develop and is usually asymptomatic or mild.[43] An interstitial lymphoplasmacytic infiltrate with variable degrees of fibrosis, including honeycombing, has been described.[48] More classic NSIP and

UIP patterns are also reported, as well as vascular changes including plexiform lesions.[45,49] The lack of a well-defined pattern of interstitial injury in MCTD may be due to the complex clinical presentation of the disease. MCTD as a separate entity from other CTD is controversial in rheumatology. Last, it is unclear if the different clinical symptoms present in MCTD link to any specific lung pathology, although a recent report suggested a link between ILD and esophageal motor dysfunction.[50] More studies are needed to appropriately define the pulmonary manifestations of MCTD.

Fig. 6. UIP. (*A*) Temporal and spatial heterogeneity are common in UIP with areas showing active fibrosis with fibroblastic foci (*black arrow*) and areas without fibroblastic foci. Also there are areas showing less involvement by fibrosis on the right of the image (stain: hematoxylin and eosin; original magnification ×40). (*B*) Fibroblastic focus (*black arrow*) in an area of active fibrosis in a patient with UIP (stain: hematoxylin and eosin; original magnification ×100).

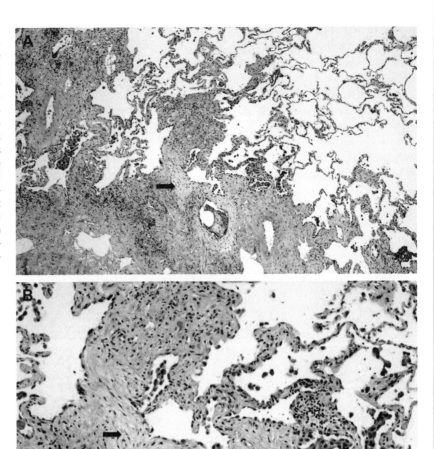

Mixed Connective Tissue Disease Interstitial Lung Disease Key Points

- ALI is rare
- Pulmonary involvement in most patients with MCTD
- Histologic patterns unclear at present

SJÖGREN SYNDROME

OVERVIEW

SS is characterized by chronic inflammation centered in the salivary glands, which results in gland fibrosis and clinical findings of xerostomia and keratoconjunctivitis sicca, as well as production of the autoantibodies, anti-SSA/Ro and anti-SSB/La. The incidence and prevalence of SS varies between the populations studied and between primary and secondary forms of the disease.[51,52] Lung involvement is not uncommon, affecting 9% to 20% of patients with SS.[53,54] Lung involvement is associated with increased morbidity in patients with SS.[55] Pulmonary involvement is not confined to the interstitial compartment; the tracheobronchial tree may also be affected leading to xerotrachea and small airway disease.[56]

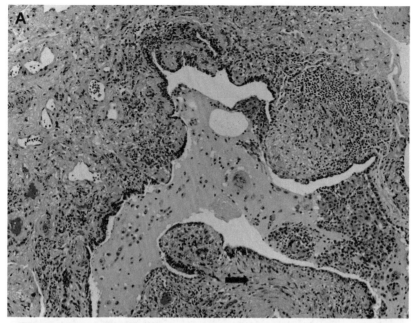

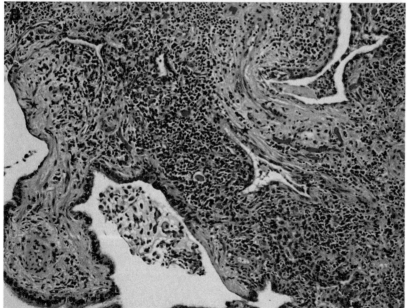

Fig. 7. Patient with UIP and CTD (*A*) Note the fibroblastic focus (*black arrow*) with admixed interstitial lymphoplasmacytic infiltrate (stain: hematoxylin and eosin; original magnification ×100) (*B*) Poorly formed, possibly early, fibroblastic foci (*black stars*) within dense lymphoplasmacytic infiltrate (stain: hematoxylin and eosin; original magnification ×200). Significant interstitial lymphoplasmacytic inflammation in a patient with ILD may suggest CTD-ILD.

FIBROSING DISEASE IN SJÖGREN SYNDROME INTERSTITIAL LUNG DISEASE

The most common appearance of ILD in SS is NSIP, and fibrotic NSIP is the most common subtype of NSIP reported.[57–60] Other patterns of ILD can be observed, including UIP and LIP. Classically, LIP was thought to be common in SS, but LIP is now understood to be a rare benign lymphoproliferative disorder (**Fig. 12**).[61] A number of these early LIP cases may have represented cellular NSIP patterns. Nonetheless, LIP accounts for approximately 15% of cases of ILD in SS.[62] Besides LIP and cellular NSIP, changes typical to most CTD-ILD can also be observed, including follicular bronchiolitis. Not surprisingly, given the discussion on the lymphoplasmacytic patterns observed in SS, there is a significantly increased

Fig. 8. Diffuse alveolar hemorrhage showing both intact red blood cells and fibrinous exudate (stain: hematoxylin and eosin; original magnification ×100).

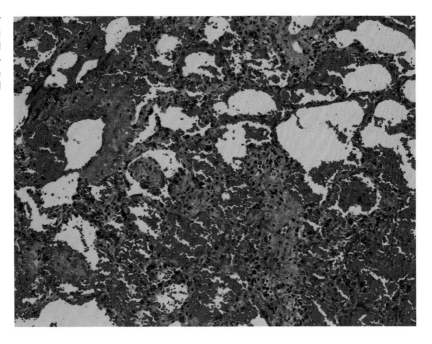

risk of development of hematologic malignancies in patients with SS (**Fig. 13**).[63] Last, there are reports of numerous other pulmonary manifestations of SS, including cystic and cavitary lung disease, amyloidosis, and Langerhans cell histiocytosis.[54,64]

DIFFERENTIAL DIAGNOSIS

The differential diagnosis obviously includes other CTD-ILD, but the preponderance of lesions with notable lymphoplasmacytic infiltration requires the pathologist to rule out malignant lymphoproliferative disorders.

Fig. 9. Patient with recent diffuse alveolar hemorrhage. A careful inspection shows focal hemosiderin deposition (*black arrows*). This finding suggests that there may be repeated episodes of alveolar hemorrhage. This raises the possibility of a vasculitic process, but at a minimum suggests that there was hemorrhage before, from some lung insult (stain: hematoxylin and eosin; original magnification ×200).

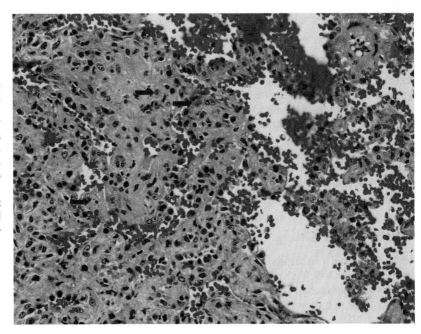

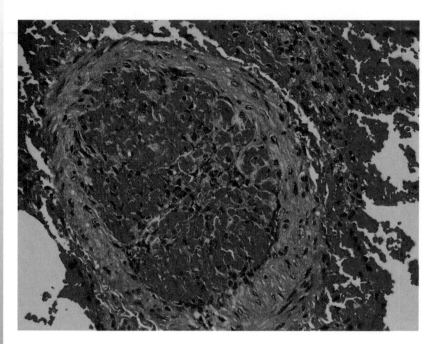

Fig. 10. Pulmonary arteriole showing organizing thrombus (stain: hematoxylin and eosin; original magnification ×200).

Sjögren Syndrome Interstitial Lung Disease Key Points

- Can involve the entire tracheobronchial tree
- Fibrotic NSIP is most common pattern of injury
- LIP may be encountered

POLYMYOSITIS AND DERMATOMYOSITIS

OVERVIEW

Polymyositis and dermatomyositis (PM/DM) are chronic inflammatory myopathies with the latter also having an integumentary component. Taking the inflammatory myopathies together, the prevalence is between 9 and 32 cases per 100,000 people.[65] Pulmonary involvement in PM/DM is less common than in other CTD-ILD with the reported incidence between 5% and 46%; regardless, the majority of patients with PM/DM show HRCT changes of ILD.[66,67]

PATTERNS OF INJURY

Acute interstitial processes are common, often showing OP or DAD (Fig. 14).[68,69] These changes can be superimposed on more chronic processes. NSIP is the most common process seen in almost 82% of patients.[70] Cellular NSIP is

most likely. OP and UIP patterns can also be found, but are less common. Pleuritis and small airway inflammation are less commonly observed. Similar to SS, there is an increased risk of malignancy in patients with PM/DM (Fig. 15). Of the many potential malignancies, lymphoma and lung cancer are most notable for the pulmonary pathologist.[71]

ANTISYNTHETASE SYNDROME

In recent years, the antisynthetase syndrome has been described and includes PM/DM with ILD and antisynthetase antibodies, of which eight have been identified.[72] It is important to recognize the antisynthetase syndrome, as there may be a more favorable outcome in these patients, especially those with anti–Jo-1, although the literature as a whole is not yet conclusive.[72] Some authors suggest that unexplained NSIP pattern with overlapping OP or ALI should prompt a search for antisynthetase antibodies.[20]

DIFFERENTIAL DIAGNOSIS

The differential diagnosis again includes many of the other CTD-ILDs, but the changes may be complicated by the increased frequency of ALI with DAD observed in these patients. Pathologists also need to be cognizant of antisynthetase syndrome.

Fig. 11. Patterns of cellular nonspecific interstitial pneumonitis. (*A, B*) Uniform thickening of alveolar septa without areas of dense fibrosis or fibroblastic foci (stain: hematoxylin and eosin; original magnification ×40).

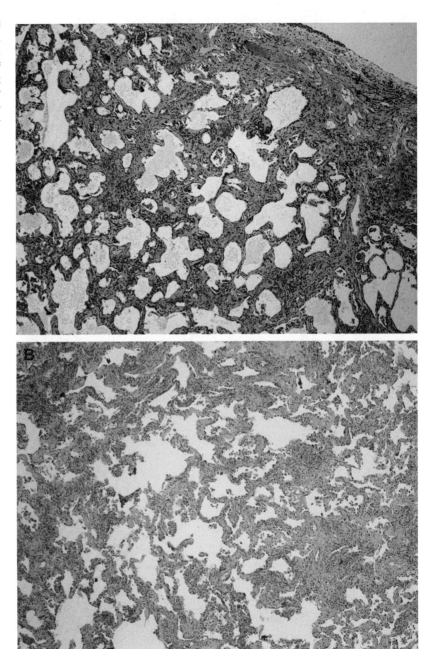

Polymyositis/Dermatomyositis Interstitial Lung Disease Key Points

- Acute processes common
  - Often superimposed on chronic fibrosing disease
- Cellular NSIP is most likely pattern observed
- Antisynthetase syndrome may be important for prognosis

SYSTEMIC SCLEROSIS

OVERVIEW

Systemic sclerosis, or SCL, is a CTD associated with chronic inflammation, vascular damage, and fibrosis of the skin (in localized disease) and visceral organs (in systemic disease). SCL is a rare disease and is seen in approximately 1 in 10,000 people globally.[73] SCL carries a higher morbidity and mortality than other CTD and

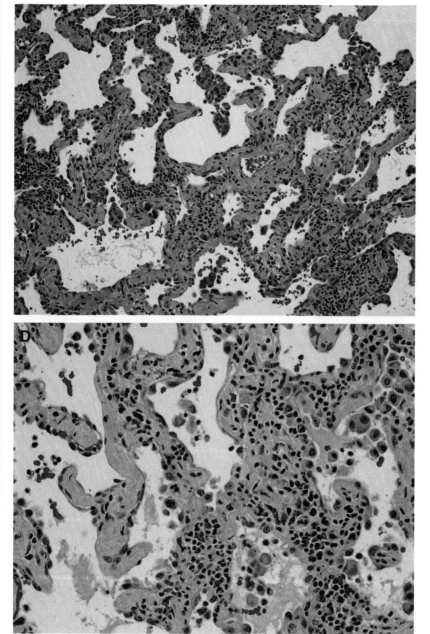

Fig. 11. (*continued*). (*C*) The alveolar septa are thickened and numerous cells are present within the interstitium (stain: hematoxylin and eosin; original magnification ×100). (*D*) The interstitial infiltrate is composed of lymphocytes and plasma cells (stain: hematoxylin and eosin; original magnification ×200).

pulmonary involvement is very common.[73,74] Pulmonary disease is considered the leading cause of death in patients with SCL.[75] Pulmonary disease in SCL is divided between the interstitial and vascular compartments. Pulmonary arterial hypertension occurs in approximately 15% of patients with SCL and is actually more common in the localized form of the disease.[73] Fortunately, early identification of pulmonary arterial hypertension is possible and treatment options are available, although contemporary treatments do not significantly alter the course of this devastating disease.[76] The vascular changes observed in SCL are beyond the scope of this review and are not further discussed here.

FIBROSING DISEASE IN SYSTEMIC SCLEROSIS INTERSTITIAL LUNG DISEASE

The predominant ILD pattern in SCL is NSIP.[77] Fibrotic NSIP is the predominant form which leads

Fig. 12. LIP. (*A*) Marked expansion of the interstitium by dense lymphoplasmacytic infiltrate (stain: hematoxylin and eosin; original magnification ×40). (*B*) The interstitium is completely packed by lymphocytes and plasma cells (stain: hematoxylin and eosin; original magnification ×200).

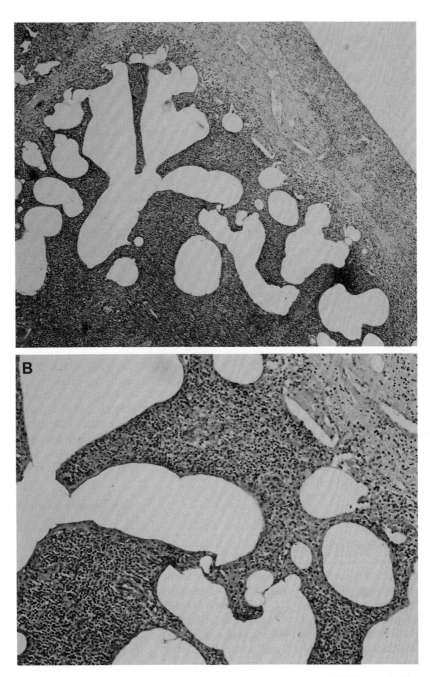

to a paucicellular, monotonous collagenization of the interstitium (**Fig. 16**). Classically, the underlying lung architecture is preserved. UIP may also be observed. OP and DAD are rare. Given the multisystem involvement common in SCL, some authors note that esophageal dysmotility may lead to subclinical aspiration (microaspiration), a finding that the pathologist should note, because these patients should be identified so aspiration precautions can be initiated (**Fig. 17**).[78] The fibrotic NSIP pattern in the appropriate clinical setting should easily yield a diagnosis of SCL-ILD, and after careful examination, one should be able to exclude idiopathic ILD patterns.

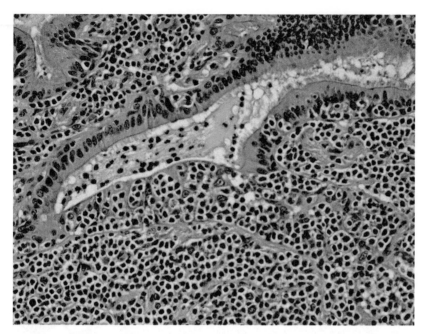

Fig. 13. Bronchial-associated lymphoid tissue lymphoma showing a monotonous population of small lymphocytes with marked involvement of the bronchiolar epithelium. These features are worrisome for lymphoma and this population was determined to be clonal (stain: hematoxylin and eosin; original magnification ×400).

Systemic Sclerosis Interstitial Lung Disease Key Points

- High morbidity and mortality
- Pulmonary hypertensive and vascular changes common
- Fibrotic NSIP common

SUPERIMPOSED CHANGES

Superimposed changes can be challenging when diagnosing ILD. As has been previously mentioned, many of the CTD-ILDs have a chronic, progressive fibrosing pattern, but can also show patterns associated with ALI. In general, acute exacerbations (or ALI) of ILD can be identified when there is clinical decline in lung function, CT changes showing new ground glass opacities, and/or consolidation that is superimposed on a fibrosing pattern.[79] Histopathologic changes associated with the acute exacerbation include DAD, OP, and DAH. Aspiration, infection, and environmental toxins all could potentially induce an acute exacerbation, but most work on classifying acute exacerbation has been done in the setting of idiopathic ILD, and how these potential insults impact CTD-ILD is currently debatable.[80] Regardless, it is the authors' personal experience that changes associated with ALI are not uncommon

in explanted and autopsy lungs in both patients with idiopathic ILD and CTD-ILD. These changes make classification of the underlying fibrosing process difficult, and careful histopathologic, clinical, and radiographic review is likely necessary to render the appropriate diagnosis.

Superimposed Changes Key Points

- Common
  - DAD
  - OP
  - DAH
- Various etiologies
  - Infection
  - Aspiration
  - Environmental toxin
  - Unknown

EMERGING ENTITIES AND CONCEPTS

INTERSTITIAL PNEUMONIA WITH AUTOIMMUNE FEATURES

Recently, a distinct entity has emerged from patients with ILD that do not meet criteria for

Fig. 14. OP superimposed upon NSIP. (*A*) Intra-alveolar Masson body diagnostic of OP. The background alveolar septa seem to be slightly thickened, but the OP obscures the underling lung parenchyma (stain: hematoxylin and eosin; original magnification ×200). (*B*) Another field from the same patient shows reactive pneumocytes lining uniformly thickened alveolar septa without fibroblastic foci, diagnostic for NSIP (stain: hematoxylin and eosin; original magnification ×200).

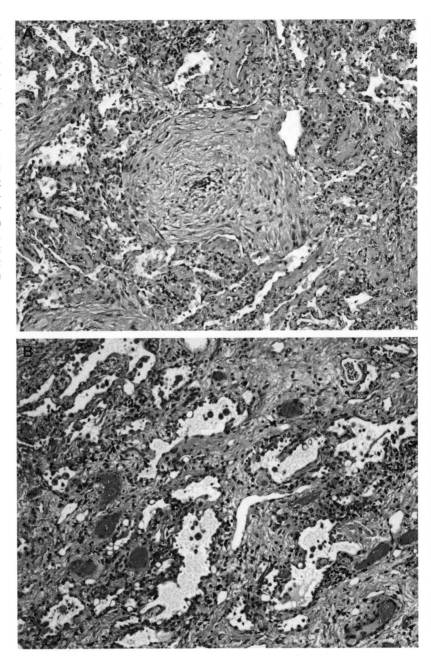

diagnosis of a CTD. This entity was descried as autoimmune-featured ILD and is now termed IPAF.[81] The histopathologic features that can be observed in IPAF include NSIP, OP, NSIP with OP overlap, LIP, interstitial lymphoid aggregates with germinal centers, and diffuse lymphoplasmacytic infiltration (with or without lymphoid follicles).[82] As more knowledge is gathered regarding understanding of IPAF, it will continue to be important for the pathologist to recognize IPAF features, because these may impact prognosis and alter treatment decisions.

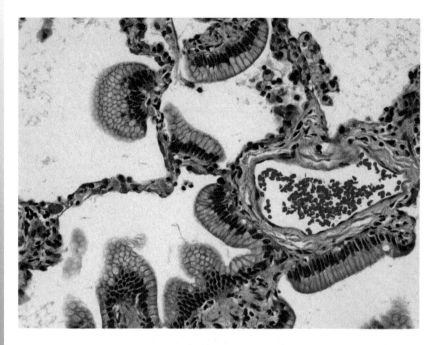

Fig. 15. Adenocarcinoma in a patient with UIP who underwent lung transplantation. Routine sections were taken of the explanted lungs. There were multiple foci of mucinous adenocarcinoma in situ (stain: hematoxylin and eosin; original magnification ×200).

ACUTE FIBRINOUS AND ORGANIZING PNEUMONIA

A more recently described pattern of ALI is acute fibrinous and OP (AFOP). AFOP is similar to DAD, except that traditional hyaline membranes are not present, but rather there is organization of hyaline material into round balls that fill the alveolar space (**Fig. 18**).[83] The process does not need to be diffuse and is often patchy. AFOP has been reported in patient with CTD.[84–87] There is etiologic and pathogenic overlap with DAD, and how similar or dissimilar are AFOP and DAD is yet to be determined.

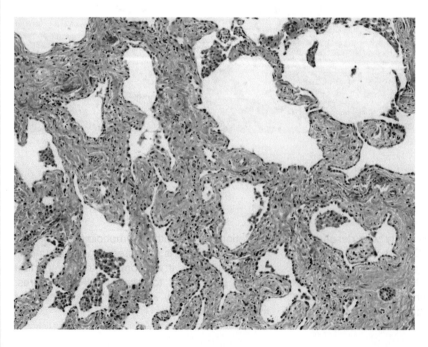

Fig. 16. Uniformly thickened alveolar septa with few interstitial lymphocytes characteristic of fibrotic NSIP pattern (stain: hematoxylin and eosin; original magnification ×100).

Fig. 17. Section from a patient with UIP showing multiple foci of multinucleated foreign body giant cells characteristic of microaspiration (stain: hematoxylin and eosin; original magnification ×200).

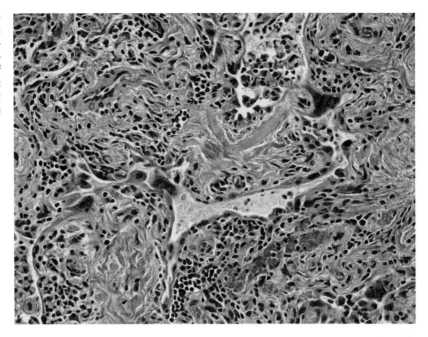

COMBINED UNUSUAL INTERSTITIAL PNEUMONITIS–NONSPECIFIC INTERSTITIAL PNEUMONIA PATTERN

Last, little is understood regarding UIP with concurrent NSIP pattern (**Fig. 19**). This finding has previously been published in a study conducted on the pathologic quantification of CTD-ILD versus idiopathic-ILD.[88] Although little data exist at the present time, this feature seems to be highly specific for CTD-ILD.

Fig. 18. AFOP showing rounded balls of fibrinous material in the intra-alveolar space. No foci of typical hyaline membranes were observed (stain: hematoxylin and eosin; original magnification ×200).

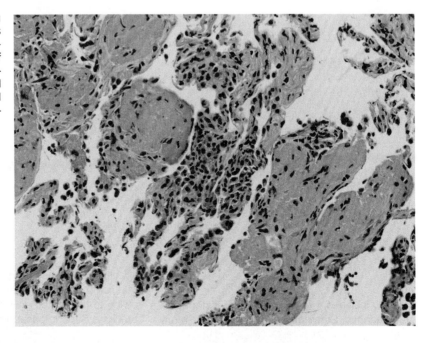

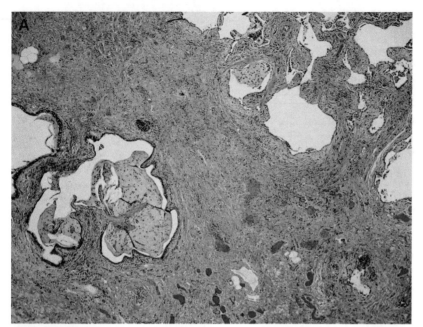

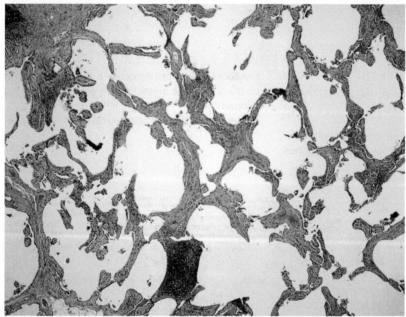

Fig. 19. A patient with mixed UIP and NSIP patterns. (*A*) Classic findings of UIP, including dense fibrosis, fibroblastic foci and honeycombing (stain: hematoxylin and eosin; original magnification ×40). (*B*) Another area of the lung from the same patient showing uniformly thickened alveolar septa without fibroblastic foci, highly suggestive of NSIP pattern. The combination of UIP and NSIP patterns in the same patient is highly suggestive of CTD-ILD.

SUMMARY

CTD-ILD includes a wide spectrum of histopathologic changes. Some of these changes are more specific, or at least suggestive, of a certain rheumatologic condition, but significant overlap exists owing to the limited ability of the lung to respond to injury. Superimposed changes can complicate

Emerging Topics Key Points

- IPAF
  - Do not meet criteria of CTD diagnosis
  - ILD patterns include
    - NSIP
    - OP
    - NSIP and OP
    - LIP
  - Increased interstitial lymphocytes/plasma cells are a clue
  - Lymphoid aggregate maybe present
- AFOP has been reported in connection with CTD-ILD
- Mixed pattern UIP-NSIP maybe specific for CTD-ILD

the histopathologic picture. Diagnosis of CTD-ILD may be suggested by the pathologist when certain features are present, including NSIP-pattern, interstitial lymphoplasmacytic inflammation with or without lymphoid follicles/germinal centers, and the presence of a mixed UIP-NSIP pattern. Ideally, the diagnosis of CTD-ILD would be made in a multidisciplinary fashion during an ILD multidisciplinary conference or similar setting.

REFERENCES

1. Wakwaya Y, Brown KK. Idiopathic pulmonary fibrosis: epidemiology, diagnosis and outcomes. Am J Med Sci 2019;357(5):359–69.
2. Mittoo S, Gelber AC, Christopher-Stine L, et al. Ascertainment of collagen vascular disease in patients presenting with interstitial lung disease. Respir Med 2009;103(8):1152–8.
3. Dellaripa PF. Interstitial lung disease in the connective tissue diseases; a paradigm shift in diagnosis and treatment. Clin Immunol 2018;186:71–3.
4. Strand MJ, Sprunger D, Cosgrove GP, et al. Pulmonary function and survival in idiopathic vs secondary usual interstitial pneumonia. Chest 2014;146(3): 775–85.
5. Ryerson CJ, Corte TJ, Lee JS, et al. A standardized diagnostic ontology for fibrotic interstitial lung disease. An International Working Group Perspective. Am J Respir Crit Care Med 2017;196(10):1249–54.
6. Wall CP, Gaensler EA, Carrington CB, et al. Comparison of transbronchial and open biopsies in chronic infiltrative lung diseases. Am Rev Respir Dis 1980;123(3):5.
7. Ferson PF, Landreneau RJ. Thoracoscopic lung biopsy or open lung biopsy for interstitial lung disease. Chest Surg Clin N Am 1998;8(4):749–62.
8. Riley DJ, Costanzo EJ. Surgical biopsy: its appropriateness in diagnosing interstitial lung disease. Curr Opin Pulm Med 2006;12:331–6.
9. American Thoracic Society, European Respiratory Society. American Thoracic Society/European Respiratory Society international multidisciplinary consensus classification of the idiopathic interstitial pneumonias. Am J Respir Crit Care Med 2002;165: 277–304.
10. Travis WD, Costabel U, Hansell DM, et al. An official American Thoracic Society/European Respiratory Society statement: update of the international multidisciplinary classification of the idiopathic interstitial pneumonias. Am J Respir Crit Care Med 2013; 188(6):733–48.
11. Jokerst C, Purdy H, Bhalla S. An overview of collagen vascular disease-associated interstitial lung disease. Semin Roentgenol 2015;50(1):31–9.
12. Chung JH, Montner SM, Adegunsoye A, et al. CT findings, radiologic-pathologic correlation, and imaging predictors of survival for patients with interstitial pneumonia with autoimmune features. AJR Am J Roentgenol 2017;208(6):1229–36.
13. Chung JH, Cox CW, Montner SM, et al. CT features of the usual interstitial pneumonia pattern: differentiating connective tissue disease-associated interstitial lung disease from idiopathic pulmonary fibrosis. AJR Am J Roentgenol 2018;210(2):307–13.
14. Raghu G, Collard HR, Egan JJ, et al. An official ATS/ERS/JRS/ALAT statement: idiopathic pulmonary fibrosis: evidence-based guidelines for diagnosis and management. Am J Respir Crit Care Med 2011;183(6):788–824.
15. Bradley B, Branley HM, Egan JJ, et al. Interstitial lung disease guideline: the British Thoracic Society in collaboration with the Thoracic Society of Australia and New Zealand and the Irish Thoracic Society. Thorax 2008;63(Suppl 5):v1–58.
16. Scott DL, Wolfe F, Huizinga TWJ. Rheumatoid arthritis. Lancet 2010;376(9746):1094–8.
17. Feldmann M, Brennan FM, Maini RN. Rheumatoid arthritis. Cell 1996;85:307–10.
18. Gabbay E, Tarala R, Will R, et al. Interstitial lung disease in recent onset rheumatoid arthritis. Am J Respir Crit Care Med 1997;156:528–35.
19. Dawson JK, Fewins HE, Desmond J, et al. Fibrosing alveolitis in patients with rheumatoid arthritis as assessed by high resolution computed tomography, chest radiography, and pulmonary function tests. Thorax 2001;56:622–7.
20. Solomon JJ, Fischer A. Connective tissue disease-associated interstitial lung disease: a focused review. J Intensive Care Med 2015;30(7):392–400.
21. Koslow M, Young JR, Yi ES, et al. Rheumatoid pulmonary nodules: clinical and imaging features compared with malignancy. Eur Radiol 2019;29(4): 1684–92.

22. Sagdeo P, Gattimallanahali Y, Kakade G, et al. Rheumatoid lung nodule. BMJ Case Rep 2015;2015, [pii: bcr2015213083].

23. Sargin G, Senturk T. Multiple pulmonary rheumatoid nodules. Reumatologia 2015;53(5):276–8.

24. Schreiber J, Koschel D, Kekow J, et al. Rheumatoid pneumoconiosis (Caplan's syndrome). Eur J Intern Med 2010;21(3):168–72.

25. Yousem SA, Colby TV, Carrington CB. Lung biopsy in rheumatoid arthritis. Am Rev Respir Dis 1985; 131(5):770–7.

26. Pratt D, Schwartz M, May J, et al. Rapidly fatal pulmonary fibrosis: the accelerated variant of interstitial pneumonitis. Thorax 1979;34:587–93.

27. Khaja M, Menon L, Niazi M, et al. Diffuse alveolar hemorrhage and acute respiratory distress syndrome during treatment of rheumatoid arthritis with etanercept. J Bronchology Interv Pulmonol 2012; 19(3):228–31.

28. Chhabra P, Law AD, Suri V, et al. Methotrexate induced lung injury in a patient with primary CNS lymphoma: a case report. Mediterr J Hematol Infect Dis 2012;4(1):e2012020.

29. Taniguchi K, Usul Y, Matsuda T, et al. Methotrexate-induced acute lung injury in a patient with rheumatoid arthritis. Int J Clin Pharmacol Res 2005;25(3):101–5.

30. Margagnoni G, Papi V, Aratari A, et al. Methotrexate-induced pneumonitis in a patient with Crohn's disease. J Crohns Colitis 2010;4(2):211–4.

31. Beasley MB. The pathologist's approach to acute lung injury. Arch Pathol Lab Med 2010;134:719–27.

32. Imokawa S, Colby TV, Leslie KO, et al. Methotrexate pneumonitis: review of the literature and histopathological findings in nine patients. Eur Respir J 2000; 15(2):373–81.

33. Lee HK, Kim DS, Yoo B, et al. Histopathologic pattern and clinical features of rheumatoid arthritis-associated interstitial lung disease. Chest 2005; 127(6):2019–27.

34. Danchenko N, Satia JA, Anthony MS. Epidemiology of systemic lupus erythematosus: a comparison of worldwide disease burden. Lupus 2006;15:308–18.

35. Mittoo S, Fischer A, Strand V, et al. Systemic lupus erythematosus-related interstitial lung disease. Curr Rheumatol Rev 2010;6(2):99–107.

36. Mittoo S, Fell CD. Pulmonary manifestations of systemic lupus erythematosus. Semin Respir Crit Care Med 2014;35(2):249–54.

37. Matthay RA, Schwarz MI, Petty TL, et al. Pulmonary manifestations of systemic lupus erythematosus: review of twelve cases of acute lupus pneumonitis. Medicine (Baltimore) 1975;54(5):397–409.

38. Cheema GS, Quismorio FP. Interstitial lung disease in systemic lupus erythematosus. Curr Opin Pulm Med 2000;6(5):424–9.

39. Swigris JJ, Fischer A, Gillis J, et al. Pulmonary and thrombotic manifestations of systemic lupus erythematosus. Chest 2008;133(1):271–80.

40. Haupt HM, Moore GW, Hutchins GM. The lung in systemic lupus erythematosus. Analysis of the pathologic changes in 120 patients. Am J Med 1981;71(5):791–8.

41. Yokoi T, Tomita Y, Fukaya M, et al. Pulmonary hypertension associated with systemic lupus erythematosus: predominantly thrombotic arteriopathy accompanied by plexiform lesions. Arch Pathol Lab Med 1998;122(5):467–70.

42. Tansey D, Wells AU, Colby TV, et al. Variations in histological patterns of interstitial pneumonia between connective tissue disorders and their relationship to prognosis. Histopathology 2004;44(6):585–96.

43. Ortega-Hernandez OD, Shoenfeld Y. Mixed connective tissue disease: an overview of clinical manifestations, diagnosis and treatment. Best Pract Res Clin Rheumatol 2012;26(1):61–72.

44. Ungprasert P, Crowson CS, Chowdhary VR, et al. Epidemiology of mixed connective tissue disease, 1985-2014: a population-based study. Arthritis Care Res 2016;68(12):1843–8.

45. Sullivan WD, Hurst DJ, Harmon CE, et al. A prospective evaluation emphasizing pulmonary involvement in patients with mixed connective tissue disease. Medicine 1984;63:92–107.

46. Prakash UB. Respiratory complications in mixed connective tissue disease. Clin Chest Med 1998; 19(4):733–46.

47. Vivero M, Padera RF. Histopathology of lung disease in the connective tissue diseases. Rheum Dis Clin North Am 2015;41(2):197–211.

48. Wiener-Kronish JP, Solinger AM, Warnock ML. Severe pulmonary involvement in mixed connective tissue disease. Am Rev Respir Dis 1981;124:499–503.

49. Kozuka T, Johkoh T, Honda O, et al. Pulmonary involvement in mixed connective tissue disease: high-resolution CT findings in 41 patients. J Thorac Imaging 2001;16(2):94–8.

50. Fagundes MN, Caleiro MT, Navarro-Rodriguez T, et al. Esophageal involvement and interstitial lung disease in mixed connective tissue disease. Respir Med 2009;103(6):854–60.

51. Alani H, Henty JR, THomson NL, et al. Systematic review and meta-analysis of the epidemiology of poly-autoimmunity in Sjögren's syndrome (secondary Sjögren's syndrome) focusing on autoimmune rheumatic diseases. Scand J Rheumatol 2018;47(2): 141–54.

52. Qin B, Wang J, Yang Z, et al. Epidemiology of primary Sjogren's syndrome: a systematic review and meta-analysis. Ann Rheum Dis 2015;74(11):1983–9.

53. Vivino FB. Sjogren's syndrome: clinical aspects. Clin Immunol 2017;182:48–54.

54. Flament T, Bigot A, Chaigne B, et al. Pulmonary manifestations of Sjogren's syndrome. Eur Respir Rev 2016;25(140):110–23.

55. Roca F, Dominique S, Schmidt J, et al. Interstitial lung disease in primary Sjogren's syndrome. Autoimmun Rev 2017;16(1):48–54.

56. Papiris S, Maniati M, Constantopoulos S, et al. Lung involvement in primary Sjogren's syndrome is mainly related to small airway disease. Ann Rheum Dis 1999;58:61–4.

57. Reina D, Vilaseca DR, Torrente-Segarra V, et al. Sjögren's syndrome-associated interstitial lung disease: a multicenter study. Reumatol Clin 2016; 12(4):201–5.

58. Parambil JG, Myers JL, Lindell RM, et al. Interstitial lung disease in primary Sjögren syndrome. Chest 2006;130:1489–95.

59. Ito I, Nagai S, Kitaichi M, et al. Pulmonary manifestations of primary Sjogren's syndrome: a clinical, radiologic, and pathologic study. Am J Respir Crit Care Med 2005;171:632–8.

60. Yamadori I, Fujita J, Bandoh S, et al. Nonspecific interstitial pneumonia as pulmonary involvement of primary Sjögren's syndrome. Rheumatol Int 2002; 22:89–92.

61. Panchabhai TS, Farver C, Highland KB. Lymphocytic interstitial pneumonia. Clin Chest Med 2016; 37(3):463–74.

62. Ramos-Casals M, Brito-Zeron P, Seror R, et al. Characterization of systemic disease in primary Sjögren's syndrome: EULAR-SS task force recommendations for articular, cutaneous, pulmonary and renal involvements. Rheumatology 2015;54: 2230–8.

63. Royer B, Cazals-Hatem D, Sibilia J, et al. Lymphomas in patients with Sjögren's syndrome are marginal zone B-cell neoplasms, arise in diverse extranodal and nodal sites, and are not associated with viruses. Blood 1997;90:766–75.

64. Gupta N, Wikenheiser-Brokamp KA, Fischer A, et al. Diffuse cystic lung disease as the presenting manifestation of Sjogren syndrome. Ann Am Thorac Soc 2016;13(3):371–5.

65. Findlay AR, Goyal NA, Mozaffar T. An overview of polymyositis and dermatomyositis. Muscle Nerve 2015;51(5):638–56.

66. Fathi M, Dastmalchi M, Rasmussen E, et al. Interstitial lung disease, a common manifestation of newly diagnosed polymyositis and dermatomyositis. Ann Rheum Dis 2004;63(3):297–301.

67. Fathi M, Lundberg IE. Interstitial lung disease in polymyositis and dermatomyositis. Curr Opin Rheumatol 2005;17(6):701–6.

68. Won Huh J, Soon Kim D, Keun Lee C, et al. Two distinct clinical types of interstitial lung disease associated with polymyositis-dermatomyositis. Respir Med 2007;101(8):1761–9.

69. Tazelaar HD, Viggiano RW, Pickersgill J, et al. Interstitial lung disease in polymyositis and dermatomyositis. Clinical features and prognosis as correlated with histologic findings. Am Rev Respir Dis 1990; 141(3):727–33.

70. Douglas WW, Tazelaar HD, Hartman TE, et al. Polymyositis-dermatomyositis-associated interstitial lung disease. Am J Respir Crit Care Med 2001; 164(7):1182–5.

71. Hill CL, Zhang Y, Sigurgeirsson B, et al. Frequency of specific cancer types in dermatomyositis and polymyositis: a population-based study. Lancet 2001;357(9250):96–100.

72. Zamora AC, Hoskote SS, Abascal-Bolado B, et al. Clinical features and outcomes of interstitial lung disease in anti-Jo-1 positive antisynthetase syndrome. Respir Med 2016;118:39–45.

73. Denton CP, Khanna D. Systemic sclerosis. Lancet 2017;390(10103):1685–99.

74. Giacomelli R, Liakouli V, Berardicurti O, et al. Interstitial lung disease in systemic sclerosis: current and future treatment. Rheumatol Int 2017;37(6):853–63.

75. Steen VD, Medsger TA. Changes in causes of death in systemic sclerosis, 1972-2002. Ann Rheum Dis 2007;66(7):940–4.

76. Cappelli S, Bellando Randone S, Camiciottoli G, et al. Interstitial lung disease in systemic sclerosis: where do we stand? Eur Respir Rev 2015;24(137): 411–9.

77. Bouros D, Wells AU, Nicholson AG, et al. Histopathologic subsets of fibrosing alveolitis in patients with systemic sclerosis and their relationship to outcome. Am J Respir Crit Care Med 2002;165(12):1581–6.

78. Ebert EC. Esophageal disease in scleroderma. J Clin Gastroenterol 2006;40(9):769–75.

79. Kolb M, Bondue B, Pesci A, et al. Acute exacerbations of progressive-fibrosing interstitial lung diseases. Eur Respir Rev 2018;27(150), [pii:180071].

80. Ryerson CJ, Collard HR. Acute exacerbations complicating interstitial lung disease. Curr Opin Pulm Med 2014;20(5):436–41.

81. Vij R, Noth I, Strek ME. Autoimmune-featured interstitial lung disease: a distinct entity. Chest 2011; 140(5):1292–9.

82. Adegunsoye A, Oldham JM, Valenzi E, et al. Interstitial pneumonia with autoimmune features: value of histopathology. Arch Pathol Lab Med 2017;141(7): 960–9.

83. Beasley MB, Franks TJ, Galvin JR, et al. Acute fibrinous and organizing pneumonia: a histological pattern of lung injury and possible variant of diffuse alveolar damage. Arch Pathol Lab Med 2002;126(9): 1064–70.

84. Wang Y, Zhao S, Du G, et al. Acute fibrinous and organizing pneumonia as initial presentation of primary Sjogren's syndrome: a case report and literature review. Clin Rheumatol 2018;37(7):2001–5.

85. Valim V, Rocha RH, Couto RB, et al. Acute fibrinous and organizing pneumonia and undifferentiated connective tissue disease: a case report. Case Rep Rheumatol 2012;2012:549298.

86. Hariri LP, Unizony S, Stone J, et al. Acute fibrinous and organizing pneumonia in systemic lupus erythematosus: a case report and review of the literature. Pathol Int 2010;60(11):755–9.

87. Prahalad S, Bohnsack JF, Maloney CG, et al. Fatal acute fibrinous and organizing pneumonia in a child with juvenile dermatomyositis. J Pediatr 2005; 146(2):289–92.

88. Cipriani NA, Strek M, Noth I, et al. Pathologic quantification of connective tissue disease-associated versus idiopathic usual interstitial pneumonia. Arch Pathol Lab Med 2012;136(10):1253–8.

Small Airway Disease
A Step Closer to Etiology-Based Classification of Bronchiolitis

Anatoly Urisman, MD, PhD*, Kirk D. Jones, MD

KEYWORDS

- Small airway disease • Bronchiolitis • Obliterative bronchiolitis • Restrictive bronchiolitis
- Follicular bronchiolitis • Diffuse panbronchiolitis • Classification

---

Key points

- Obliterative bronchiolitis, follicular bronchiolitis, and diffuse panbronchiolitis are distinct histologic patterns of primary bronchiolar injury.
- When identified in a lung biopsy, each of the above 3 patterns provides a clinically useful differential diagnosis.
- Further subclassification according to underlying cause or associated condition is best accomplished through clinical and radiologic correlation.
- Similar to the diagnosis of interstitial lung disease, classification of small airway disease is best accomplished in the multidisciplinary discussion setting.

ABSTRACT

Three major histologic patterns of bronchiolitis: obliterative bronchiolitis, follicular bronchiolitis, and diffuse panbronchiolitis, are reviewed in detail. These distinct patterns of primary bronchiolar injury provide a useful starting point for formulating a differential diagnosis and considering possible causes. In support of the aim toward a cause-based classification system of small airway disease, a simple diagnostic algorithm is provided for further subclassification of the above 3 bronchiolitis patterns according to the major associated etiologic subgroups.

BACKGROUND AND TERMINOLOGY

The term *small airway disease* (SAD) refers to a set of pathologic conditions that affect small airways and are typically associated with obstructive physiology on pulmonary function testing (PFT). Small airways are noncartilaginous airways of less than 2 mm in diameter, which include membranous (terminal) bronchioles and respiratory bronchioles. Histologically, several patterns of bronchiolar injury (bronchiolitis) have been recognized over the last few decades, which form the basis for classifying SAD. In addition, because surgical lung biopsy cannot be performed in all patients, classification schema based on both clinical and radiological findings have also been proposed. However, no single classification of SAD has been widely accepted.[1–4]

In this review, the authors focus on the major histologic patterns of bronchiolitis, which intrinsically involve the bronchioles and have sufficiently distinct (nonoverlapping) features: *obliterative bronchiolitis* (OB), *follicular bronchiolitis* (FB), and *diffuse panbronchiolitis* (DPB). These patterns appear to represent unique mechanisms of injury and thus provide the most useful point of reference in further subclassification according to possible causes or associated clinical syndromes. In addition, these histologic patterns are more likely to be encountered in patients with subtle or

---

Department of Pathology, University of California San Francisco, 505 Parnassus Avenue, Box 0102, San Francisco, CA 94143, USA
* Corresponding author.
E-mail address: Anatoly.Urisman@ucsf.edu

Surgical Pathology 13 (2020) 189–196
https://doi.org/10.1016/j.path.2019.10.004

"unclassifiable" findings on chest imaging, often prompting a surgical biopsy for diagnosis.

Although *organizing pneumonia* (OP) and *acute bronchopneumonia* (PNA) are often considered under the general umbrella of SAD, these histologic patterns are primarily airspace filling (by fibroblast-rich plugs of granulation tissue in OP or neutrophils in acute PNA) with bronchiolar involvement present largely as a secondary finding. Furthermore, both OP and acute PNA are generally well recognized based on clinical and imaging findings and generally do not require a biopsy. Likewise, *respiratory bronchiolitis* (RB), a ubiquitous finding in smokers (and sometimes in association with other inhalation exposures), is most often encountered alongside other findings of smoking-related interstitial lung disease (ILD) (eg, emphysema with or without fibrosis) and typically does not represent a diagnostic challenge based on clinical and imaging findings alone. Therefore, OP, acute PNA, and RB will not be discussed further.

Peribronchiolar metaplasia (PM) is characterized by metaplastic replacement of the normal flat epithelium of the alveolar ducts and adjacent alveolar septa by bronchiolar-type cuboidal, columnar, or ciliated columnar epithelium. Although PM is a useful histologic marker of chronic bronchiolar injury to recognize in both surgical and transbronchial biopsies, it is rare as an isolated finding. Instead, PM is often encountered in association with other injury patterns, often with interstitial fibrosis, which become the focus of histologic classification.[5] Therefore, PM as a sole histologic finding is rather nonspecific.

The term *lymphocytic bronchiolitis* is sometimes used to refer collectively to the histologic patterns of SAD characterized by lymphocyte-predominant inflammation within the bronchiolar walls. Three main patterns of lymphocytic bronchiolitis have been recognized: (i) cellular bronchiolitis; (ii) FB; and (iii) DPB. Cellular bronchiolitis is the least specific pattern, which may be encountered occasionally as a sole finding, particularly in transbronchial biopsies. However, in surgical biopsies, other associated findings, such as granulomas, different patterns of interstitial fibrosis, smoking-related changes, neutrophilic inflammation, bacterial or fungal microorganisms, viral cytopathic changes, or exogenous material, often point to a more specific diagnostic category. In contrast, both FB and DPB histologic patterns provide higher specificity when considering the associated conditions or underlying causes.

Acute bronchiolitis is primarily a clinical diagnosis used to describe an acute respiratory illness in infants. It is classically caused by respiratory syncytial virus (RSV), but numerous other viruses as well as some bacteria have been implicated in both pediatric and adult cases.[6,7] Lung biopsy is rarely performed, but the classic histologic changes include bronchiolar intraepithelial and subepithelial lymphocytic and neutrophilic inflammation and epithelial necrosis in more severe cases.[7] Features of diffuse alveolar damage (DAD), PNA, or even necrotizing pneumonia are also common. When evaluating surgical biopsy or autopsy specimens from such cases, the authors advocate the use of histologic diagnoses describing the primary pattern of injury, such as DAD, acute PNA, or necrotizing PNA. Furthermore, if bronchiolar injury is the dominant finding, then *neutrophilic bronchiolitis* and *necrotizing bronchiolitis* are preferable to avoid confusion with the clinical diagnosis of acute bronchiolitis. Aside from infectious causes, necrotizing bronchiolitis can be observed in cases of toxic fume inhalation and drug toxicity. Some of these patients may develop constrictive bronchiolitis as a late complication.

Although the term *granulomatous bronchiolitis* is sometimes used to describe bronchiolar involvement by granulomatous inflammation, the use of more specific histologic diagnoses that attempt to subclassify the findings into more clinically useful categories should be attempted whenever possible. Specifically, the presence or absence of necrotizing granulomas must be mentioned, and cases with necrosis should trigger an appropriate infectious workup. Features of bronchiectasis or neutrophilic inflammation are also important to note, as both are more likely to be associated with an infectious cause. Conversely, in cases dominated by sarcoid-type nonnecrotizing granulomas, other features of pulmonary sarcoidosis, such as the classical perilymphatic distribution, clustering of the granulomas, and associated fibrosis, are helpful. Because both infectious granulomatous airway disease and pulmonary sarcoidosis typically show concurrent and often more prominent involvement of large airways, the authors do not advocate the use of *granulomatous bronchiolitis* among primary bronchiolitis patterns.

OBLITERATIVE BRONCHIOLITIS

OB, also known as constrictive bronchiolitis, is histologically characterized by distinctive progressive remodeling of bronchiolar walls that leads to narrowing and obliteration of bronchiolar lumens (**Fig. 1**). Active lesions show subepithelial fibroblastic proliferation, often with edematous myxoid appearance, which in many cases may

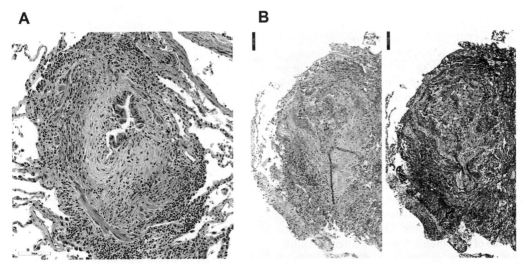

Fig. 1. OB. (*A*) Bronchiole with a well-developed active scarring lesion of OB in a surgical biopsy from a patient with GVHD. Note prominent accumulation of myxoid fibroblast-rich tissue between the respiratory epithelium and smooth muscle resulting in marked narrowing of the bronchiolar lumen (hematoxylin and eosin [H&E]; scale bar = 100 μm) (*B*) An early OB lesion in a transbronchial biopsy from a lung allograft recipient with declining expiratory flows and evidence of segmental air trapping on imaging. Note subtle subepithelial scarring and accumulation of foamy macrophages within the lumen. Fragmentation of the bronchiolar elastica by the developing scar is best appreciated on the EVG stain (H&E, left, and EVG, right; scale bars = 100 μm).

not be associated with significant inflammation. Advanced lesions show progressive replacement by collagenous fibrosis with obliteration of the lumens. Although early lesions can be difficult to recognize because they are often subtle and focal, advanced lesions may be easily mistaken for small interstitial scarlike nodules. The presence of bronchiolectasis, luminal mucus plugging, or giant cell granulomas (often with cholesterol clefts) in peribronchiolar airspaces is an important clue to bronchiolar obstruction and should increase the level of suspicion for possible OB. Multiple level sections may be necessary to visualize the diagnostic lesions, and elastic tissue stains, such as Verhoeff-van Gieson (EVG), are often helpful in visualizing collapsed bronchiolar lumens and remnant smooth muscle in advanced lesions.[8,9] Of note, artifactual collapse of the bronchiolar lumens may occur as a result of ex vivo smooth muscle contraction in surgical biopsy and autopsy specimens.[10] This artifact should not be confused with true subepithelial scarring lesions of OB.

Although detailed molecular mechanisms of bronchiolar injury in OB are not well understood, the histologic features of OB and the known causes associated with OB suggest that airway remodeling in response to bronchiolar epithelial cell injury may be the primary driver in the pathogenesis of OB. This view is supported by the association of OB with numerous substances thought to induce chemical injury in respiratory epithelial cells,[11,12] including a growing list of occupational toxins, environmental pollutants, and therapeutic agents.[13,14] OB is also a well-documented complication of cellular rejection in lung allografts[15,16] and a rare manifestation of graft-versus-host disease (GVHD) following bone marrow stem cell transplantation.[17,18] In these cases, bronchiolar epithelial cell injury is attributed to alloimmune mechanisms mediated by cytotoxic CD8[+] and helper CD4[+] T cells.[19] Outside of transplant populations, OB is most often encountered in autoimmune connective tissue disease (ACTD), particularly in rheumatoid arthritis (RA), and rarely, in other types of ACTD,[20,21] where autoimmune mechanisms are likely responsible for the observed bronchiolar epithelial injury. Similarly, viral cytotoxic injury to the bronchiolar epithelial cells is likely the initial injury responsible for the rare cases of OB, which develop as a delayed complication of viral bronchiolitis or viral pneumonia. Adenovirus is the classical association, particularly in children, but other viruses and bacteria have been implicated.[9]

The diagnosis of OB can be challenging and often requires correlation with clinical and radiological findings, best accomplished in a formal multidisciplinary conference setting.[22,23] High-resolution computed tomography (HRCT) features most commonly associated with OB include mosaic perfusion, air-trapping on expiratory views, and bronchiectasis in more advanced cases.[24,25] Thorough exposure history is key to identifying possible cases of exposure-associated OB. Similarly, clinical or serologic evidence of ACTD is helpful in identifying cases of ACTD-associated OB. In fact, recent studies show that up to one-half of the cases of idiopathic OB are associated with ACTD on further diagnostic workup.[26,27] The presence of superimposed interstitial fibrosis, identified histologically or on imaging, should also point to possible ACTD-associated OB. In a recent study of RA-associated OB, approximately 30% of the patients had evidence of superimposed interstitial fibrosis on imaging.[28] In lung transplant patients, OB manifests as bronchiolitis obliterans syndrome (BOS) and is usually diagnosed clinically based on the evidence of spirometric flow obstruction not attributable to other causes.[29,30] Although allograft transbronchial biopsies have relatively low (29%–70%) sensitivity for OB, they are helpful in establishing a definitive diagnosis when features of OB are identified.[31–33]

FOLLICULAR BRONCHIOLITIS

Follicular bronchiolitis (FB) is defined by the presence of prominent peribronchiolar inflammation with the formation of subepithelial lymphoid aggregates with or without germinal centers (Fig. 2).[34–36] Bronchiolectasis and mucostasis are also commonly present and develop as result of luminal obstruction. Some of the airways may show cellular bronchiolitis (less prominent inflammation without lymphoid follicles). Cases with additional heavy diffuse lymphocytic inflammation within alveolar septa should be diagnosed as lymphocytic interstitial pneumonia (LIP).[37,38] The presence of significant neutrophilic inflammation should arouse suspicion for airway infection. Conversely, large nodular or masslike lymphoid lesions, prominent perivascular infiltrates, or tissue-destructive lymphoid infiltrates should raise concern for a possible lymphoid neoplasm.

The clinical conditions associated with FB are diverse but chiefly consist of those with inherited or acquired immune deficiency or immune dysregulation. These conditions include ACTDs (particularly Sjogren syndrome and RA), severe combined immunodeficiency, various forms of hypogammaglobulinemia, and human immunodeficiency virus/AIDS.[34–36] In these conditions, a histologic overlap with LIP is common. FB is also observed in patients with severe chronic obstructive pulmonary disease and in conditions associated with chronic airway infection, such as cystic fibrosis, right middle lobe syndrome, or primary

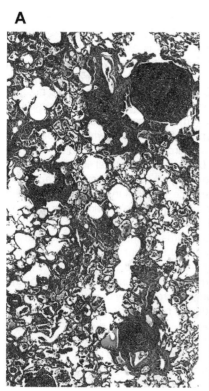

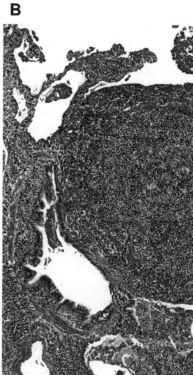

A   **B**

Fig. 2. FB. Surgical biopsy from a 60-year-old woman with mixed connective tissue disease. (*A*) Low-magnification view shows prominent bronchiolocentric interstitial inflammation with large peribronchiolar lymphoid follicles (H&E, ×20 magnification). (*B*) High-magnification view of a large peribronchiolar lymphoid follicle shows a germinal center in the center of the follicle. Note the diffuse lymphocytic interstitial inflammation involving the bronchiole and peribronchiolar alveolar septa (H&E, ×100 magnification).

ciliary dyskinesia. These cases typically show concurrent bronchiectasis and accumulation of neutrophils in the airway lumens.

The pathogenesis of FB is poorly understood, but the histologic appearance of persistent peribronchiolar lymphoid follicles, with or without germinal centers, suggests dysregulation of mechanisms normally involved in antigen presentation. In support of this view, animal models of autoimmune FB show that antigen-specific regulatory T (Treg) cells are required to counteract and keep in check the expansion of the follicular infiltrates.[39] Conversely, several genetic alterations that disrupt the normal function of Treg cells, such as mutations in CD25,[40] CTLA4,[41,42] and STAT3,[43,44] have been implicated in familial forms of autoimmune disease that often have lung involvement and show histologic features of FB. COPA syndrome is another rare form of familial autoimmune disease with lung involvement and prominent FB. Abnormal skewing of the T-helper cell profile toward Th17 phenotype in COPA syndrome[45] suggests immune dysregulation as the underlying mechanism for FB. In cases of FB associated with chronic infection, pathogen-derived antigens are likely driving the formation and persistence of peribronchiolar follicles.[46] Similarly, FB associated with various types of immunodeficiency may be the result of ineffective pathogen clearance and persistence of pathogen-derived antigens.[47]

DIFFUSE PANBRONCHIOLITIS

DPB was initially described as a new clinicopathologic entity in the 1960s by Japanese clinicians who reported a series of cases from Japan.[48,49] By 1980 to the 1990s, cases of DPB were recognized more widely around the world.[50,51] *Diffuse* in the name DPB refers to bilateral lung distribution of the bronchiolar lesions, and *pan* denotes involvement of all layers of the respiratory bronchiole. Histologically, DPB defines a subtype of lymphocytic bronchiolitis, which primarily affects respiratory bronchioles and is characterized by a combination of lymphocytic bronchiolar and peribronchiolar inflammation and distinctive accumulation of foamy macrophages within the peribronchiolar interstitium (**Fig. 3**). Bronchiolar lumens and adjacent alveoli also often contain foamy macrophages as well as variable numbers of lymphocytes and neutrophils. Associated bronchiolocentric fibrosis is usually present, particularly in advanced cases.

Clinical features of DPB include presentation between the second and fifth decade of life with chronic cough and copious sputum production. More than 80% of patients have associated chronic

Fig. 3. DPB. (*A*) Low-magnification view shows bronchiolocentric interstitial inflammation and bronchiolectasis. The lumens are filled by a cellular exudate (H&E, ×20 magnification). (*B*) High-magnification view demonstrates prominent accumulation of foamy macrophages in the peribronchiolar interstitium. The lumens contain large numbers of neutrophils (H&E, ×100 magnification).

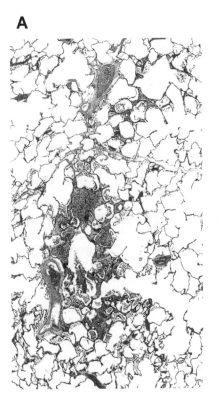

A

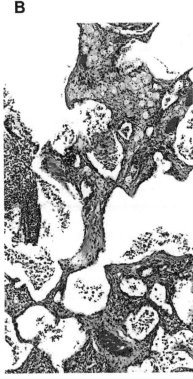

B

paranasal sinusitis.[51] There is a slight male predominance (~5:3 male-to-female ratio). Although special stains for microorganisms performed on the biopsy tissue are virtually always negative, chronic bacterial infection with *Haemophilus influenzae*, *Streptococcus pneumoniae*, *Moraxella catarrhalis*, or *Pseudomonas aeruginosa* can be detected in sputum cultures, particularly in advanced cases with bronchiectasis. Radiologically, DPB usually shows bilateral centrilobular nodules and branching linear densities. Airway thickening and bronchiectasis with "tree-in-bud" opacities are observed in advanced cases.[24] Better recognition of the disease and long-term treatment with low-dose macrolide antibiotics have substantially improved the clinical outcomes and prognosis in DPB.[52,53]

The cause and pathogenesis of DPB are not well understood. Bronchiolar accumulation and persistent activation of neutrophils as well as hypersecretion of mucus appear to be important contributors to small airway injury.[51] Although evidence of bacterial infection (most often *H influenzae* or *P aeruginosa*) is detected in up to one-half of the patients at presentation and more often later in the disease,[54,55] whether persistent low-level bacterial infection is the primary driver of small airway injury remains unresolved. The increased frequency of several HLA alleles in DPB, which are more common in Asia, may explain the higher prevalence of the disease in patients from Asia. The most notable examples are HLA-Bw54[56] and HLA-A11.[57] However, it is unknown whether these HLA alleles mark pathogenic differences in antigen presentation and antibacterial adaptive immunity or whether additional susceptibility genes are involved. The role of foamy macrophages in the pathogenesis of DPB is also unknown at present. However, the appearance of similar tissue-infiltrating foam cells in other conditions associated with chronic bacterial infections, particularly by gram-negative rods (eg, malakoplakia or xanthogranulomatous pyelonephritis), is intriguing.

It is important to note that not all cases with the DPB pattern of bronchiolitis on histology will show clinical findings typically observed in DPB. In fact, an alternative cause, such as a drug reaction, aspiration, or even hypersensitivity pneumonitis (HP), may have a significant histologic overlap with DPB. Therefore, the authors tend to use a descriptive histologic diagnosis, such *lymphocytic bronchiolitis with interstitial macrophages*, and suggest the differential diagnosis, including DPB, in the discussion.

APPROACH TO DIAGNOSIS

Over the last decade, multidisciplinary discussion (MDD) involving pulmonologists, radiologists, and pathologists has emerged as the gold standard for diagnosis of ILD.[22] Similarly, MDD is highly desirable when considering a diagnosis of SAD. If histologic evaluation of a biopsy reveals a bronchiolitis pattern, careful correlation with clinical findings (eg, obstructive physiology on PFT) and imaging results (eg, air-trapping on HRCT expiratory views) is imperative for confident diagnosis. Furthermore, clinical-radiologic-pathologic correlation often makes it possible to go from a histologic pattern of injury with its differential diagnosis to a more specific likely underlying cause.

The following algorithm can be used when considering a diagnosis of SAD:

1. Is bronchiolitis the dominant pattern of injury?
   In cases with bronchiolitis superimposed on a pattern of ILD (eg, nonspecific interstitial pneumonia (NSIP), emphysema, desquamative interstitial pneumonia (DIP), LIP), evaluation should focus on classifying the primary pattern of ILD. In such cases, ILD and SAD are likely due to a common cause.
2. Is one of the 3 most distinctive patterns of bronchiolitis present? If present, use clinical findings to subgroup according to possible cause/associated condition.
   a. **OB**
      i. **Alloimmune injury (BOS, GVHD)**
      ii. **Chemical exposure**
      iii. **ACTD**
      iv. **Postinfectious**
      v. **Idiopathic**
   b. **FB**
      i. **Immunodeficiency (inherited or acquired)**
      ii. **ACTD**
      iii. **Chronic infection**
      iv. **Idiopathic**
   c. **DPB (lymphocytic bronchiolitis with interstitial macrophages)**
      i. **DPB**
      ii. **Other (drug toxicity, aspiration, HP)**

In the above approach, the 3 primary histologic patterns of bronchiolitis identify broad but unique categories of SAD. Combined with the clinical and imaging data (ideally in an MDD setting) and aided by additional serologic or molecular/genetic studies, these general categories can be further subclassified, taking us a step closer to a cause-based rather than histology-based classification system of SAD.

DISCLOSURE

The authors have nothing to disclose.

REFERENCES

1. Wright JL, Cagle P, Churg A, et al. Diseases of the small airways. Am Rev Respir Dis 1992;146(1): 240–62.

2. Ryu JH, Myers JL, Swensen SJ. Bronchiolar disorders. Am J Respir Crit Care Med 2003;168(11): 1277–92.

3. Visscher DW, Myers JL. Bronchiolitis: the pathologist's perspective. Proc Am Thorac Soc 2006;3(1): 41–7.

4. Allen TC. Pathology of small airways disease. Arch Pathol Lab Med 2010;134(5):702–18.

5. Fukuoka J, Franks TJ, Colby TV, et al. Peribronchiolar metaplasia: a common histologic lesion in diffuse lung disease and a rare cause of interstitial lung disease: clinicopathologic features of 15 cases. Am J Surg Pathol 2005;29(7):948–54.

6. Aherne W, Bird T, Court SD, et al. Pathological changes in virus infections of the lower respiratory tract in children. J Clin Pathol 1970;23(1):7–18.

7. Kindt GC, Weiland JE, Davis WB, et al. Bronchiolitis in adults. A reversible cause of airway obstruction associated with airway neutrophils and neutrophil products. Am Rev Respir Dis 1989;140(2):483–92.

8. Myers JL, Colby TV. Pathologic manifestations of bronchiolitis, constrictive bronchiolitis, cryptogenic organizing pneumonia, and diffuse panbronchiolitis. Clin Chest Med 1993;14(4):611–22.

9. Schlesinger C, Meyer CA, Veeraraghavan S, et al. Constrictive (obliterative) bronchiolitis: diagnosis, etiology, and a critical review of the literature. Ann Diagn Pathol 1998;2(5):321–34.

10. Thunnissen E, Blaauwgeers HJ, de Cuba EM, et al. Ex vivo artifacts and histopathologic pitfalls in the lung. Arch Pathol Lab Med 2016;140(3):212–20.

11. Palmer SM, Flake GP, Kelly FL, et al. Severe airway epithelial injury, aberrant repair and bronchiolitis obliterans develops after diacetyl instillation in rats. PLoS One 2011;6(3):e17644.

12. O'Koren EG, Hogan BL, Gunn MD. Loss of basal cells precedes bronchiolitis obliterans-like pathological changes in a murine model of chlorine gas inhalation. Am J Respir Cell Mol Biol 2013; 49(5):788–97.

13. Kreiss K. Occupational causes of constrictive bronchiolitis. Curr Opin Allergy Clin Immunol 2013;13(2): 167–72.

14. Rosenow EC 3rd, Myers JL, Swensen SJ, et al. Drug-induced pulmonary disease. An update. Chest 1992;102(1):239–50.

15. Tazelaar HD, Yousem SA. The pathology of combined heart-lung transplantation: an autopsy study. Hum Pathol 1988;19(12):1403–16.

16. Abernathy EC, Hruban RH, Baumgartner WA, et al. The two forms of bronchiolitis obliterans in heart-lung transplant recipients. Hum Pathol 1991; 22(11):1102–10.

17. Clark JG, Crawford SW, Madtes DK, et al. Obstructive lung disease after allogeneic marrow transplantation. Clinical presentation and course. Ann Intern Med 1989;111(5):368–76.

18. Marras TK, Chan CK. Obliterative bronchiolitis complicating bone marrow transplantation. Semin Respir Crit Care Med 2003;24(5):531–42.

19. Jaramillo A, Fernandez FG, Kuo EY, et al. Immune mechanisms in the pathogenesis of bronchiolitis obliterans syndrome after lung transplantation. Pediatr Transplant 2005;9(1):84–93.

20. Colby TV. Pulmonary pathology in patients with systemic autoimmune diseases. Clin Chest Med 1998; 19(4):587–612, vii.

21. Urisman A, Jones KD. Pulmonary pathology in connective tissue disease. Semin Respir Crit Care Med 2014;35(2):201–12.

22. American Thoracic S, European Respiratory S. American Thoracic Society/European Respiratory Society International Multidisciplinary Consensus Classification of the Idiopathic Interstitial Pneumonias. This joint statement of the American Thoracic Society (ATS), and the European Respiratory Society (ERS) was adopted by the ATS board of directors, June 2001 and by the ERS Executive Committee, June 2001. Am J Respir Crit Care Med 2002; 165(2):277–304.

23. Rice A, Nicholson AG. The pathologist's approach to small airways disease. Histopathology 2009;54(1): 117–33.

24. Hansell DM. Small airways diseases: detection and insights with computed tomography. Eur Respir J 2001;17(6):1294–313.

25. Hansell DM. HRCT of obliterative bronchiolitis and other small airways diseases. Semin Roentgenol 2001;36(1):51–65.

26. Arcadu A, Ryu J. Constrictive (obliterative) bronchiolitis as presenting manifestation of connective tissue disease. Eur Respir J 2016;48(suppl 60): PA4882.

27. Callahan SJ, Vranic A, Flors L, et al. Sporadic obliterative bronchiolitis: case series and systematic review of the literature. Mayo Clin Proc Innov Qual Outcomes 2019;3(1):86–93.

28. Lin E, Limper AH, Moua T. Obliterative bronchiolitis associated with rheumatoid arthritis: analysis of a single-center case series. BMC Pulm Med 2018; 18(1):105.

29. Heng D, Sharples LD, McNeil K, et al. Bronchiolitis obliterans syndrome: incidence, natural history, prognosis, and risk factors. J Heart Lung Transplant 1998;17(12):1255–63.

30. Estenne M, Maurer JR, Boehler A, et al. Bronchiolitis obliterans syndrome 2001: an update of the

diagnostic criteria. J Heart Lung Transplant 2002; 21(3):297–310.

31. Kramer MR, Stoehr C, Whang JL, et al. The diagnosis of obliterative bronchiolitis after heart-lung and lung transplantation: low yield of transbronchial lung biopsy. J Heart Lung Transplant 1993;12(4): 675–81.

32. Cagle PT, Brown RW, Frost A, et al. Diagnosis of chronic lung transplant rejection by transbronchial biopsy. Mod Pathol 1995;8(2):137–42.

33. Reichenspurner H, Girgis RE, Robbins RC, et al. Stanford experience with obliterative bronchiolitis after lung and heart-lung transplantation. Ann Thorac Surg 1996;62(5):1467–72, [discussion: 1472–3].

34. Fortoul TI, Cano-Valle F, Oliva E, et al. Follicular bronchiolitis in association with connective tissue diseases. Lung 1985;163(5):305–14.

35. Romero S, Barroso E, Gil J, et al. Follicular bronchiolitis: clinical and pathologic findings in six patients. Lung 2003;181(6):309–19.

36. Aerni MR, Vassallo R, Myers JL, et al. Follicular bronchiolitis in surgical lung biopsies: clinical implications in 12 patients. Respir Med 2008;102(2): 307–12.

37. Morris JC, Rosen MJ, Marchevsky A, et al. Lymphocytic interstitial pneumonia in patients at risk for the acquired immune deficiency syndrome. Chest 1987; 91(1):63–7.

38. Nicholson AG. Lymphocytic interstitial pneumonia and other lymphoproliferative disorders in the lung. Semin Respir Crit Care Med 2001;22(4):409–22.

39. Schmitt EG, Haribhai D, Jeschke JC, et al. Chronic follicular bronchiolitis requires antigen-specific regulatory T cell control to prevent fatal disease progression. J Immunol 2013;191(11):5460–76.

40. Bezrodnik L, Caldirola MS, Seminario AG, et al. Follicular bronchiolitis as phenotype associated with CD25 deficiency. Clin Exp Immunol 2014; 175(2):227–34.

41. Kuehn HS, Ouyang W, Lo B, et al. Immune dysregulation in human subjects with heterozygous germline mutations in CTLA4. Science 2014;345(6204): 1623–7.

42. Schubert D, Bode C, Kenefeck R, et al. Autosomal dominant immune dysregulation syndrome in humans with CTLA4 mutations. Nat Med 2014;20(12): 1410–6.

43. Flanagan SE, Haapaniemi E, Russell MA, et al. Activating germline mutations in STAT3 cause early-onset multi-organ autoimmune disease. Nat Genet 2014;46(8):812–4.

44. Milner JD, Vogel TP, Forbes L, et al. Early-onset lymphoproliferation and autoimmunity caused by germline STAT3 gain-of-function mutations. Blood 2015; 125(4):591–9.

45. Watkin LB, Jessen B, Wiszniewski W, et al. COPA mutations impair ER-Golgi transport and cause hereditary autoimmune-mediated lung disease and arthritis. Nat Genet 2015;47(6):654–60.

46. Yadava K, Bollyky P, Lawson MA. The formation and function of tertiary lymphoid follicles in chronic pulmonary inflammation. Immunology 2016;149(3): 262–9.

47. Maglione PJ, Ko HM, Beasley MB, et al. Tertiary lymphoid neogenesis is a component of pulmonary lymphoid hyperplasia in patients with common variable immunodeficiency. J Allergy Clin Immunol 2014;133(2):535–42.

48. Yamanaka A, Saiki S, Tamura S, et al. Problems in chronic obstructive bronchial diseases, with special reference to diffuse panbronchiolitis. Naika 1969; 23(3):442–51, [in Japanese].

49. Iwata M, Colby TV, Kitaichi M. Diffuse panbronchiolitis: diagnosis and distinction from various pulmonary diseases with centrilobular interstitial foam cell accumulations. Hum Pathol 1994;25(4):357–63.

50. Fitzgerald JE, King TE Jr, Lynch DA, et al. Diffuse panbronchiolitis in the United States. Am J Respir Crit Care Med 1996;154(2 Pt 1):497–503.

51. Poletti V, Casoni G, Chilosi M, et al. Diffuse panbronchiolitis. Eur Respir J 2006;28(4):862–71.

52. Tanimoto H. A review of the recent progress in treatment of patients with diffuse panbronchiolitis associated with Pseudomonas aeruginosa infection in Japan. Antibiot Chemother (1971) 1991;44:94–8.

53. Kudoh S, Azuma A, Yamamoto M, et al. Improvement of survival in patients with diffuse panbronchiolitis treated with low-dose erythromycin. Am J Respir Crit Care Med 1998;157(6 Pt 1):1829–32.

54. Homma H, Yamanaka A, Tanimoto S, et al. Diffuse panbronchiolitis. A disease of the transitional zone of the lung. Chest 1983;83(1):63–9.

55. Sugiyama Y. Diffuse panbronchiolitis. Clin Chest Med 1993;14(4):765–72.

56. Keicho N, Tokunaga K, Nakata K, et al. Contribution of HLA genes to genetic predisposition in diffuse panbronchiolitis. Am J Respir Crit Care Med 1998; 158(3):846–50.

57. Park MH, Kim YW, Yoon HI, et al. Association of HLA class I antigens with diffuse panbronchiolitis in Korean patients. Am J Respir Crit Care Med 1999; 159(2):526–9.

Transbronchial Cryobiopsy in the Diagnosis of Diffuse Lung Disease

Alberto Cavazza, MD[a],*, Thomas V. Colby, MD[b],
Alessandra Dubini, MD[c], Sara Tomassetti, MD[d],
Claudia Ravaglia, MD[d], Venerino Poletti, MD[d],
Maria Cecilia Mengoli, MD[a], Elena Tagliavini, MD[a],
Giulio Rossi, MD[e]

KEYWORDS

- Interstitial lung disease • Diffuse lung disease • Transbronchial cryobiopsy
- Idiopathic pulmonary fibrosis • Usual interstitial pneumonia • Nonspecific interstitial pneumonia
- Multidisciplinary diagnosis

Key points

- Transbronchial cryobiopsy provides larger and better-preserved specimens compared with traditional (forceps) transbronchial biopsy.
- In diffuse lung disease, the diagnostic yield of transbronchial cryobiopsy is much better than that of forceps transbronchial biopsy and slightly lower than that of surgical lung biopsy, but with a lower complication rate than the latter (including a lower procedure-related mortality).
- In the setting of multidisciplinary discussion of patients with diffuse lung disease, cryobiopsy provides diagnostic and prognostic information comparable with surgical lung biopsy.

ABSTRACT

Transbronchial cryobiopsy, a new diagnostic procedure in patients with diffuse lung disease, provides larger and better-preserved lung specimens compared to forceps biopsy. The diagnostic yield of cryobiopsy is much better than that of forceps biopsy and slightly lower than that of surgical lung biopsy, but with a lower complication rate compared to the latter. Literature suggests that in the multidisciplinary approach to patients with diffuse lung disease cryobiopsy provides diagnostic and prognostic information similar to surgical lung biopsy. Cryobiopsy can also be performed in some patients unsuitable for surgical biopsy, yet in whom histologic input is needed.

OVERVIEW

Transbronchial cryobiopsy entered the arena of diffuse lung disease because both traditional invasive techniques (transbronchial biopsy with conventional forceps and surgical lung biopsy) have limitations. In particular, transbronchial forceps biopsy is a relatively safe technique with high specificity but with an unacceptably low sensitivity ($\cong 30\%$) for the diagnosis of usual interstitial pneumonia (UIP).[1–3] When idiopathic pulmonary fibrosis (IPF) is a clinico-radiologic possibility and transbronchial biopsy suggests fibrotic nonspecific interstitial pneumonia (NSIP) or smoking-related changes or shows normal lung, the probability of unsampled UIP is high. Surgical lung biopsy, on

a Pathology Unit, Azienda USL/IRCCS di Reggio Emilia, Viale Risorgimento 80, Reggio Emilia 42100, Italy;
b Department of Pathology and Laboratory Medicine (Emeritus), Mayo Clinic Arizona, 13400 East Shea Boulevard, Scottsdale, AZ 85259, USA; c Pathology Unit, Azienda USL Romagna, GB Morgagni Hospital, via C. Forlanini 34, Forlì, Italy; d Department of Diseases of the Thorax, Azienda USL Romagna, GB Morgagni Hospital, via C. Forlanini 34, Forlì, Italy; e Pathology Unit, Azienda USL Romagna, St. Maria delle Croci Hospital, Ravenna, Italy
* Corresponding author.
E-mail address: cavazza.alberto@ausl.re.it

the contrary, has both high specificity and sensitivity ($\cong$95%), but suffers from significant side effects, including infections, prolonged air leak, and persistent pain. In a large, retrospective study of surgical lung biopsies performed for diffuse lung disease in the United States,[4] in-hospital death occurred in 1.7% of patients following elective procedures and in 16% following nonelective procedures. Of note, mortality risk increased with age, comorbidities, male sex, and provisional diagnosis of IPF or connective tissue diseases, all common conditions in this group of patients. Although complications are also probably related to the experience of the surgeon[5] and clinical practice varies, in many centers only a minority of patients, in whom the guidelines[6] recommend histology for multidisciplinary diagnosis, undergo a surgical lung biopsy because of risk-benefit considerations or patient refusal. With this background in mind, Margaritopoulos and Wells[7] wrote in 2012: "... an alternative mode of biopsy that overcomes these problems without substantial loss of diagnostic accuracy would be invaluable."

TRANSBRONCHIAL CRYOBIOPSY: THE TECHNIQUE

Cryobiopsy was originally used for the debulking of endobronchial tumors, and in this setting cryobiopsy has also been shown to increase the diagnostic yield of biopsies of endobronchial lesions compared with forceps biopsies.[8] More recently, cryobiopsy has been used to sample lung tissue, both in localized lesions[9] and, for the reasons outlined, in diffuse lung disease. The methods used to perform transbronchial cryobiopsy in diffuse lung disease vary in different centers, but in most it is performed in intubated patients under deep sedation or general anesthesia.[10–13] In brief, a cryoprobe (1.9 or 2.4 mm in diameter) is introduced into the lung under fluoroscopic guidance through the working channel of a flexible bronchoscope. At a distance of $\cong$1 cm from the thoracic wall the probe is cooled for a few seconds and then removed with the lung tissue attached ("stuck") to it en bloc with the bronchoscope (en bloc removal is necessary because the size of the specimen is larger than the working channel of the bronchoscope). A bronchial blocker (eg, Fogarty balloon) previously inserted in the target bronchial segment is immediately inflated after each biopsy to control bleeding. The specimen is thawed in physiologic saline and quickly (and very gently) transferred to formalin.

If properly performed, cryobiopsy is safer than surgical lung biopsy, with lower contraindications (including no age limits), lower hospitalization time, and lower costs.[14] Given the lower complication rate cryobiopsy can be performed in many patients not fit for surgical biopsy. The main complications of transbronchial cryobiopsy are pneumothorax and bleeding. In a recent large series of 699 patients,[15] pneumothorax occurred in 19.2% (requiring

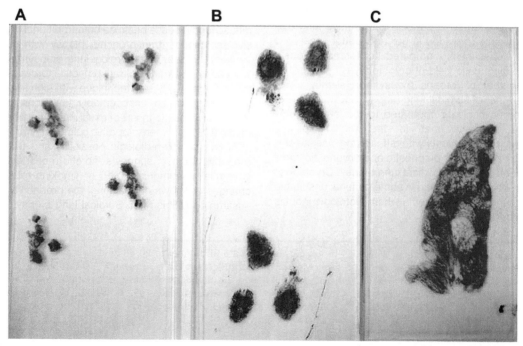

Fig. 1. A cryobiopsy (typically $\cong$0.5 cm in long axis) (*B*) is compared at the same magnification with a traditional transbronchial biopsy (typically 0.1–0.3 cm in long axis) (*A*) and with a surgical lung biopsy (typically $\cong$4 cm in long axis) (*C*).

chest tube drainage in 70.1%), severe hemorrhage in 0.7%, and death within 30 days of the procedure in 0.4% (2 from acute exacerbation of IPF, and 1 from neoplastic thrombotic microangiopathy).

TRANSBRONCHIAL CRYOBIOPSY: THE SPECIMENS

Transbronchial cryobiopsies are generally larger than conventional transbronchial biopsies but smaller than surgical lung biopsies, as shown in **Fig. 1.** The mean size of cryobiopsy specimens is reported in several studies[15–24] and varies from 9 to 64.2 mm^2. The technique is operator-dependent and requires an experienced bronchoscopist. A good cryobiopsy should be *at least* 5 mm in longest axis and reflective of pathologic regions seen radiologically: a small cryobiopsy (eg, 2–3 mm diameter) may be no better than a conventional transbronchial biopsy in terms of diagnostic utility.

Cryobiopsy specimens are processed routinely.[11,13,25] As for any fragile specimen, an important issue is to minimize tissue manipulation both in the bronchoscopic room and in the pathology laboratory. The specimens should not be sectioned grossly and should be embedded in

Fig. 2. Main artifacts that can be found in cryobiopsy specimens. (*A*) Artifactual acute lung injury secondary to trauma of the procedure, consisting in airspace accumulation of blood and fibrin/proteinaceous material. This artifact is common as a focal finding, but occasionally it is quite extensive. Hematoxylin-eosin, 40×. (*B*) Intra-alveolar displacement of normal bronchial epithelium by the cryoprobe. Hematoxylin-eosin, 100×.

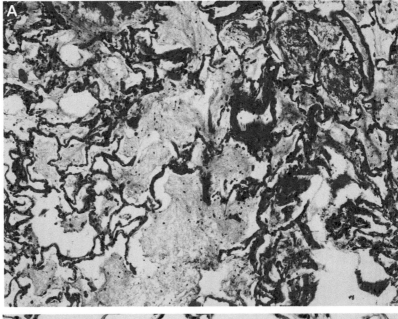

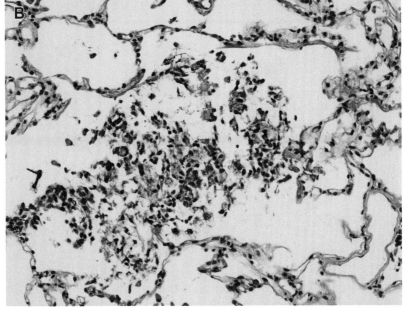

paraffin along the long axis to maximize surface area on the slide. At least 2 slides at different levels stained with hematoxylin-eosin are recommended, leaving some tissue in the block for further stains/studies as needed.

ARTIFACTS AND TISSUES OTHER THAN LUNG ENCOUNTERED ON TRANSBRONCHIAL CRYOBIOPSY SPECIMENS

Compared with forceps transbronchial biopsy, the tissue obtained with cryobiopsy is not only larger but also better preserved, lacking the crush artifacts invariably present in the former. Cryobiopsies also lack the typical artifacts found in cryostat frozen sections. The main artifacts and nonlung tissues encountered on cryobiopsies are shown in **Figs. 2** and **3**.

PATHOLOGIST'S INTERPRETATION OF CRYOBIOPSIES

Cryobiopsies should be interpreted like any other lung biopsy performed for diffuse lung disease.[11,13,25] Ideally a specific histologic diagnosis

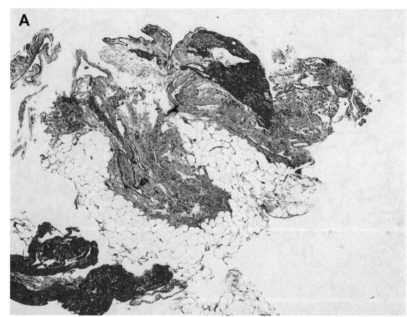

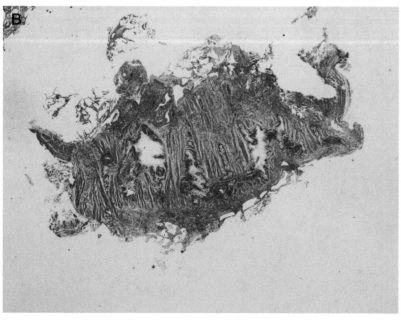

Fig. 3. Main nonpulmonary tissues that can be found in cryobiopsy specimens. (*A*) Parietal pleura/thoracic wall. Pleura (visceral and/or parietal) was present in 25.3% of cryobiopsies in a large series.[15] (*B*) Bronchial wall. A cryobiopsy consisting exclusively or mostly in bronchial wall is one of the main reasons of inadequacy of the procedure.

Fig. 3. (continued). (C) Medium-sized vessel. Hematoxylin-eosin, 20×.

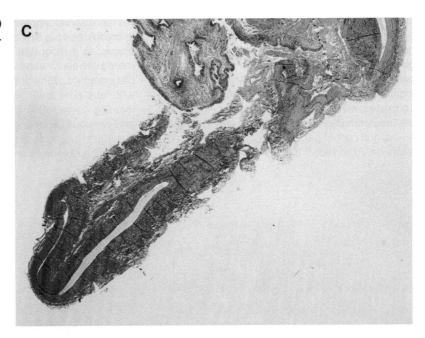

should be achieved (eg, neoplastic cells, microorganisms, Langerhans cells in pulmonary Langerhans cell histiocytosis), but failing that the pathologist should address the abnormalities present (eg, inflammation, fibrosis, granulomas) and try to identify a histologic pattern or an anatomic distribution and then develop a differential diagnosis that can be discussed at a multidisciplinary meeting. Although cryobiopsies are smaller than surgical lung biopsies and the diagnostic yield is

Fig. 4. A cryobiopsy showing UIP in a patient with a multidisciplinary diagnosis of IPF, consisting in the combination of patchy fibrosis and fibroblastic foci. Note the absence of ancillary findings suggestive of secondary UIP (eg, significant cellularity, granulomas). In these cases, the level of diagnostic confidence is high, similar to surgical lung biopsy. In cryobiopsy, as in surgical lung biopsy, honeycombing is not necessary for the diagnosis of UIP: in a recent study on 63 patients with UIP on cryobiopsy and a final diagnosis of IPF, honeycombing was present in 28.6% of the cases and was not correlated with a different outcome or with a specific clinico-radiologic phenotype.[28] Hematoxylin-eosin, 20×.

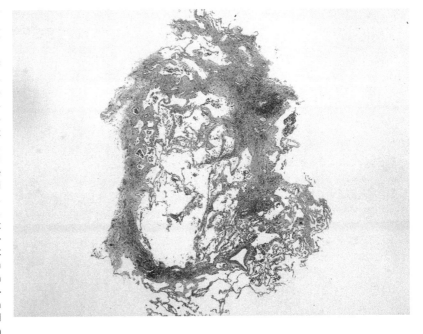

lower (see later discussion), many are "large enough" to reach a specific diagnosis or to allow pattern recognition, including UIP. We suggest giving a level of confidence (high vs low) for the pathologic interpretation,[26] and then both pathologic interpretation and level of confidence are correlated with clinical and radiologic findings at the time of multidisciplinary discussion, becoming an integral part of patient management. Recently, a standardized report has been proposed.[27]

Interobserver agreement between pathologists in cryobiopsies is similar to that of surgical lung biopsies: in a recent series,[15] interpersonal agreement between 3 experienced pathologists for the diagnosis of UIP versus non-UIP was 0.72. As with any new pathologic specimen, there is a learning curve in the interpretation of cryobiopsy and previous experience with diffuse lung disease in surgical lung biopsies is important. Some examples of cryobiopsies are illustrated in **Figs. 4–9.**

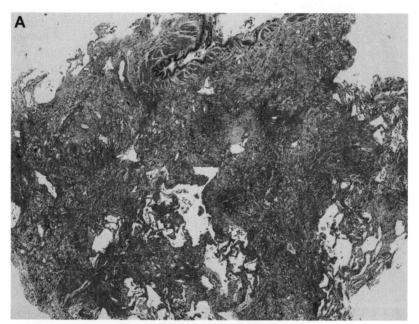

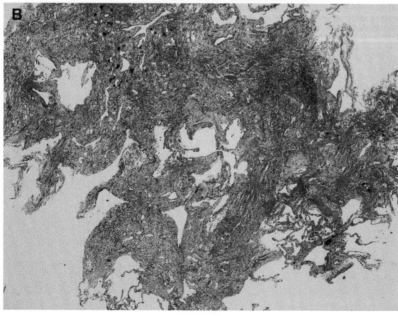

Fig. 5. Two cryobiopsies in the same patient (*A*) from the lower lobe and (*B*) from the upper lobe, both showing dense, patchy fibrosis and fibroblastic foci. In the upper lobe an elastotic tissue was also present, a combination of findings raising the possibility of pleuroparenchymal fibroelastosis combined with UIP (radiologically confirmed). Hematoxylin-eosin, 40×.

Fig. 6. Fibrosing NSIP, consisting in uniform interstitial fibrosis with mild cellularity and without fibroblastic foci. Hematoxylin-eosin, 40×.

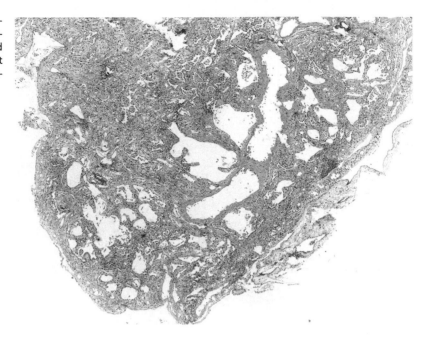

DIAGNOSTIC YIELD OF CRYOBIOPSY IN DIFFUSE LUNG DISEASE

The diagnostic yield of transbronchial cryobiopsy in diffuse lung disease (including specific settings, such as lung transplantation,[29] immunocompromised patients,[30] and small airway disease[31]) varies from 51% to more than 90%, with an average of 80% to 85%.[14,15,18,19,21,23,32–37] This diagnostic rate is maintained even when the studied population is enriched with UIP cases[18] and is much better than that of conventional transbronchial biopsy and lower than that of surgical lung biopsy for fibrotic diffuse lung disease (~30% and ~95%, respectively). In a recent large series of cryobiopsy in patients with diffuse lung disease,[15] the yield for histologic diagnosis was 87.8%, and multidisciplinary diagnosis was achieved in 90.1%. Importantly, the diagnostic yield was influenced by the number of samples taken and by the number of sites biopsied; it significantly increased when at least 2 samples were obtained from 2 different sites (either in the same lobe or in different lobes). Considering only patients with fibrotic diffuse lung disease undergoing cryobiopsy in 2 sites, discordant histology (for example, NSIP in the upper lobe and UIP in the lower lobe) was seen in 27.9% of the cases. A sampling strategy similar to that suggested for surgical lung biopsies seems to be adequate to reduce the risk of sampling errors due to histologic variability (ie, discordant histology).

Studies comparing the diagnostic yield of transbronchial cryobiopsy and surgical lung biopsy in the same patients are few: in most the latter was performed after the former only when cryobiopsy results were considered insufficient to reach a firm diagnosis. Summing the data of these limited studies,[26,38,39] surgical lung biopsy confirmed the diagnostic impression of the previous cryobiopsy in 15 of 22 patients (68%). The small number of cases and the selection bias strongly limits the value of these data. A recent study[40] evaluated the first-choice diagnoses performed blindly by an expert pathologist in a series of 21 patients with diffuse lung disease who underwent cryobiopsies immediately followed by surgical lung biopsies in the same anatomic locations. The diagnoses performed on cryobiopsies and surgical lung biopsies were concordant in 8 cases (38%) and discordant in 9 (42.8%), whereas in the remaining 4 cases cryobiopsies were nondiagnostic/inadequate. However, based on the data presented in Table 2 of Romagnoli and colleagues[40] and considering only the cases in which cryobiopsies were adequate (the only in which in the routine practice a subsequent surgical lung biopsy would not be proposed), the concordance of the 2 techniques with the original multidisciplinary diagnoses was comparable (42.8% for cryobiopsies, 47.6% for surgical lung biopsies). As correctly pointed out by the authors the study has some limitations, particularly the small number of patients and the possibility for the involved

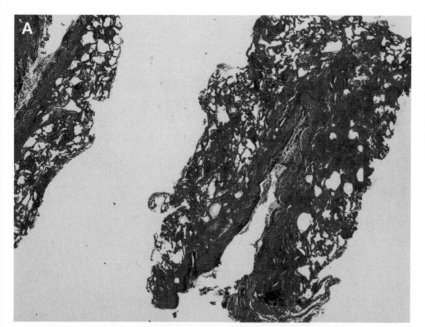

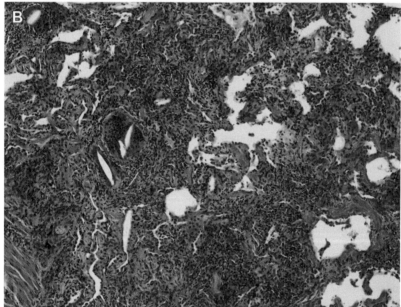

Fig. 7. A quite small cryobiopsy showing cellular NSIP with a vague bronchiolocentric accentuation (*A*) (hematoxylin-eosin, 40×) and inconspicuous granulomas (*B*) (hematoxylin-eosin, 200×), suggestive of subacute hypersensitivity pneumonitis (clinically confirmed).

pathologist to register just 1 diagnosis per case without multidisciplinary discussion, a situation very different from routine practice.

The 2 main explanations for an inadequate/nondiagnostic cryobiopsy are (1) the presence of only bronchial wall with minimal or no peribronchial alveolar tissue, a relatively frequent phenomenon with inexperienced operators due to inadequate penetration of the probe into the lung parenchyma and (2) the presence of only normal lung tissue or

lung tissue with focal/mild nonspecific changes (such as minimal inflammation, minimal fibrosis); this finding is more common with small cryobiopsies, but sometimes observed also with large specimens that did not succeed in sampling the radiologic abnormalities. As in surgical lung biopsy, cryobiopsy should also target abnormal computed tomography (CT) findings. In the near future, integration of new endoscopic guidance tools for the cryoprobe may be helpful to target the best biopsy

Fig. 8. Bronchiolocentric stellate scars with emphysema, suggestive of healed Langerhans cell histiocytosis (clinically-radiologically confirmed). Hematoxylin-eosin, 20×.

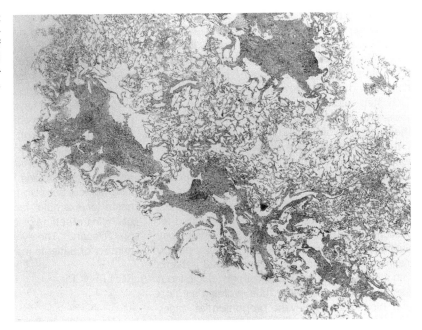

areas with greater precision, potentially further increasing the diagnostic yield and reducing the complication rate of the technique.[41–43]

VALUE OF CRYOBIOPSY FOR THE PATIENT WITH DIFFUSE LUNG DISEASE

Several studies have evaluated the diagnostic utility of transbronchial cryobiopsy in the setting of the multidisciplinary diagnosis of diffuse lung disease.[15,18,21,23,35,37,39] Probably the most significant is that by Tomassetti and colleagues,[26] in which 117 patients with diffuse lung disease underwent either transbronchial cryobiopsy (58) or surgical lung biopsy (57). Each case was evaluated by 2 clinicians, radiologists, and pathologists in a stepwise fashion, similar to the methodology originally used by Flaherty and colleagues[44] for

Fig. 9. A cryobiopsy showing foci of organizing pneumonia in the background of chronic smoking changes. In these sorts of cases, the differential diagnosis with early UIP/IPF can be difficult and requires the support of the clinical and radiologic data. This biopsy refers to a 35-year-old man, heavy smoker, presenting with fever and pulmonary consolidations that were resolving at the time of biopsy. Hematoxylin-eosin, 40×.

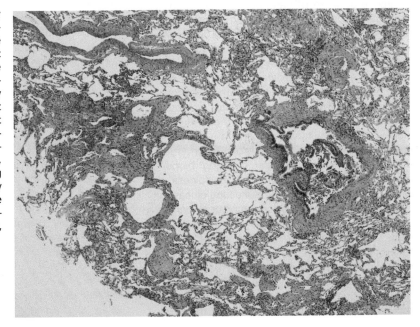

surgical lung biopsies. In brief, at each step the participants received more information: first clinical-radiological data, then BAL data, then biopsy data (sometimes obtained through cryobiopsy and sometimes through surgical lung biopsy), and finally follow-up data. At the end of each step each participant made his/her diagnosis, with a level of confidence for that diagnosis. The main result of the study was that cryobiopsies and surgical lung biopsies had statistically the same effect on the diagnosis of IPF in terms of level of confidence and interpersonal agreement, 2 surrogate parameters of diagnostic accuracy. Similar results were obtained in a recent prospective multicenter study (Hetzel et al, submitted for publication), in which transbronchial cryobiopsy significantly increased the level of multidisciplinary diagnostic confidence in a series of 128 patients with diffuse lung disease in whom histologic input was needed for diagnosis, thus avoiding surgical lung biopsy in a relevant proportion of cases (65.3%).

Studies on the prognostic value of cryobiopsy in patients with diffuse lung disease are just coming out. In Tomassetti and colleagues (submitted for publication), cryobiopsies performed in 310 consecutive patients with diffuse lung disease were evaluated blindly by 3 pathologists, and the results integrated into the multidisciplinary discussion. After a mean follow-up of 54 months, a significant prognostic separation was found both between the blind histologic diagnosis of UIP versus non-UIP (including UIP vs NSIP) and between the multidisciplinary diagnosis of IPF versus non-IPF. These results recapitulate the prognostic difference between UIP and non-UIP obtained in historical studies with surgical lung biopsies.[45] In a series of 174 consecutive patients diagnosed with IPF between September 2006 and June 2017 and treated either with pirfenidone or nintedanib, there was no significant difference in survival between patients in whom the diagnosis was performed through transbronchial cryobiopsy and surgical lung biopsy.[46] If confirmed in further studies, these results will demonstrate the prognostic equivalence of a diagnosis of IPF performed through cryobiopsy and surgical lung biopsy, providing the ultimate proof of the usefulness of cryobiopsy in the setting of diffuse lung disease.

Given the above discussion, cryobiopsy can be considered as a first diagnostic step in many patients with diffuse lung disease in whom clinico-radiologic data are not sufficient for a firm diagnosis, limiting surgical lung biopsy to those patients in whom cryobiopsy is nondiagnostic.[47–49] Such a sequential approach could significantly reduce the complications in terms of morbidity and mortality compared with the approach in which surgical lung biopsy is the sole diagnostic procedure.

In summary, transbronchial cryobiopsy provides enough histologic information to reach a multidisciplinary diagnosis in most patients with diffuse lung disease, with lower risk compared with surgical lung biopsy. Cryobiopsy also affords more patients with diffuse lung disease to have the benefit of histology compared with surgical lung biopsy, including patients in whom the severity of disease and/or complications would preclude a surgical lung biopsy, but also patients with mild/early disease, for example, facilitating an early diagnosis of IPF in the setting of interstitial lung abnormalities on CT scan.[50] The availability of tissue in a higher number of patients may also facilitate research.

REFERENCES

1. Tomassetti S, Cavazza A, Colby TV, et al. Transbronchial biopsy is useful in predicting UIP pattern. Respir Res 2012;13:96.
2. Shim HS, Park MS, Park IK. Histopathologic findings of transbronchial biopsy in usual interstitial pneumonia. Pathol Int 2010;60:373–7.
3. Sheth JS, Belperio JA, Fishbein MC. Utility of transbronchial vs surgical lung biopsy in the diagnosis of suspected fibrotic interstitial lung disease. Chest 2017;151:389–99.
4. Hutchinson JP, Fogarty AW, McKeever TM, et al. In-hospital mortality following surgical lung biopsy for interstitial lung disease in the United States: 2000 to 2011. Am J Respir Crit Care Med 2016;193:1161–7.
5. Fisher JH, Shapera S, To T, et al. Procedure volume and mortality after surgical lung biopsy in interstitial lung disease. Eur Respir J 2019;53:1801164.
6. Raghu G, Remy-Jardin M, Myers JL, et al. Diagnosis of idiopathic pulmonary fibrosis. An official ATS/ERS/JRS/ALAT clinical practice guideline. Am J Respir Crit Care Med 2018;198:e44–68.
7. Margaritopoulos GA, Wells AU. The role of transbronchial biopsy in the diagnosis of diffuse parenchymal lung diseases: con. Rev Port Pneumol 2012;18:61–3.
8. Hetzel J, Eberhardt R, Herth FJ, et al. Cryobiopsy increases the diagnostic yield of endobronchial biopsy: a multicentre trial. Eur Respir J 2012;39:685–90.
9. Schumann M, Bostanci K, Bugalho A, et al. Endobronchial ultrasound-guided cryobiopsies in peripheral pulmonary lesions: a feasibility study. Eur Respir J 2014;43:233–9.
10. Poletti V, Ravaglia C, Tomassetti S. Transbronchial cryobiopsy in diffuse parenchymal lung diseases. Curr Opin Pulm Med 2016;22:289–96.

11. Lentz RJ, Argento AC, Colby TV, et al. Transbronchial cryobiopsy for diffuse parenchymal lung disease: a state-of-the art review of procedural techniques, current evidence, and future challenges. J Thorac Dis 2017;9:2186–203.

12. Colella S, Haentschel M, Shah P, et al. Transbronchial lung cryobiopsy in interstitial lung diseases: best practice. Respiration 2018;95:289–300.

13. Hetzel J, Maldonado F, Ravaglia C, et al. Transbronchial cryobiopsy for the diagnosis of diffuse parenchymal lung diseases: expert statement from the cryobiopsy working group on safety and utility and a call for standardization of the procedure. Respiration 2018;95:188–200.

14. Ravaglia C, Bonifazi M, Wells AU, et al. Safety and diagnostic yield of transbronchial lung cryobiopsy in diffuse parenchymal lung disease: a comparative study versus video-assisted thoracoscopic lung biopsy and a systematic review of the literature. Respiration 2016;91:215–27.

15. Ravaglia C, Wells AU, Tomassetti S, et al. Diagnostic yield and risk/benefit analysis of trans-bronchial lung cryobiopsy in diffuse parenchymal lung diseases: a cohort of 699 patients. BMC Pulm Med 2019;19:16.

16. Babiak A, Hetzel J, Krishna G, et al. Transbronchial cryobiopsy: a new tool for lung biopsies. Respiration 2009;78:203–8.

17. Griff S, Ammenwerth W, Schonfield N, et al. Morphometrical analysis of transbronchial cryobiopsy. Diagn Pathol 2011;6:53.

18. Casoni GL, Tomassetti S, Cavazza A, et al. Transbronchial lung cryobiopsy in the diagnosis of fibrotic interstitial lung diseases. PLoS One 2014;9:e86716.

19. Griff S, Schonfeld N, Ammenwerth W, et al. Diagnostic yield of transbronchial cryobiopsy in non-neoplastic lung disease: a retrospective case series. BMC Pulm Med 2014;14:171.

20. Fruchter O, Fridel L, Rosengarten D, et al. Transbronchial cryobiopsy in lung transplantation patients: first report. Respirology 2013;18:669–73.

21. Pajares V, Puzo C, Castillo D, et al. Diagnostic yield of transbronchial cryobiopsy in interstitial lung disease: a randomized trial. Respirology 2014;19:900–6.

22. Kropski JA, Pritchett JM, Mason WR, et al. Bronchoscopic cryobiopsy for the diagnosis of diffuse parenchymal lung disease. PLoS One 2013;8:e78674.

23. Bango-Alvarez A, Ariza Prota M, Torres-Rivas H, et al. Transbronchial cryobiopsy in interstitial lung disease: experience in 106 cases—how to do it. ERJ Open Res 2017;3, [pii:00148-2016].

24. Fruchter O, Fridel L, El Raouf BA, et al. Histological diagnosis of interstitial lung diseases by cryo-transbronchial biopsy. Respirology 2014;19:683–8.

25. Colby TV, Tomassetti S, Cavazza A, et al. Transbronchial cryobiopsy in diffuse lung disease. Update for the pathologist. Arch Pathol Lab Med 2017;141:891–900.

26. Tomassetti S, Wells AU, Costabel U, et al. Bronchoscopic lung cryobiopsy increases diagnostic confidence in the multidisciplinary diagnosis of idiopathic pulmonary fibrosis. Am J Respir Crit Care Med 2016;193(7):745–52.

27. Ravaglia C, Rossi G, Tomassetti S, et al. Report standardization in transbronchial lung cryobiopsy. Arch Pathol Lab Med 2019;143:416–7.

28. Ravaglia C, Bosi M, Wells AU, et al. Idiopathic pulmonary fibrosis: prognostic impact of histologic honeycombing in transbronchial lung cryobiopsy. Multidiscip Respir Med 2019;14:3.

29. Montero MA, de Garcia J, Amigo MC, et al. The role of transbronchial cryobiopsy in lung transplantation. Histopathology 2018;73:593–600.

30. Fruchter O, Fridel L, Rosengarten D, et al. Transbronchial cryobiopsy in immunocompromised patients with pulmonary infiltrates: a pilot study. Lung 2013;191:619–24.

31. Lentz RJ, Fessel JP, Johnson JE, et al. Transbronchial cryobiopsy can diagnose constrictive bronchiolitis in veterans of recent conflicts in the Middle East. Am J Respir Crit Care Med 2016;193:806–8.

32. Johannson KA, Marcoux VS, Ronksley PE, et al. Diagnostic yield and complications of transbronchial lung cryobiopsy for interstitial lung disease. A systematic review and metaanalysis. Ann Am Thorac Soc 2016;13:1828–38.

33. Sharp C, McCabe M, Adamali H, et al. Use of transbronchial cryobiopsy in the diagnosis of interstitial lung disease—a systematic review and cost analysis. QJM 2017;110:207–14.

34. Iftikhar IH, Alghothani L, Sardi A, et al. Transbronchial lung cryobiopsy and video-assisted thoracoscopic lung biopsy in the diagnosis of diffuse parenchymal lung disease. A meta-analysis of diagnostic test accuracy. Ann Am Thorac Soc 2017;14:1197–211.

35. Ussavarungsi K, Kern RM, Roden AC, et al. Transbronchial cryobiopsy in diffuse parenchymal lung disease. Retrospective analysis of 74 cases. Chest 2017;151:400–8.

36. Walscher J, Gross B, Eberhardt R, et al. Transbronchial cryobiopsies for diagnosing interstitial lung disease: real-life experience from a tertiary referral center for interstitial lung disease. Respiration 2019;97:348–54.

37. Kronborg-White S, Folkersen B, Rasmussen TR, et al. Introduction of cryobiopsy in the diagnostics of interstitial lung disease-experience in a referral center. Eur Clin Respir J 2017;4:1274099.

38. Hagmejer L, Theegarten D, Treml M, et al. Validation of transbronchial cryobiopsy in interstitial lung disease—interim analysis of a prospective trial and

critical review of the literature. Sarcoidosis Vasc Diffuse Lung Dis 2016;33:2–9.

39. Bondue B, Pieters T, Alexander P, et al. Role of trans-bronchial lung cryobiopsies in diffuse parenchymal lung diseases: interest of a sequential approach. Pulm Med 2017;2017:6794343.

40. Romagnoli M, Colby TV, Berthet JP, et al. Poor concordance between sequential transbronchial lung cryobiopsy and surgical lung biopsy in the diagnosis of diffuse interstitial lung diseases. Am J Respir Crit Care Med 2019;199:1249–56.

41. Gupta A, Youness H, Dhillon SS, et al. The value of using radial endobronchiale ultrasound to guide transbron-chial lung cryobiopsy. J Thorac Dis 2019;11:329–34.

42. Wijmans L, Bonta PI, Rocha-Pinto R, et al. Confocal laser endomicroscopy as a guidance tool for trans-bronchial lung cryobiopsy in interstitial lung disor-ders. Respiration 2019;97:259–63.

43. Hariri LP, Adams DC, Wain JC, et al. Endobronchial optical coherence tomography for low-risk micro-scopic assessment and diagnosis of idiopathic pul-monary fibrosis in vivo. Am J Respir Crit Care Med 2018;197:949–52.

44. Flaherty KR, King TE, Raghu G, et al. Idiopathic interstitial pneumonia: what is the effect of a multidisciplinary approach to diagnosis? Am J Re-spir Crit Care Med 2004;170:904–10.

45. Bjoraker JA, Ryu JH, Edvin MK, et al. Prognostic sig-nificance of histopathologic subsets in idiopathic pulmonary fibrosis. Am J Respir Crit Care Med 1998;157:199–203.

46. Pannu JK, Hewlett JC, Smith AB, et al. Survival impli-cations of transbronchial cryobiopsy and other diag-nostic modalities in idiopathic pulmonary fibrosis. J Thorac Dis 2019;11:E20–3.

47. Poletti V, Ravaglia C, Dubini A, et al. How might transbronchial cryobiopsy improve diagnosis and treatment of diffuse parenchymal lung disease pa-tients? Expert Rev Respir Med 2017;11:913–7.

48. Ravaglia C, Tomassetti S, Poletti V. New idiopathic pulmonary fibrosis guidelines: are cryobiopsy and surgery competitive in clinical practice? Am J Respir Crit Care Med 2019;199:666–7.

49. Maldonado F, Kropski JA. Should transbronchial cry-obiopsy be considered the initial biopsy of choice in patients with a possible interstitial lung disease? Yes. Chest 2019;155:893–5.

50. Hatabu H, Hunninghake GM, Lynch DA. Interstitial lung abnormality: recognition and perspectives. Radiology 2019;291:1–3.

Moving?

Make sure your subscription moves with you!

To notify us of your new address, find your **Clinics Account Number** (located on your mailing label above your name), and contact customer service at:

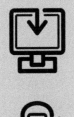

Email: journalscustomerservice-usa@elsevier.com

800-654-2452 (subscribers in the U.S. & Canada)
314-447-8871 (subscribers outside of the U.S. & Canada)

Fax number: 314-447-8029

Elsevier Health Sciences Division
Subscription Customer Service
3251 Riverport Lane
Maryland Heights, MO 63043

*To ensure uninterrupted delivery of your subscription, please notify us at least 4 weeks in advance of move.

Printed and bound by CPI Group (UK) Ltd, Croydon, CR0 4YY

03/10/2024

01040371-0001